# Diseases of Skeletal Muscle

# Diseases of Skeletal Muscle

Editor

**ROBERT L. WORTMANN,** M.D.
Professor and Chair
Department of Internal Medicine
University of Oklahoma College of Medicine
Tulsa, Oklahoma

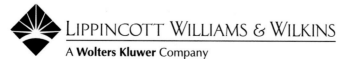
LIPPINCOTT WILLIAMS & WILKINS
A **Wolters Kluwer** Company
Philadelphia · Baltimore · New York · London
Buenos Aires · Hong Kong · Sydney · Tokyo

*Acquisitions Editor:* Richard Winters
*Developmental Editor:* Erin O'Connor
*Production Editor:* Melanie Bennitt
*Manufacturing Manager:* Kevin Watt
*Cover Designer:* Christine Jenny
*Compositor:* Lippincott Williams & Wilkins Desktop Division
*Printer:* Edwards Brothers

© 2000 by LIPPINCOTT WILLIAMS & WILKINS
227 East Washington Square
Philadelphia, PA 19106-3780 USA
LWW.com

Printed in the USA

**Library of Congress Cataloging-in-Publication Data**
Diseases of skeletal muscle / [edited by] Robert L. Wortmann.
     p.   cm.
  Includes bibliographical references and index.
  ISBN 0-7817-1614-4
  1. Muscles—Diseases.  I. Wortmann, Robert.
  [DNLM: 1. Muscle, Skeletal.  2. Muscular Diseases.  WE 550 D611 2000]
RC925.D526   2000
616.7′4—dc21
DNLM/DLC                                     99-31927
for Library of Congress                      CIP

10  9  8  7  6  5  4  3  2  1

This work is dedicated to my wife Dottie.

# Contents

## Part III. Approach to the Patient

# Contributing Authors

**Paul Bolin Jr.,** M.D.   *Associate Professor and Section Head, Department of Medicine, Section of Nephrology, East Carolina University School of Medicine, 2355 Arlington Boulevard, Greenville, North Carolina 27858*

**Edward H. Bossen,** M.D.   *Professor, Department of Pathology, Duke University School of Medicine; Associate Director, Department of Pathology, Duke University Medical Center, Box 3712, Room 3095 Yellow Zone, Durham, North Carolina 27710*

**William S. David,** M.D., Ph.D.   *Assistant Professor, Department of Neurology, University of Minnesota Medical School, Minneapolis, Minnesota 55455; Associate Physician, Department of Neurology, Hennepin County Medical Center, 701 Park Avenue South, Minneapolis, Minnesota 55415*

**Dennis D. Dykstra,** M.D., Ph.D.   *Chairman, Department of Physical Medicine and Rehabilitation, Fairview—University of Minnesota Hospital and Clinics; Associate Professor, Department of Physical Medicine and Rehabilitation, University of Minnesota Medical School, Mayo Memorial Building, Box 297, 420 Delaware Avenue SE, Minneapolis, Minnesota 55455*

**David B. Hellmann,** M.D., F.A.C.P.   *Mary Betty Stevens Professor, Department of Medicine, Johns Hopkins University School of Medicine, 1830 East Monument Street, Room 9030, Baltimore, Maryland 21205*

**Joseph A. Houmard,** Ph.D.   *Director, Human Performance Laboratory, Department of Exercise and Sport Science, East Carolina University, 371 Ward Sports Medicine Building, Greenville, North Carolina 27858*

**Lawrence J. Kagen,** M.D.   *Professor, Department of Medicine, Weill Medical College of Cornell University, New York, New York; Attending Physician, Department of Medicine, Division of Rheumatology, Hospital for Special Surgery, 535 East 70th Street, New York, New York 10021*

**David Lacomis,** M.D.   *Associate Professor, Departments of Neurology and Pathology, University of Pittsburgh School of Medicine; Staff Neurologist and Neuromuscular Pathologist, Departments of Neurology and Pathology, University of Pittsburgh Medical Center Health System, Presbyterian University Hospital, 200 Lothrop Street, Room F878, Pittsburgh, Pennsylvania 15213*

**Maren L. Mahowald,** M.D.   *Professor, Department of Medicine, University of Minnesota Medical School; Chief, Department of Rheumatology, Veterans Affairs Medical Center, One Veterans Drive, Room 111-R, Minneapolis, Minnesota 55417*

**Ronald P. Messner,** M.D.   *Rheumatologist, Department of Medicine, Fairview—University of Minnesota Hospital and Clinics; Professor and Director, Department of Medicine, University of Minnesota Medical School, Mayo Memorial Building, Box 108, 420 Delaware Street SE, Minneapolis, Minnesota 55455*

**Chester V. Oddis, M.D.**   *Associate Professor, Department of Medicine, University of Pittsburgh Medical Center and University of Pittsburgh School of Medicine, Kaufmann Building, Suite 502, 3471 Fifth Avenue, Pittsburgh, Pennsylvania 15213*

**Nancy J. Olsen, M.D.**   *Associate Professor, Department of Medicine, Vanderbilt University, T-3219 Medical Center North, Nashville, Tennessee 37232-2681*

**Lauren M. Pachman, M.D.**   *Professor, Department of Pediatrics, Northwestern University Medical School, Chicago, Illinois; Chief, Division of Immunology and Rheumatology, The Children's Memorial Medical Center, 2300 Children's Plaza, #50, Chicago, Illinois 60614*

**Jane H. Park, Ph.D.**   *Professor, Department of Molecular Physiology and Biophysics and Department of Medicine, Vanderbilt University, T-3219 Medical Center North, Nashville, Tennessee 37232-2681*

**Robert W. Simms, M.D.**   *Associate Professor and Clinical Director, Department of Medicine, Section of Rheumatology, Boston University Arthritis Center, 715 Albany Street, K5, Boston, Massachusetts 02118*

**Ira N. Targoff, M.D.**   *Staff Physician, Department of Medicine, Veterans Affairs Medical Center, Oklahoma City, Oklahoma; Associate Professor, Department of Medicine, University of Oklahoma Health Sciences Center, 920 Stanton L. Young Boulevard, Oklahoma City, Oklahoma 73014*

**Robert L. Wortmann, M.D.**   *Professor and Chair, Department of Internal Medicine, University of Oklahoma College of Medicine, 2808 South Sheridan Road, Tulsa, Oklahoma 74129-1077*

# Preface

This work is an expression of my interest and understanding of diseases of skeletal muscle. This interest began more than 20 years ago during my rheumatology fellowship when I first encountered patients with polymyositis. That was shortly after Bohan and Peter had published their landmark work suggesting criteria for that diagnosis and providing criteria for classifying the idiopathic inflammatory myopathies. Because of their creativity, the evaluation of patients with inflammatory muscle disease seemed entirely rational.

Upon completing my training, I felt confident in dealing with polymyositis. However, I soon learned that not all muscle weakness was caused by that disease and that I really did not know much about the other causes. Several factors contributed to my predicament. First, as a rheumatology trainee, I felt that if I saw a patient with muscle weakness, the differential diagnosis was limited: either polymyositis or a problem cared for by another specialist. Second, the understanding of most diseases of skeletal muscle was primitive. In addition, the study of skeletal muscle tissue did not fall into any particular medical discipline. Finally, a collection of information or an organization that addressed the full spectrum of afflictions of the tissue did not exist.

Over the last two decades, some things have changed. I have seen more patients with myopathy who do not have polymyositis and I have become more familiar with other causes of muscle weakness. During this time, an explosion of new information has emerged, allowing us to more easily link pathophysiology and molecular defects with diseases. Finally, an excellent encyclopedic text that covers the field is available, Drs. Engel and Franzini-Armstrong's comprehensive text, *Myology*. Nevertheless, I find that many physicians still have a limited view of myopathies, which they derive, at least in part, from the biases of their specialty training.

The purpose of this text is to provide a broader review of the disorders of skeletal muscle than is available in subspecialty texts and in greater depth than is available in general texts. I hope that by imparting information about the normal tissue, a discussion of disease, manifestations, and treatments linked with their underlying pathophysiology, and a detailed review of evaluation tools, the reader will become a better clinician and teacher.

# Acknowledgments

I thank each contributor for their excellent work. I give special thanks to Suzanne Godley, whose personal devotion and skills allowed this text to be completed so effectively and allowed me to continue the rest of my work throughout the editing process. I thank the many students, co-workers, and teachers who have taught me so much throughout my career. I also acknowledge four of my mentors: Robert F. Wortmann, M.D., my father, who by example taught me about the professional aspects of medicine; Douglas W. Voth, M.D., who, more than anyone, stimulated me to be the clinician I am; William N. Kelley, M.D., who introduced me to science and demonstrated the value of administration in academic medicine; and Robert W. Lightfoot, Jr., M.D., who is one of the best and most caring teachers I have known.

*Robert L. Wortmann*

# PART I

## Characteristics of Normal Muscle

*Diseases of Skeletal Muscle,*
edited by Robert L. Wortmann.
Lippincott Williams & Wilkins, Philadelphia © 2000

# 1

# Muscle Structure and Development

## Edward H. Bossen

*Department of Pathology, Duke University School of Medicine and Duke University Medical Center, Durham, North Carolina 27710*

Normal skeletal muscle is composed of multinucleated cells called fibers arranged in fascicles surrounded by connective tissue called the perimysium. The space between individual muscle fibers, normally insignificant, is referred to as the endomysium (Fig. 1). Within the fibers are contractile proteins, called filaments. These proteins are responsible for the transduction of chemical energy into mechanical work during muscle contraction and relaxation. The contractile filaments are configured in structures called myofilaments.

Electron microscopy discloses alternating dark and light bands in the muscle fiber. The dark band is referred to as the A band and the light band as the I band. The A band is 1.5 µm in length, but the I band length varies with the state of contraction because the filaments of the I band slide into the A band with fiber shortening (contraction) and out of the A band with lengthening (relaxation). In the middle of the I band is a thin dark band called the Z line. A thin M line is present in the middle of the A band and is bound by pale H zones on either side. The A band and two I bands between two Z lines comprise the sarcomere, the basic unit of skeletal muscle fibers, which is 2.5 to 3.0 µm in length (1) (Figs. 2 and 3). Muscle fibers grow by adding sarcomeres at the myotendon junction (2).

The dark A band is composed primarily of myosin filaments 15 to 18 µm thick, whereas the I band is composed predominately of actin filaments 7 to 10 µm thick. Proteins other than myosin and actin are also present. Myomesin, M protein, and creatine kinase are present at the M line. C, H, and X proteins are also present in the A band. Troponin, tropomyosin, and nebulin are in the I band. The Z line includes α-actinin (3). The giant protein titin is anchored at the Z line and can reach to the M line (4). Titin and nebulin, together with M- and Z-line proteins, form a complex scaffolding that maintains the organization of the sarcomere during contraction and relaxation.

The external envelope of the muscle fiber is the sarcolemma. The sarcolemma is composed of two layers. The inner layer is the plasma membrane of the muscle fiber and the outer layer is the adjacent basal lamina. The myoneural junction is found on the surface of the fiber (Fig. 4). The early muscle fiber is innervated by a single myelinated axon. Until innervation, other nuclei produce mRNAs of subunits of acetylcholine receptors. This ceases with innervation but recurs after denervation (5). If a muscle fiber is denervated, reinneration occurs at the original site of the myoneural junction (6). A Schwann cell covers the axon at the myoneural junction. The muscle fiber, at this point sometimes referred to as a sole plate, is composed of many folds and secondary clefts that contain acetylcholine receptors and acetylcholinesterase (7).

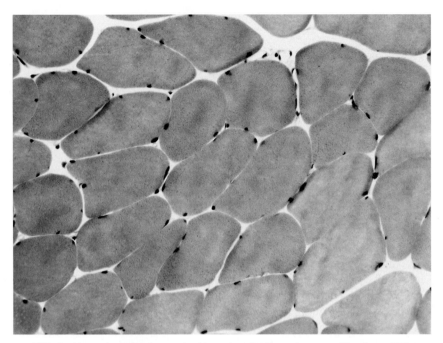

**FIG. 1.** Normal skeletal muscle. Hemotoxylin & eosin, magnification ×250.

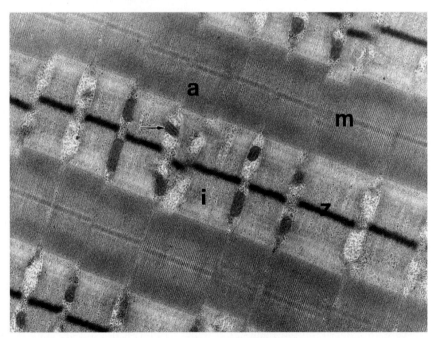

**FIG. 2.** Electron micrograph of skeletal muscle illustrating the A and I bands and the Z and M lines. Mitochondria (*arrow*) are located in the I band. Magnification ×18,200.

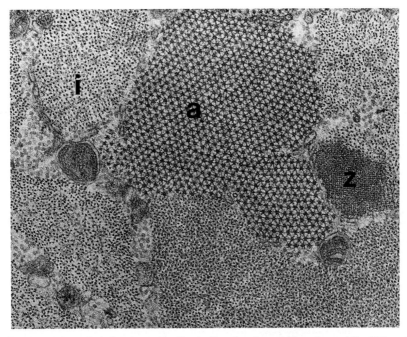

**FIG. 3.** Cross-section of skeletal muscle illustrating the A and I bands and the Z line. Magnification ×87,500.

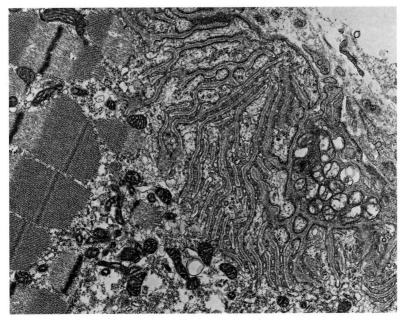

**FIG. 4.** A myoneural junction is illustrated. Note the prominent clefts on the muscle side of the junction. Magnification ×5,250.

The stimulation for contraction involves two tubular systems in addition to the myoneural junction. The transverse tubular system, often referred to as T tubules, is a network of invaginations of the plasma membrane into the muscle fiber and connects by way of junctional processes to another network, the sarcoplasmic reticulum, at terminal cisternae of the sarcoplasmic reticulum (Fig. 5). The peripheral junctional sarcoplasmic reticulum is also connected directly to the plasmalemma (8). The transverse tubular system and the sarcoplasmic reticulum are involved in the excitation contraction cycle of the muscle. Discussions of muscle physiology can be found in Chapter 2.

Mitochondria, the principal source of chemical energy for the fiber, are located in the I band on either side of the Z line (Fig. 2). Muscle fibers also contain glycogen, which is dispersed in the cytoplasm (sarcoplasm), and lipid, which is concentrated adjacent to mitochondria.

Satellite cells are another constituent of muscle (9). These are found beneath the basal lamina of muscle fibers and outside the plasmalemma of the fiber (Fig. 6). Satellite cells seem to occupy a grove in the fiber so that the basal lamina that covers both cells is continuous. Satellite cells are presumptive myoblasts and are more prominent in children than adults (10). They differ, however, from the fetal myoblasts (11). Satellite cells contribute to the growth of muscle fibers (12) and respond to muscle damage by differentiating into a myoblast, which proliferate and participate in the repair process when fibers are damaged by overuse or disease (13).

Other normal structures include intramuscular nerve twigs and muscle spindles (Fig. 7). The muscle spindle is a tension-sensing structure composed of nuclear bag and nuclear chain fibers, so named because of the organization of their nuclei.

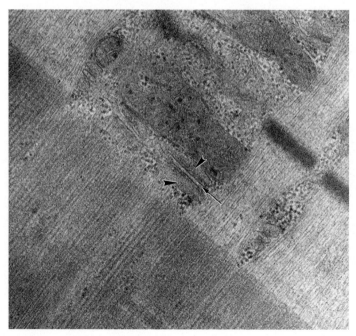

**FIG. 5.** The transverse tubular system (*arrow*) is in continuity with the cell surface. It interfaces with the sarcoplasmic reticulum at the terminal cisternae (*arrowheads*).

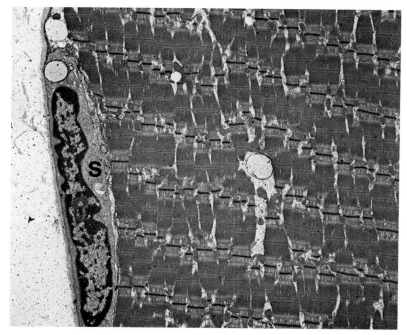

**FIG. 6.** The satellite cell (*S*) is beneath the basal lamina of the muscle fiber but has its own plasma membrane. Magnification ×8,750.

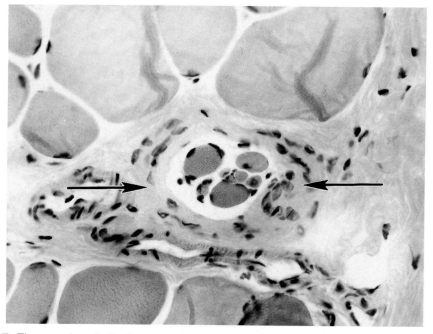

**FIG. 7.** The muscle spindle (between the *arrows*) contains nuclear bag and nuclear chain fibers. It is a tension-sensing organ. Hemotoxylin & eosin, magnification ×400.

## DEVELOPMENT

Despite many recent advances in the ability to experimentally manipulate skeletal muscle cells and in the understanding of skeletal muscle molecular biology, so many questions about human skeletal muscle development and differentiation remain unanswered (14).

Briefly, skeletal muscle is derived from somites (15). Committed mononuclear cells known as myoblasts fuse to form primary myotubes. Secondary myotubes then form. Innervation is generally considered necessary for secondary myotubule formation (16), but this has been disputed (17). Myotubes and muscle fibers are mosaics of paternal and maternal genes (18).

At the molecular level, myogenic factors are important for development. The myogenic regulatory gene *myf-5* is important for maintenance of proliferating muscle cells. The genes *MyoD* and *myogenin* are key factors in muscle differentiation and *MRF4* is critical for maturation of the fiber (19). At the protein level, components develop in the sequence desmin > titin > α-actinin > myosin, actin, and myomesin > nebulin (3). Fiber type differentiation begins at about 15 to 20 weeks of gestation and is complete by 26 to 30 weeks (20).

## AGING

Radiographic studies indicate that muscle mass decreases by approximately 25% and strength by 39% between youth and old age (21) (see Chapter 3). Autopsy studies have demonstrated a 40% reduction in the vastus lateralis of men between the ages of 20 and 80 years, primarily due to both the loss of fibers and the reduction in size of type II (fast-twitch) fibers (22). The loss is greatest for type IIB fibers (23). The loss of fibers is thought to result from the loss of spinal cord motor neurons, particularly type 2 motor neurons, with age (24).

## REFERENCES

1. Landon DN. Skeletal muscle—normal morphology, development, and innervation. In: Mastaglia FL, Detchant LW, eds. *Skeletal muscle pathology*, 2nd ed. New York: Churchill Livingstone, 1992:1–94.
2. Williams PE, Goldspink G. Longitudinal growth of striated muscle fibers. *J Cell Sci* 1971;9:751–767.
3. Craig R. The structure of the contractile filaments. In: Engel AG, Franzini-Armstrong C, eds. *Mycology*. New York: McGraw-Hill, 1992:134–175.
4. Fürst DO, Gautel M. The anatomy of a molecular giant: how the sarcomere cytoskeleton is assembled from immunoglobulin superfamily molecules. *J Mol Cell Cardiol* 1995;27:951–959.
5. Merlie JP, Isenberg KE, Russell SD, Sanes JR. Denervation supersensitivity in skeletal muscle: analysis with a cloned cDNA probe. *J Cell Biol* 1984;99:332–335.
6. Letinsky MS, Fischbeck KH, McMahan UJ. Precision of reinnervation of original postsynaptic sites in frog muscle after a nerve crush. *J Neurocytol* 1976;5:691–718.
7. Salpeter MM. Electron microscope radioautography as a quantitative tool in enzyme cytochemistry. I. The distribution of acetylcholinesterase at motor end plates of a vertebrate twitch muscle. *J Cell Biol* 1967;32:379–389.
8. Alexander CB, Bossen EH. Peripheral couplings in human skeletal muscle. *Lab Invest* 1978;39:17–20.
9. Mauro A. Satellite cell of skeletal muscle fibers. *J Biophys Biochem Cytol* 1961;9:493–494.
10. Allbrook DB, Han MF, Hellmuth AE. Population of muscle satellite cells in relation to age and mitotic activity. *Pathology* 1971;3:233–243.
11. Yablonka-Reuveni Z. Development and postnatal regulation of adult myoblasts. *Microsc Res Tech* 1995;30:366–380.
12. Moss FP, Leblond CP. Satellite cells as the source of nuclei in muscles of growing rats. *Anat Rec* 1971;170:421–436.
13. Hall-Craggs ECB. The regeneration of skeletal muscle fibres per continuum. *J Anat* 1974;117:171–178.
14. Hauschka SK. The embryonic origin of muscle. In: Engle AG, Frangini-Armstrong C, eds. *Myology,* 2nd ed. New York: McGraw-Hill, 1994:3–73.

15. Chevallier A, Kieny M, Mauger A. Limb-somite relationship: origin of the limb musculature. *J Embryol Exp Morph* 1977;41:245–258.
16. Harris AJ. Embryonic growth and innervation of rat skeletal muscles. I. Neural regulation of muscle fibre numbers. *Philos Trans R Soc Lond* 1981;293:257–277.
17. Fredette BJ, Landmesser LT. A reevaluation of the role of innervation in primary and secondary myogenesis in developing chick muscle. *Dev Biol* 1991;143:19–35.
18. Gearhart JD, Mintz B. Clonal origins of somites and their muscle derivatives: evidence from allophenic mice. *Dev Biol* 1972;29:27–37.
19. Montarras D, Chelly J, Bober E, et al. Developmental patterns in the expression of Myf5, MyoD, myogenin, and MRF4 during myogenesis. *New Biol* 1991;3:592–600.
20. Martin L, Joris C. Histoenzymological and semiquantitative study of the maturation of the human muscle fibre. In: Walton N, Canal N, Scarlato G, eds. *Muscle Diseases*. Amsterdam: Excerpta Medica, 1970:657–661.
21. Young A, Stokes M, Crowe M. The size and strength of the quadriceps muscles of old and young men. *Clin Physiol* 1985;5:145–154.
22. Lexell J. Human aging, muscle mass, and fiber type composition. *J Gerontol* 1995;50A:11–16.
23. Grimby G. Muscle performance and structure in the elderly as studied cross-sectionally and longitudinally. *J Gerontol* 1995;50A:17–22.
24. Tomlinson BE, Irving D. The numbers of limb motor neurons in the human lumbosacral cord throughout life. *J Neurol Sci* 1977;34:213–219.

*Diseases of Skeletal Muscle,*
edited by Robert L. Wortmann.
Lippincott Williams & Wilkins, Philadelphia © 2000

# 2

# Skeletal Muscle Biology, Physiology, and Biochemistry

## Robert L. Wortmann

*Department of Internal Medicine, University of Oklahoma College of Medicine, Tulsa, Oklahoma 74129*

### SKELETAL MUSCLE FIBERS

Skeletal muscle makes up over 40% of the body's mass and is crucial for function and survival. To perform properly, this tissue requires large quantities of energy. It must be able to contract and relax efficiently and must be capable of generating a wide range of forces and movements. Skeletal muscle has been able to successfully meet these demands through adaptation and the development of specialized fibers that vary in their properties and capacities.

Individual human muscles are composed of mixtures of fiber types. Within a muscle, the fibers are functionally grouped in motor units (1,2). A motor unit consists of all fibers innervated by an individual motor neuron. The fibers within each motor unit have common histochemical and electrophysiologic properties (3).

Fibers can be divided into two types based of the differences in their speed of contraction (4). Slower contracting fibers are red in color, reflecting a higher concentration of the oxygen-carrying protein myoglobin. These cells also contain higher activities of enzymes involved in aerobic metabolism, larger lipid stores, and more mitochondria (5). Although they contract more slowly, they are more metabolically efficient in terms of energy generated per mole of substrate. In addition, they are better able to sustain constant loads for longer periods of time and are relatively fatigue resistant. In contrast, the faster contracting fibers are more susceptible to fatigue. Their content of glycogen and activity of myophosphorylase is higher. Faster contracting muscle fibers can also be further subdivided between those with more or less myoglobin.

Recognition of the heterogeneity of muscle fibers has led to a variety of classification schemes (Table 1). They can be defined as fast- or slow-twitch fibers or red or white, described histochemically for the activity of myofibrillar actinomyosin ATPase (Fig. 1), aerobic enzyme or glycolytic enzyme content, or selected by the pattern of contractile protein isoforms (3–5). No individual scheme adequately describes the nature of muscle fibers, but taken together, these schemes demonstrate the complexity of the tissue and reflect the specialization required to generate the forces and endurances necessary for the efficient function.

**TABLE 1.** *Classifications of muscle fibers*

|  | Fiber type[a] | | |
| --- | --- | --- | --- |
|  | I | IIa | IIb |
| Contraction speed | Slow | Fast | Fast |
| Color[b] | Red | Red | White |
| Motor unit properties | | | |
|   Twitch speed | Slow | Intermediate | Fast |
|   Tetanic force | Small | Large | Largest |
|   Fatigue resistance | Highest | High | Low |
| Biochemical properties | | | |
|   Enzyme activity | | | |
|     ATPase pH 4.3 | High | High | Low |
|     ATPase pH 4.6 | Low | Low | High |
|     ATPase pH 10.4 | Low | Moderate | High |
|     Hypophosphorylase | Low | High | High |
|     NADH dehydrogenase | High | Intermediate | Low |
|     AMP deaminase | Low | High | High |
|   Substrate contact | | | |
|     Glycogen | Low | High | High |
|     Lipid | High | Variable | Low |
|   Myosin heavy chain isoform[c] | Cardiac β | IIa | IIb |

[a]Nomenclature most commonly applied in discussions of muscle fiber type. Derived from variations in histochemical staining for myosin ATPase activities at pH 4.3, 4.6, and 10.4 (see Fig. 1).
[b]Color is related to the concentration of the oxygen-sequestering molecule myoglobin.
[c]At least ten different isoforms of myosin heavy chain have been described.

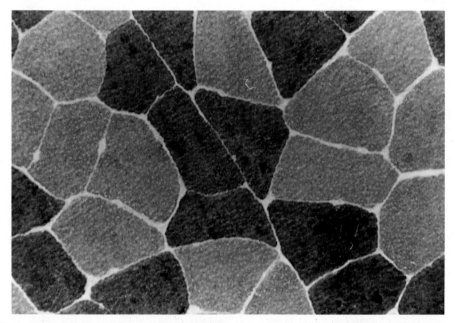

**FIG. 1.** Histochemical staining of normal skeletal muscle for ATPase activity at pH 9.4. Type II fibers are the darkest, type I fibers are the lightest.

## CONTRACTION AND RELAXATION

The function of skeletal muscle relates to the efficiency of muscle contraction and its resistance to fatigue. The process of contraction can be initiated by electrical, chemical, or mechanical stimuli that result in an action potential transmitted along the cell membrane (Table 2) (6). Electrical stimulation results when an action potential moves along a motor neuron to a presynaptic nerve terminal. There, depolarization causes the release of acetylcholine that diffuses to the postsynaptic membrane of the muscle cell and binds to specific receptors. Such binding causes conformational changes, opening channels permeable to sodium and potassium. As a result, potassium moves out of the cell and sodium moves in, depolarizing the muscle fiber and generating an endplate potential. As the wave of depolarization spreads, the resting state of the membrane is restored and maintained by an active sodium potassium exchanger, an Na-K–dependent ATPase.

The wave of depolarization spreads from the membrane to the interior of the muscle fiber through the system of transverse or T tubules, connecting the cell surface and the sarcoplasmic reticulum (7) (Fig. 2). The T tubules and sarcoplasmic reticulum are atomically separated but functionally related systems. T tubules are invaginations of the surface membrane. The sarcoplasmic reticulum is intracellular with no continuity with external plasma membrane. The sarcoplasmic reticulum plays a critical role in the contractile activity of the fiber by actively pumping and sequestering calcium. Thus, when the signal reaches the sarcoplasmic reticulum, calcium is released from the lateral sacs to diffuse among the fibrils, initiating contraction (Fig. 3).

Muscle contraction is controlled by the concentration of calcium surrounding the myofilaments and occurs as a consequence of a magnesium-dependent actomyosin ATPase (8). Activation of that enzyme results in the rapid formation of cross-bridges between actin and myosin, causing the filaments to slide and to shorten.

At rest, actomyosin ATPase is inhibited and there are no cross-bridges between the thick filaments (myosin) and thin filaments (troponin, tropomyosin, and actin). Troponin is a complex of three proteins: troponin C, which serves as the calcium-binding site; troponin I, which interacts with the magnesium ATPase of actomyosin; and troponin T, which interacts with tropomyosin (9). Troponin, along with tropomyosin, inhibits the interaction of actin and myosin. As calcium concentrations around myofibrils increase, calcium binds to troponin, causing conformational changes that release the inhibition of the enzyme. With the hydrolysis of ATP, actin-containing filaments bridge with and slide along myosin, shortening the fiber and creating tension. Skeletal muscle has the ability to develop high tension in extremely short periods of time. This requires rapid hydrolysis of ATP to ADP and inorganic phosphorous and loss of those products from the myosin. The loss of the hydrolytic products appears to be the rate-limiting event in how fast shortening can occur (10).

**TABLE 2.** *Steps in excitation-contraction and relaxation*

1. Depolarization of surface membrane
2. Spread of depolarization to interior of fiber along network of T tubules
3. Transmission across T tubules and sarcoplasmic reticulum junctions
4. Release of calcium through the now permeable sarcoplasmic reticulum membranes
5. Binding of calcium to troponin releasing inhibition of actinomyosin ATPase, which allows cross-bridging between actin and myosin and fiber shortening
6. Active pumping of calcium back into sarcoplasm reticulum, breaking the cross-links and allowing the muscle to lengthen or relax

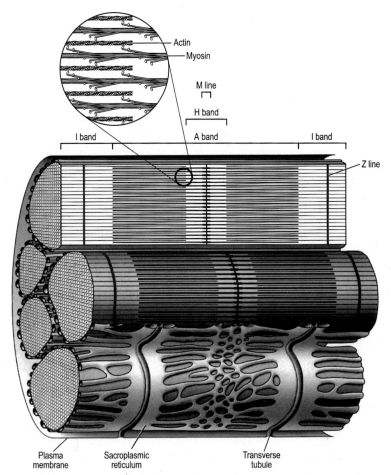

**FIG. 2.** Cross-sectional structure of a skeletal muscle fiber. Each fiber is a multinucleated cell composed of fibrils that contain the contractile proteins called myofilaments. Communication between the surface membrane, the sarcolemma, and the myofilaments is provided by the T tubule system and sarcoplasm reticulum. The T tubules are invaginations of the surface membranes that run along the boundaries of the sarcomeres. The sarcoplasmic reticulum invests the fibrils. The term triad is used to represent the area formed by two cisternal enlargements of the sarcoplasmic reticulum and adjacent T tubules. Sarcomeres are the functional contractile units of the muscle wall and are defined as the areas between Z lines. The A band is made up of thick filaments (myosin). The M line, the midpoint of a sarcomere, is formed by bulges in the centers of the thick filaments. The I band is the area of thin filaments (troponin, tropomyosin, and actin) not overlapped by thick filaments. With contraction, I bands become smaller as Z lines move toward the M lines.

The above scheme holds for each muscle fiber type. However, the speed of contraction is related to the activity of its myosin ATPase (11). It also correlates with the presence of specific isoforms for the myofibrillar proteins, including the myosin heavy chain, myosin light chains, troponins, actinins, and C proteins and the calcium-sequestering enzymes of the sarcoplasmic reticulum.

Muscle fiber relaxation is also the consequence of an active process. Shortly after calcium is released, it is pumped back into the sarcoplasmic reticulum by a calcium-depen-

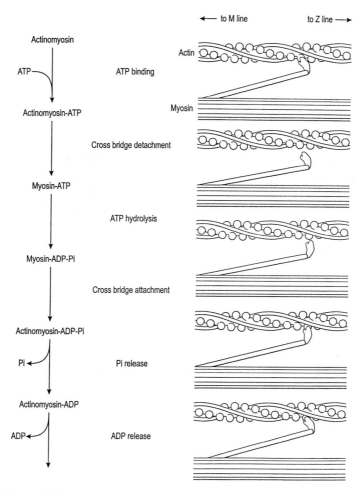

**FIG. 3.** Reactions of ATP hydrolysis that provide energy for the formation of cross-bridging between myosin and actin. Through this mechanism, muscle fiber shortening (muscle contraction) occurs.

dent ATPase. Once the concentration of calcium around the fibrils is lowered, calcium is displaced from troponin and the interaction between actin and myosin ceases, cross-links are broken, and fiber lengthening occurs.

## ENERGY METABOLISM IN SKELETAL MUSCLE

Most energy necessary for muscle contraction is provided by the hydrolysis of ATP. Intracellular concentrations of ATP are normally maintained by the action of enzymes such as creatine kinase, adenylate kinase, and myoadenylate deaminase. The energy needed to replenish ATP when it is consumed during muscle contraction is provided by the intermediary metabolism of carbohydrate and lipid by the pathways of glycolysis, the tricarboxylic acid cycle, β-oxidation, and oxidative phosphorylation (12–14).

The immediate source of energy for skeletal muscle is found in preformed compounds containing high-energy phosphate such as ATP and creatine phosphate. At rest, ATP is continuously generated through the reactions of intermediary metabolism. But despite continuous production, ATP levels remain constant because the terminal phosphate of ATP is transferred to creatine, forming creatine phosphate and ADP in a reaction catalyzed by creatine kinase. Creatine phosphate thus provides a reservoir of high-energy phosphate immediately available to reform ATP on demand and acts to buffer changes in cytoplasmic ATP concentrations. Creatine kinase and its products, creatine and creatine phosphate, also play a significant role in the transport of energy from the mitochondrial matrix to myofibrils in the sarcoplasm. This latter action is referred to as the creatine–creatine phosphate shuttle (Fig. 4) (15).

During rest and less strenuous exercise, the activity of creatine kinase renders the concentration of ATP within cells constant at the expense of creatine phosphate. When metabolic requirements, such as those that occur during prolonged contraction, exceed the capacity of oxidative phosphorylation to regenerate ATP, creatine phosphate is used to replenish ATP. When approximately 50% of the creatine phosphate has been converted to creatine, ATP levels begin to fall and inosine monophosphate (IMP) levels rise. ATP is hydrolyzed to ADP and then to AMP by adenylate kinase, and the AMP is converted to IMP by myoadenylate deaminase. During recovery from exercise, IMP is converted back to AMP by a two-step process. The conversion of AMP to IMP and back to AMP has been called the purine nucleotide cycle (Fig. 5) (16). The reactions of the purine nucleotide cycle reduce AMP levels, which are inhibitory to ATP-generating reactions; generate ammonia, which stimulates glycolysis; and release fumarate, which is converted to malate, an intermediate of the citric acid cycle and promoter of oxidative phosphorylation. Thus, the action of this cycle serves to restore ATP levels by a variety of mechanisms.

Most cellular energy is produced in mitochondria. Each mitochondria consists of two membranes. The outer portion is limiting and provides the interface with the cytoplasm. The inner membrane is folded and invaginated into cristae. The space between the membranes is termed the intermembrane space and the space inside the inner membrane is called the

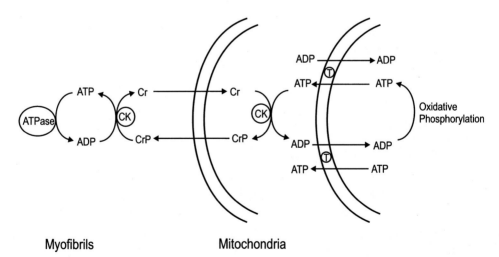

Myofibrils            Mitochondria

**FIG. 4.** Creatine–creatine phosphate shuttle. Creatine kinase activities are located on the inner mitochondrial membrane, on the myofibrils, and in the cytoplasm and play an important role in energy transfer. This shuttle allows ATP generated in the mitochondria to reach the myofibrillar contractile proteins where its hydrolysis by actinomyosin ATPase leads to muscle contraction. CK, creatine kinase; ATPase, actinomyosin ATPase; Cr, creatine; CR-P, creatine phosphate; T, adenine nucleotide translocase.

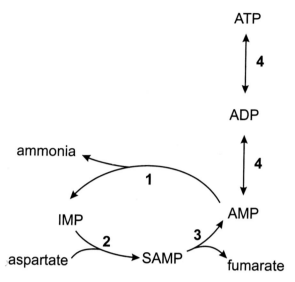

**FIG. 5.** Purine nucleotide cycle. When muscle contraction occurs under conditions that lead to insufficient creatine phosphate levels to buffer ATP concentrations adequately, ATP levels decline, forming AMP. Under these conditions, anaerobic glycolysis becomes the major route of ATP generation and the purine nucleotide cycle plays a pivotal role. The activity of myoadenylate deaminase converts AMP to IMP with the release of ammonia. Ammonia stimulates phosphofructokinase, a rate-limiting glycolytic enzyme. IMP increases stoichiometrically as ATP decreases. When oxidative conditions are restored, AMP is regenerated with the release of fumarate. Fumarate is converted to malate, an intermediate of the tricarboxylic acid cycle. The increased levels of malate "drive" the cycle, increasing the generation of ATP through oxidative phosphorylation. *1*, myoadenylate deaminase; *2*, adenylsuccinate synthetase; *3*, adenylsuccinate lyase; *4*, adenylate synthetase.

matrix. Larger quantities of creatine kinase are localized to the inner membrane space. The respiratory chain and energy-transducing processes are associated with the inner membrane. The enzymes of the tricarboxylic acid cycle and β-oxidation are found in the matrix.

Mitochondria contain their own DNA and the necessary machinery for transcription, translation, and replication (17–19). Mitochondrial DNA differs from nuclear DNA in several ways: It is circular, it is derived entirely for the maternal parent, and it lacks repair mechanisms. In addition, it codes for only a portion of its structural and enzyme proteins. In fact, the bulk of mitochondrial proteins is encoded by nuclear genes, synthesized in the cytoplasm, and transported into the mitochondrial membrane or matrix (Table 3).

**TABLE 3.** *Gene products from mitochondrial DNA*

| Components of mitochondria genoma | Genes | Number |
|---|---|---|
| Respiratory chain subunits | | 13 |
| | Complex I (ND1, ND2, ND3, ND4, ND4L, ND5, ND6) | |
| | Complex III (cytochrome *b*) | |
| | Complex IV (COXI, COXII, COXIII) | |
| | Complex V (subunit 6, subunit 8) | |
| Mitochondria translation apparatus | | 2 |
| | Ribosomal RNA 12S | |
| | Ribosomal RNA 16S | |
| Transfer RNA | | 22 |

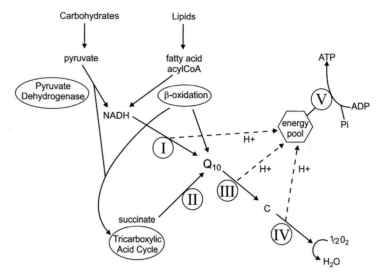

**FIG. 6.** Oxidative phosphorylation occurs on the inner membrane of mitochondria by the action of a series of enzyme complexes termed the respiratory chain. Reduced NADH is oxidized by complex I and succinate is oxidized by complex II. The resulting electrons are transformed first to cytochrome Q10 (ubiquinone) and then sequentially to complex III, cytochrome *c*, complex IV, and oxygen. The energy released is used to pump hydrogen ions out of the mitochondrial inner membrane through complexes I, III, and IV, producing an electrochemical gradient that established conditions for the condensation of ADP and inorganic phosphorous, forming ATP by complex V (ATP synthase).

Mitochondrial metabolism primarily provides for the liberation of energy from the aerobic oxidation of substrates (13). Products of the aerobic degeneration of carbohydrate and fatty acids enter the tricarboxylic acid cycle, generating reducing equivalents. The respiratory chain consists of a series of enzymes and coenzymes that function as hydrogen and electron carriers responsible for transferring reducing equivalents derived from the tricarboxylic acid cycle or fatty acid metabolism to molecular oxygen (Fig. 6 and Table 4). The large amount of free energy released is captured and conserved in the form of ATP through a process called oxidative phosphorylation. Factors that influence the rel-

**TABLE 4.** *Components of respiratory chain complexes*

| Complex | Enzyme activity | Prosthetic groups |
|---------|-----------------|-------------------|
| I | NADH dehydrogenase | FMN |
| | Iron sulfur proteins | |
| II | Succinate dehydrogenase | FAD |
| | Cytochrome $b_{560}$ | |
| | Iron sulfur proteins | |
| III | Cytochrome Q dehydrogenase | Cytochrome $b_{562}$ |
| | Cytochrome $b_{566}$ | |
| | Cytochrome $c_1$ | |
| | Iron sulfur protein center | |
| IV | Cytochrome *c* oxidase | Cytochrome *a* |
| | Cytochrome $a_3$ | |
| | Copper | |
| V | ATP synthase | Magnesium |

FMN, flavin mononucleotide; FAD, flavin adenine dinucleotide.

ative amounts of carbohydrate and lipids used for ATP production include the oxygen concentration of blood, muscle blood flow, plasma free fatty acid levels, and the number of mitochondria and levels of glycogen stores in muscle.

Intracellular glycogen stores provide the major source of carbohydrate available for energy production in skeletal muscle. Glycogen is a major storage form of carbohydrate in the body and is distributed evenly between slow- and fast-twitch muscle fibers at rest. Glycogen is a branched homopolymer of glucose in which α-1,4-linked glucose residues constitute the linear portions of the molecule and points of branching occur when α-1,6-glucosidic bonds connect on linear chains to another. It appears that there are essentially equal numbers of branched and unbranched chains in muscle glycogen. There is a uniform distribution of unit chain lengths ranging from 11 to 14, and each branched chain has two chains attached to it (20).

The pathways of glycogen synthesis and degeneration are distinct from each other. Most glucose entering the fibers from the blood is converted to glycogen, although glucose itself can be metabolized directly to pyruvate under certain conditions.

The synthesis of glycogen requires glucose to move from the blood into the muscle fiber. This occurs via a transport system that is believed to use a mobile carrier within the cell membrane. This system is stimulated by insulin. Once inside the cell, glucose is phosphorylated to form glucose-6-phosphate by the activity of hexokinase. Glycogen synthesis then proceeds by the sequence of actions of phosphoglucomutase, uridine diphosphate-glucose phosphorylase, glycogen synthase, and branching enzyme. These reactions result in polymers with molecular weights of 10 million, each containing approximately 55,000 glucose units.

During exercise of short duration and high intensity, the major source of energy is glycogen, not glucose. On demand, glucose units are enzymatically split from glycogen and are degraded through a series of reactions to pyruvate (Fig. 7). Although this pathway involves a series of enzymes, the amount of pyruvate formed is regulated primarily by the activities of phosphorylase and phosphofructokinase. Glycogen phosphorylase, termed myophosphorylase in muscle, catalyzes the phosphorolysis of glycogen to form glucose 1-phosphate glycogen. Glycogen phosphorylase exists in two forms, phosphorylase a and phosphorylase b. The latter is active in the presence of AMP. Thus, its role may be more important when AMP begins to accumulate under conditions of excessive ATP breakdown. In addition, phosphorylase b can be converted to phosphorylase a by the action of phosphorylase b kinase. Phosphorylase b kinase is activated by calcium when it is released from the sarcoplasmic reticulum. It can also be controlled by β-adrenergic agonists. This control is mediated through cyclic AMP. Glycogen phosphorylase alone can degrade only about 35% of glycogen to glucose-1-phosphate. The activity of debranching enzyme (amylo-1,6-glucosidase) together with glycogen phosphorylase can completely degrade glycogen.

The enzymes of the glycolytic pathway are found in the sarcoplasm (20). Under aerobic conditions, pyruvate is the end product of glycolysis. The formed pyruvate enters the tricarboxylic acid cycle and is metabolized by that cycle and by oxidative phosphorylation to carbon dioxide and water. In the process, large amounts of energy are liberated in the form of ATP. The metabolism of 1 molecule of glucose by aerobic glycolysis yields a net gain of 38 molecules of ATP. Under anaerobic conditions, the formed pyruvate does not enter the tricarboxylic acid cycle. Instead, it is converted to lactate. This process produces smaller quantities of ATP, only two molecules of ATP per molecule of glucose. Muscle glycogen stores are limited and can be depleted after 90 minutes of exercise at an intensity level at 70% maximum oxygen uptake.

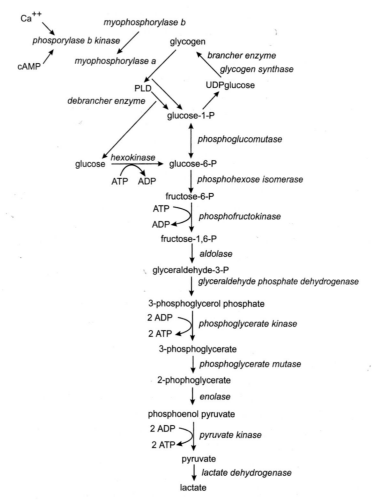

**FIG. 7.** Pathways for glycogen metabolism and glycolysis. Under most conditions, most glucose that enters the cell is converted to glycogen. When carbohydrate is used for energy, glycogen is degraded. Under aerobic conditions, pyruvate is the end product of glycolysis. The pyruvate generated is processed through the tricarboxylic acid cycle and oxidation phosphorylation. Under anaerobic conditions, pyruvate is converted to lactate.

In contrast to the limited supply of carbohydrate, the supply of lipid is plentiful. However, the speed at which lipids can be mobilized and the rate of energy production from them is slow compared with glycogen (21). Lipids in the form of fatty acids constitute the major substrates for energy production for muscles at rest, during contraction at lower intensity or of longer duration, and during recovery (22). Plasma free fatty acids provide the largest source of lipids, with intracellular stores providing very small contributions. Long-chain fatty acids move through the bloodstream from adipose tissue bound to albumin. These, plus smaller fatty acids, move across endothelial cells and into muscle cells, where they are available for energy production, storage, or synthesis into membrane components (Fig. 8). Each process requires activation of the fatty acids to acyl-coenzyme A (CoA) derivatives. The resulting activated long-chain fatty

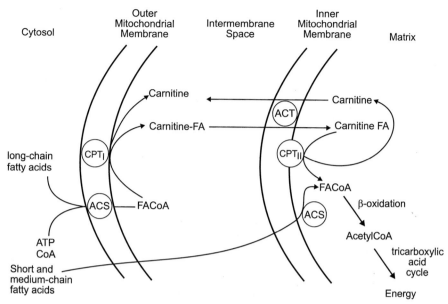

**FIG. 8.** Fatty acid metabolism in mitochondria. Short- and medium-chain fatty acids enter mitochondria by diffusion. Long-chain fatty acids enter by a multistep process that is initiated by activation by a reaction catalyzed by acyl-CoA synthetase (ACS). Next, the fatty acid-CoA is combined with a carrier molecule, carnitine, by the action of carnitine palmitoyltransferase (CPT) I. These first two enzymes are localized to the mitochondrial outer membrane. The fatty acid carnitine is then "passed" through the inner membrane to CPT II. CPT II removes the carnitine, which is transferred back into the intermembrane space by acylcarnitine translocase (ACT) and makes the fatty acid available for metabolism to acetyl-CoA molecules by β-oxidation. Five molecules of ATP are generated for each acetyl-CoA molecule generated by β-oxidation.

acids can undergo esterification, leading to the formation of cytosolic triglyceride droplets that provide a depot of lipid for future use, or oxidation after carnitine-mediated transport into mitochondria catalyzed by carnitine palmitoyltransferase activities. Once in the mitochondria, fatty acyl-CoA units are converted to acetyl-CoA by the process of β-oxidation, and acetyl-CoA is processed through the tricarboxylic acid cycle. By these processes, 1 molecule of palmitate will result in the production of 131 molecules of ATP.

## REFERENCES

1. Burke RE. Motor unit types of cat triceps surae muscle. *J Physiol (Lond)* 1967;193:141–150.
2. Burke RE. Physiology of motor units. In: Engel AG, Franzini-Armstrong C, eds. *Myology*, 2nd ed. New York: McGraw-Hill, 1994:464–483.
3. Kelly AM, Rubinstein NA. The diversity of muscle fiber types and its origin during development. In: Engel AG, Franzini-Armstrong C, eds. *Myology*, 2nd ed. New York: McGraw-Hill, 1994:119–133.
4. Barany M. ATPase activity of myosin correlated with speed of muscle shortening. *J Gen Physiol* 1967;50: 197–203.
5. Staudte H, Pette D. Correlation between enzymes of energy-supplying metabolism as a basic pattern of organization in muscle. *Comp Biochem Physiol B Biochem Mol Biol* 1972;41:533–541.
6. Sandow A. Excitation-contraction coupling in skeletal muscle. *Pharmacol Rev* 1965;17:265–279.
7. Franzini-Armstrong C. The sarcophasmic reticulum and the transverse tubuler. In: Engel AG, Franzini-Armstrong C, eds. *Myology,* 2nd ed. New York: McGraw-Hill, 1994:176–199.

8. Perry SV. Activation of contractile mechanism by calcium. In: Engel AG, Franzini-Armstrong C, eds. *Myology*, 2nd ed. New York: McGraw-Hill, 1994:529–552.
9. Greaser ML, Gregory J. Reconstitution of troponin activity from three protein components. *J Biol Chem* 1971; 246:4226–4231.
10. Awdemard E, Betrand R, Bonet A, et al. Pathways for the communication between ATPase and actin sites in myosin. *J Muscle Res Cell Motil* 1988;9:197–203.
11. Szent-Györgmi AG, Chantler PD. Control of contraction by calcium binding to myosin. In: Engel AG, Franzini-Armstrong C, eds. *Myology*, 2nd ed. New York: McGraw-Hill, 1994:506–528.
12. Kushmerick MJ. Patterns in mammalian muscle energetics. *J Exp Biol* 1985;115:165–177.
13. Layzer RB. How muscles use fuel. *N Engl J Med* 1991;324:411–412.
14. Lee CP, Martens ME. Mitochondrial respiration and energy metabolism in muscle. In: Engel AG, Franzini-Armstrong C, eds. *Myology*, 2nd ed. New York: McGraw-Hill, 1994:624–647.
15. Bessman SP, Carpenter CL. The creatine-creatine phosphate shuttle. *Annu Rev Biochem* 1985;54:831–862.
16. Lowenstein JM, Goodman MN. The purine nucleotide cycle in skeletal muscle. *Federation Proc* 1978;37: 2308–2312.
17. Giles RE, Blanc H, Cann HM, Wallace DC. Maternal inheritance of human mitochondrial DNA. *Proc Natl Acad Sci USA* 1980;7:6715–6719.
18. Anderson S, Bankier AT, Barrell BG, et al. Sequence and organization of human mitochondrial genome. *Nature* 1981;290:457–465.
19. Clayton DA. Structure and function of mitochondrial genome. *J Inherit Metab Dis* 1992;15: 439–447.
20. Brown DH. Glygogen metabolism and glycolysis in muscle. In: Engel AG, Franzini-Armstrong C, eds. *Myology*, 2nd ed. New York: McGraw-Hill, 1994:648–664.
21. Haller RG, Bertocci LA. Exercise evaluation of metabolic myopathies. In: Engel AG, Franzini-Armstrong C, eds. *Myology*, 2nd ed.. New York: McGraw-Hill, 1994:807–821.
22. Ontko JA. Lipid metabolism in muscle. In: Engel AG, Franzini-Armstrong C, eds. *Myology*, 2nd ed. New York: McGraw-Hill, 1994:665–682.

*Diseases of Skeletal Muscle,*
edited by Robert L. Wortmann.
Lippincott Williams & Wilkins, Philadelphia © 2000

# 3

# Muscle Function

## Joseph A. Houmard

*Department of Exercise and Sport Science, East Carolina University, Greenville,
North Carolina 27858*

A variety of factors, separate from those caused by disease, influence skeletal muscle function. Those that adversely affect muscle function generally cause fatigue or weakness. Several mechanisms lead to neuromuscular fatigue. Physical conditioning is perhaps the most effective means for maximizing muscle function because skeletal muscle can adapt to both endurance- and resistance-oriented training. Aging involves unique problems that cause decreased muscle function, but physical conditioning can exert a positive influence on aged muscle. An understanding of these factors as they pertain to healthy or normal individuals will enhance one's ability to appreciate the changes that occur in clinical disorders that affect skeletal muscle.

## NEUROMUSCULAR FATIGUE

Fatigue is defined as the point when a muscle fails to maintain the required or expected force to perform a given activity (1). Fatigue is thus not total exhaustion or a complete inability to exert tension but rather a more subtle phenomenon where impaired muscle function is manifest. Although the development of fatigue is a hindrance to being physically active or during rehabilitation, it may serve as a protective function against muscle damage (2).

Although the definition of fatigue is simplistic, the underlying mechanisms are complex and not 34well understood (3,4). This is largely due to the multifactoral nature of the condition. Factors related to fatigue include, but are not limited to, impairments within the muscle, at neuromuscular junctions, and within the central nervous system and training, health, and hydration status (3–6). The lack of understanding coupled with the complexity of the processes involved have allowed several theories to be developed. Most hold that fatigue results from a combination of events that occur during any given activity and that a single mechanism is often not solely responsible.

### Central Fatigue

The elements of the central nervous system that are likely involved in neuromuscular fatigue are the sites where the muscular movement is initiated, including the cerebral cortex, basal ganglia, cerebellum, and the motor neurons. It is difficult to obtain direct measurements of these pathways during motor tasks. Thus, there is relatively little direct evidence for the involvement of the central nervous system in fatigue. The simplest support for central fatigue is that in the exercising subject, force can often be increased or maintained with verbal encouragement (2). Perhaps the best evidence for central fatigue comes from the observation that an exhausted limb recovers more rapidly if the contralateral limb is exercised at a mild workload (7–9). This recovery effect is called the "Setchenov phenomenon" and is attributed to sensory input from the mildly exercising limb facilitating the function of motor centers of the brain and alleviating central fatigue. This theory could explain how "diverting activities" may be an effective means for increasing work output during rehabilitation efforts where central fatigue is a factor (8).

Central fatigue may become more important during prolonged physical activity (10,11). Depletion of branched-chain amino acids by muscle metabolism during prolonged activity can lead to increased tryptophan concentrations within the brain. The elevated tryptophan, the chemical hypothesized to promote drowsiness, depresses brain function by inducing an excess of the neurotransmitter 5-hydroxy-tryptamine, which in turn can promote fatigue. In support, consumption of beverages containing branched-chain amino acids may improve performance and reduce perceived effort during prolonged activity (11). Central exhaustion may also play a role in well-motivated individuals, although peripheral mechanisms seem to be the main cause of fatigue (1–6,12). Central fatigue must, however, be strongly considered in clinical states where central cognition is altered. These conditions include neuroasthenia, hysterical paralysis, and other situations where motivation for voluntary motor activity is impaired (1).

### Peripheral Fatigue

Although central mechanisms may be involved, fatigue is more commonly attributed to an impairment within the muscle itself. This theory stems from the work of Merton (13). In classic experiments, maximal voluntary isometric contractions were performed by the thumb adductor muscles (adductor pollicis) to fatigue. Electric shocks were then applied to the motor nerve to stimulate the muscle. The shocks generated clear action potentials to the muscle but no corresponding increase in tension, indicating that the source of fatigue resided within the muscle (Fig. 1).

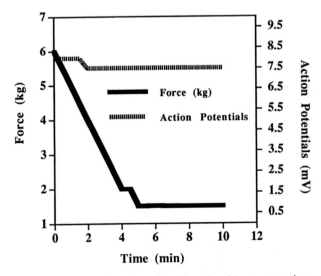

**FIG. 1.** Maximal isometric contraction strength of thumb adductor muscles and corresponding action potentials. (From Ref. 13.) When electrical shocks were imposed to the motor nerve, action potentials were maintained, supporting failure in the contractile apparatus rather than the nervous system.

A variety of mechanisms may account for fatigue within skeletal muscle. During short-duration high-intensity muscle contractions, the main energy source is endogenous ATP. As the supply is limited (only enough for 1 to 2 seconds of activity), the repletion of ATP must take place for muscle contraction to continue. The source for the resynthesis of ATP is stored creatine phosphate with the dephosphorylation reaction rapidly catalyzed by creatine kinase. During short-duration maximal muscle contractions, fatigue is reached when creatine phosphate levels are virtually depleted (14–16). At this point, ATP levels also begin to decrease, resulting in a decrement in tension-generating ability. The depletion of creatine phosphate is thus a mechanism promoting fatigue in maximal activities lasting 8 to 20 seconds. This can be dramatically illustrated by studying the dynamics of the 100-m sprint finals in events such as the Summer Olympics. World class athletes are actually slowing down in the final segments of the event due to creatine phosphate depletion in skeletal muscle.

The important role of creatine is provided by observations that creatine supplementation can increase resting muscle creatine phosphate stores and have a positive effect on muscle power (17). An elevation in fasting creatine with supplementation also correlates with an extension of the time until fatigue develops. This results in a potentiation of gains in strength and muscle mass with repeated days of physical training using resistance exercise (18). An accumulation of inorganic phosphate inherent with the consumption of ATP may directly inhibit cross-bridge interaction between actin and myosin and lead to fatigue (16,19,20). Thus, a combination of factors inherent with the rapid depletion of creatine phosphate and ATP can contribute to fatigue during intense muscle contractions.

ATP and creatine phosphate concentrations can be rapidly replenished when oxygen is available. Both levels recover to approximately resting levels in skeletal muscle within 10 to 15 minutes after intense contractions, as long as blood flow is sufficient (21). In contrast, occlusion of the vessels leading to the active muscle bed delays the resynthesis of both ATP and creatine phosphate. This emphasizes the importance of oxygen delivery and a well-developed cardiovascular system for skeletal muscle function. The ability of muscle to rapidly replete creatine phosphate allows healthy individuals to perform repeated muscle contraction of 1 to 12 seconds duration at intense workloads with relatively little decline in force generation as long as recovery time is adequate. Therefore, the importance of adequate recovery should be emphasized when attempting to maintain muscle tension at high levels.

During high-intensity muscle activity of longer duration (more than 1 to 2 minutes), additional mechanisms related to energy generation play roles in neuromuscular fatigue. Lactic acid is produced during more prolonged activity as the result of increased carbohydrate utilization through glycolysis. Lactic acid rapidly dissociates into a lactate ion and a hydrogen ion. Some of the produced hydrogen ions are buffered by various proteins within the cell. Eventually, as glycolysis continues, hydrogen ions accumulate from lactic acid and other glycolytic intermediates (1–5,16,22). The production of hydrogen ions is positively related to the intensity of the contractile activity. Consequently, the more intense the activity, the higher the rate of lactic acid production (16,23–25).

The accumulation of hydrogen ions can contribute to muscular fatigue in several ways. The energy-generating enzymes of glycolysis, particularly the rate-limiting enzyme phosphofructokinase, are inhibited at a lower pH (5,11,16,20,21). The production of lactic acid through glycolysis thus essentially serves as a negative feedback mechanism for energy production. This may be a protective device against placing excessive stress on the muscle. The hydrogen ions also physically impair actin–myosin cross-bridge interaction by competitively displacing calcium from troponin (5). This direct inhibition of the contractile apparatus may contribute to a perception of rigor during intense muscular activity. Finally, the acid accumulation stimulates pain receptors, producing sensations in the muscle often described as burning. For individuals with a low pain tolerance, this may be an important mechanism contributing to fatigue. Hydrogen ions that diffuse into the blood and enter the brain can cause symptoms of nausea and confusion (5).

Lactic acid accumulates during continuous muscular activity at an intense workload. This accumulation coincides with the development of fatigue, typically within 2 to 10 minutes. Lactic acid concentrations also progressively increase when repeated (intermittent) bouts of intense contractile work are performed with relatively short intervals for recovery. Recovery intervals should be an important consideration in rehabilitative efforts, which often involve repeated intense muscle contractions with rest between the work bouts. Both the nature and duration of the rest interval are important in reducing blood and muscle lactic acid levels. For example, complete rest actually increases the susceptibility of the muscle to fatigue compared with performing very mild exercise during recovery (23–25). This is attributed to the increased blood flow caused by mild exercise. As a result, the hydrogen ions diffuse out of the muscle into the relatively large buffering pool of plasma (23–25). If the recovery workload is too intense, however, hydrogen ion concentration will, instead, increase due to the stimulation of glycolysis. Therefore, relatively mild muscular activity rather than complete rest is recommended between bouts of exercise during intermittent work. However, during intense intermittent work, lactic acid still accumulates and contributes to fatigue unless a complete return to the resting state is reached with a lengthy rest interval (24,25).

The use of intermittent work to build tolerance and improve muscle function is thus an interplay between the activity and recovery periods. If this ratio is well selected, then considerable positive adaptations that enhance muscle function can be achieved. Repeated work bouts with moderate recoveries will stimulate adaptations in both the oxidative and glycolytic energy-producing pathways (25). In contrast, full recovery between bouts may provide relative comfort but results in less adaptive stimulus to the tissue.

The nature of fatigue during long-duration low-intensity muscle contractions involves mechanisms that are related to energy depletion. During prolonged contractile activity (45 to 60 minutes), the energy to meet the demand of the work is derived from the combination of protein, carbohydrate, and fat sources. Although a topic of debate, the relative contribution of protein to total energy production during prolonged submaximal contractile activity is approximately 10% or less (26). At work intensity of relatively low levels, up to 30% to 50% of the energy is derived from lipid stores, in adipose tissue, and intramuscular cytoplasmic triglycerides (27). This source is effective for prolonged muscle contraction. For example, lipid stores in a relatively lean individual can supply energy for approximately 120 hours of activity. The limiting factor with lipid oxidation is the relatively slow rates of energy-production compared with carbohydrate utilization. Nevertheless, lipid oxidation can produce ATP at a rapid enough rate to meet the energy demands for low to moderate level activities for sustained intervals.

The remainder of the energy requirements during moderate activity must be met with carbohydrate utilization. Although carbohydrate can be catabolized at a fairly rapid rate and supply adequate amounts of energy, storage is limited. In a normal sedentary individual, muscle and liver glycogen stores generally become depleted after approximately 90 to 120 minutes of moderate intensity muscular work (16,23,24). When these carbohydrate stores are depleted, fatigue ensues as contractile activity decreases due to the limiting and slower rate of fat metabolism. The depletion of carbohydrate is thus a major

60% to almost 95% type I. In sprinters the opposite is evident, as only 10% to 20% of the fibers are slow twitch, with the remainder of type II fibers (24,45). This type of disparity may also be evident in disease states. Type II, and more specifically type IIb muscle fibers, predominate in muscle of obese and obese individuals with non–insulin-dependent diabetes mellitus (46–49). Conditions such as hyperthyroidism (41,42,50) and chronic heart failure (51) may also promote the increased expression of type II muscle fibers.

A predominance of type II fibers may present a practical problem in relation to muscle function and development of fatigue. The IIb fiber is thought to be a "default" fiber that is primarily expressed in the absence of physical activity due to its inefficient contractile characteristics (52). An individual initiating physical activity with a high amount of type IIb fibers is thus relatively prone to fatigue. This may explain, at least in part, why obese individuals find contractile activity so uncomfortable and difficult to maintain. The plasticity of muscle, however, allows transition in fiber type from the IIb to the more fatigue-resistant IIa fibers within 6 to 8 weeks of either endurance- or resistance-oriented training (42,49,53). In fact, there are very few type IIb fibers in trained athletes (24,49). This change in the contractile characteristics is concomitant with other alterations that produce a more fatigue-resistant fiber. Thus, contractile activity may become perceptually less stressful if an individual can continue past 6 to 8 weeks of conditioning. The attainment of a type IIa to type I (fast to slow) fiber transition, however, is debatable and may only be evident after years of intense training (24,53). Initial muscle fiber type and the time course for muscle fiber type transition are thus important factors that influence muscle function.

Resistance training provides an effective method for improving muscle function. Effective resistance training produces two important functional outcomes. First, the ability to generate maximal force increases. Second, muscular endurance, the number of times a given mass can be lifted, also increases. These adaptations are associated with dramatic changes in skeletal muscle morphology.

The major adaptation with resistance-oriented physical conditioning is a pronounced hypertrophy of the recruited muscle fibers (54,55). The increase in cross-sectional area of the fiber is primarily due to an accompanying increase in the number and size of the myofibrils, which produces an enhanced ability to produce force (Fig. 3). There is also

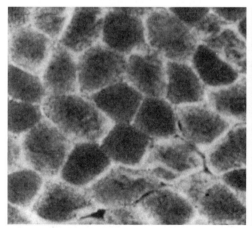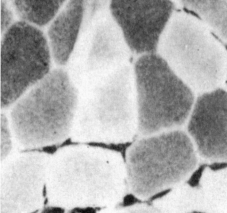

**FIG. 3.** Example of relative increase in muscle fiber cross-sectional area with resistance training in human skeletal muscle. Individual fibers often increase their cross-sectional area by approximately 10% to 20% or more with an adequate overload stimulus.

an increase in connective tissue, which aids in providing a framework for the increased force production.

The magnitude of the hypertrophy with resistance training depends on the nature of the physical activity. As much as 100 years ago, it was realized that the overload principal was an essential part of enhancing muscle function (56). The overload principal simply involves periodically assessing strength gains and increasing the workload accordingly to produce a maximal training stimulus. Thus, periodic assessment and adjustment of the conditioning plan is essential in providing an adequate stimulus for optimal gains in muscle function.

The type of muscle contraction is also important. With resistance training three exercise modalities are commonly used. Isometric training involves exerting tension with no change in muscle length. Isotonic training involves lifting (concentric portion) and then lowering (eccentric portion) a specific mass. The term isotonic is used as the same mass or weight is moved through the range of motion of the lift. Isokinetic training involves the muscle contracting at the same speed while exerting tension. This type of training uses specialized equipment because accommodating resistance must be applied through the range of motion due to the different amounts of force produced at various joint angles.

Although isometric contractions enhance muscle strength, any gains are highly specific to the joint angle used during the contractile activity (57,58). Isometric training also produces relatively small increases in muscle strength and endurance compared with other types of contractions (58). The more common type of resistance training (isotonic) involves moving a mass against gravity (concentric contraction) and then lowering the mass with gravity (eccentric contraction). The impact of various permutations of this type of training has been extensively examined and summarized (54–58), and both muscular endurance and force-generating ability increase when the overload principle is practiced.

The stimulus for hypertrophy and functional gains may differ between the concentric and eccentric portions of the lift due to inherent differences in the activities (59–61). For example, the eccentric component involves muscle lengthening against tension and produces muscle damage and soreness. In contrast, concentric contractions are more typical in terms of the classic concept of muscle shortening and are not associated with overt cellular disruption and soreness after training. The neural activation patterns of eccentric and concentric muscle contractions are also quite specific, and improvements in strength seems to carry over primarily to the respective contraction mode. It thus appears that using training where both concentric and eccentric contractions are used will produce the greatest functional gains relative to normal every day activities.

In isokinetic training, speed is kept constant through the range of motion despite differences in force-generating ability at the various joint angles. The consistent speed is often accomplished with the use of a hydraulic system. Consequently, isokinetic exercise results in the maximal development of muscular tension throughout the range of motion and the greatest overall activation of motor units. The effectiveness of this type of training for stimulating improved muscle function (endurance and strength) has been demonstrated repeatedly (57,58,62,63) (Fig. 4). Because of the maximal involvement of motor units, improvements in muscle function can be accomplished within 7 weeks with as little as 1 minute of exercise per day (62). The speed of contraction during training is important because strength gains are relatively specific to the training speed (62,63).

The adaptations that occur in skeletal muscle with resistance-oriented training are not limited to hypertrophy. The ability to produce ATP through the oxidative pathways is improved by relatively small increases in capillary density and oxidative enzymes. These changes may contribute to enhanced endurance by promoting lactic acid removal and facilitating ATP production (54,55). Repeated elevations of lactic acid with training also ap-

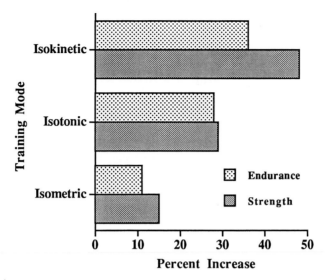

**FIG. 4.** Comparison of isokinetic, isotonic, and isometric strength-training programs on muscle strength (one repetition maximum) and endurance (ability to lift a given mass). All programs were performed for 4 days per week over 8 weeks. The data indicate the relative effectiveness of isokinetic training. (From Ref. 58.)

pear to stimulate production of muscle proteins, which serve as buffers and increase subjective pain tolerance. Alterations in muscle glycogen stores occur with resistance training. ATP and creatine phosphate stores do not, however, appear to increase (54,55,64). There is also some evidence that hyperplasia (an increase in muscle fiber number) occurs, although this may be limited to unique experimental paradigms (65). Adaptations in the central nervous system are also important. With repeated days of resistance training, the central nervous system begins to recruit additional motor units, resulting in increased generation force. It appears that the initial increases in muscle strength with training are primarily due to this central nervous system adaptation because very little muscle hypertrophy occurs before 6 to 8 weeks of a conditioning program (54,66). These factors, in combination with hypertrophy, contribute to the marked ability to generate tension and increase endurance in skeletal muscle with progressive resistance training.

As with resistance training, the alterations that occur with endurance-oriented physical conditioning are numerous. A primary adaptation with endurance training is an enhanced ability of the muscle fiber to extract and use oxygen. Increases in muscle capillary and mitochondrial densities are largely responsible for this adaptation (3–5,23,24,39,67–70). The increased capacity for oxygen use results in a relatively greater recruitment of the oxidative pathways in trained muscle that minimizes lactic acid production and prolongs the onset of fatigue. The utilization of both intramuscular and extracellular lipid is also promoted, decreasing the reliance on the more limited muscle glycogen supplies.

The plasticity of muscle with endurance training is marked. Muscle enzymes associated with the oxidative processes can increase twofold or more with capillary density increasing as well. Glycogen and triglyceride stores also increase in the trained muscle fibers (71,72). These alterations contribute to an increase in whole body maximum oxygen consumption ($Vo_2max$). This increase may generally reach 10% to 20%, or more, with 14 weeks of endurance training, although changes among individuals on a similar exercise program are quite variable. Factors such as genetics and cardiac function contribute to the variability (73). Some types of training modalities, such as intermittent contractile activity combined with short rest periods (interval training), can produce more dramatic changes in the muscle cell (24).

For enhanced muscle function and general overall health, a combination of both resistance- and endurance-oriented training is typically recommended. The impact of the type of training on muscle function, specifically the ability to generate force, should be considered. In one experiment, healthy subjects trained on a cycle ergometer (endurance), performed resistance training (strength), or a combination of both (74). The ability to produce tension was then measured by torque-producing ability on an isokinetic device during leg extension (Fig. 5). Endurance training produced no increase in leg strength, whereas resistance training markedly improved strength. The interesting finding concerned the combination group. The ability to produce torque was actually impaired in the combination group compared with the resistance training-only individuals. These and other data suggest that endurance training can actually impede the ability to exert force (74,75). Why this occurs, however, is not understood. Consideration of these results should be given when designing a physical conditioning program.

Although individuals can work for months, if not years, to develop improved muscle function, unfortunately many adaptations are rapidly lost when the training ceases. These losses occur regardless of the degree of time devoted to the conditioning program. This phenomenon is all too dramatically demonstrated with endurance training (Fig. 6). In one study, athletes who were training for years were studied at various time points after a training cessation (76). A significant compromise (7% to 10%) in maximal oxygen uptake became apparent after as little as 14 to 24 days of no training. The activities of many oxidative enzymes begin to decrease dramatically after approximately 14 days of training cessation (77). This leads to a decrement in oxygen extraction ability as evident by a reduction in arterial-venous oxygen difference during exercise. The ability to use oxygen is

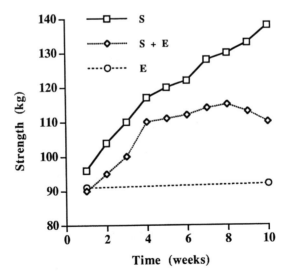

**FIG. 5.** Leg strength (knee extension) changes in response to three types of training: strength (S), endurance (E), and strength and endurance (S + E). Strength was tested weekly in S and S + E and before and after 10 weeks of training in E. The data indicate that endurance-oriented contractile activity can actually impair the development of muscular strength. (From Ref. 68.)

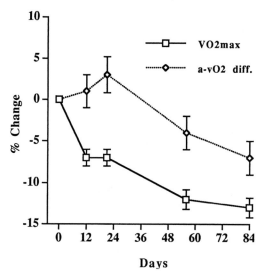

**FIG. 6.** Impact of training cessation on $V_{O_2}$max and arterial-mixed venous oxygen difference (a–$vO_2$ diff) at maximal exercise. These data indicate the rapid rate at which training adaptations are lost in skeletal muscle with training cessation in even highly trained individuals who have been exercising for years. (From Ref. 76.)

thus dramatically compromised with a relatively acute cessation of training despite years of the contractile stimulus. This is associated with a concomitant decrease in functional capacity of the muscle and general exercise tolerance.

A similar phenomenon is evident with resistance training (Fig. 7). There are relatively rapid gains in the ability to generate force that result from adaptations in the central nervous system and within the muscle itself with resistance training. When training ceases,

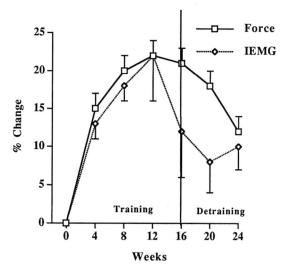

**FIG. 7.** Relative alterations in maximal isometric quadriceps force and integrated electromyographic (IEMG) activity during leg extension with 16 weeks of training and 8 weeks of training cessation. The data indicate that adaptations gained with resistance training are rapidly lost when the training ceases. (From Ref. 78.)

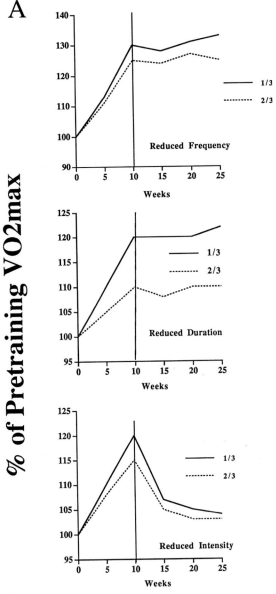

**FIG. 8.** Effects of training and 15 weeks of either a one-third (solid lines) or two-thirds (broken lines) reduction in exercise frequency, duration, and intensity on maximal oxygen uptake (**A**). The training adaptation is largely maintained despite considerable reductions in training volume; however, when intensity is reduced, maximal oxygen consumption is compromised. This relationship is demonstrated in **B** in relation to muscle citrate synthase activity (81). Activity of this enzyme increased with training and was maintained when the same training was performed for the ensuing 2 weeks (maintained group) or when training frequency decreased from 4 days to 2 days per week (reduced). When training ceased for 2 weeks (detraining), citrate synthase declined.

a rapid reversion toward pretraining values occurs. This loss in strength parallels a reduction in integrated muscle electromyographic activity, suggesting a loss in the ability of the central nervous system to recruit the required motor units (78). Muscular atrophy also begins to develop with as little as 2 weeks after cessation of training, contributing to a loss in force-generating ability (79).

It is unreasonable to expect any individual to maintain a consistent overload situation in terms of a conditioning stimulus. Fortunately, once a training adaptation is gained, a minimal amount of the training stimulus can maintain positive changes (Fig. 8). Hickson et al. (80) reported that up to a 75% reduction in either training frequency (number of training sessions per week) or training duration (duration of each training session) allowed maintenance of $Vo_2max$ for up to 15 weeks. Because $Vo_2max$ is a function of the ability of skeletal muscle to extract and use oxygen, these data suggest that muscle function is also preserved when training volume is diminished. In keeping with this is the observation that citrate synthase activity, a marker of mitochondrial function, is preserved with a 50% reduction in training duration (81). When training totally ceases, however, the activity of this enzyme virtually returns to sedentary levels. In addition, when training intensity is reduced, there is a reduction in $Vo_2max$, suggesting a compromise in muscle oxidative function (80).

Similar findings are evident in relation to resistance training. A 50% reduction in training volume will maintain force-generating ability, whereas training cessation results in a rapid decrement to pretraining levels (82). Together, these findings indicate that muscle function can be maintained with a reduced training stimulus but is negatively affected with the cessation of contractile activity.

## IMPACT OF AGING ON SKELETAL MUSCLE FUNCTION

Normal biologic aging involves a variety of changes in skeletal muscle. Muscle function, particularly force-generating ability, is compromised with the aging process (Fig. 9).

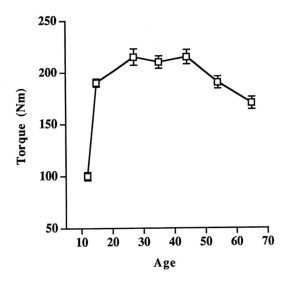

**FIG. 9.** Maximal isometric strength during knee extension exercise for subjects of various age groups. These data indicate that strength begins to decline at approximately age 50 years. (From Ref. 80.)

This decrement is largely due to a reduction in muscle mass from decreases in both muscle fiber size and muscle fiber number. A variety of other mechanisms, such as changes in the energy-producing machinery, may also contribute to the decline in muscle function with aging. Data from the Framingham study (83) indicated that approximately 40% of the female population aged 55 to 64 years, 45% aged 65 to 74 years, and 65% aged 75 to 84 years were unable to lift 4.5 kg. These same women also reported that they were unable to perform many aspects of everyday activities due to poor strength. It is difficult to discern whether these changes result from biologic consequences of aging or are secondary to a reduction in physical activity (67,68,84,85).

It appears that muscle strength is largely maintained up to the fifth decade of life, declines by about 15% per decade in the sixth and seventh decade, and decreases at a much faster rate (perhaps 30% per decade) thereafter (2,17,68,86). This decline in strength has been attributed to several mechanisms. An absolute loss in muscle mass is a primary culprit (67,68,87). This conclusion is primarily derived from measuring strength in older versus younger individuals and correcting for relative muscle mass. Many studies have observed no differences between young and old subjects in strength per unit of muscle but a marked reduction in overall strength. Other studies suggest that the loss in strength with aging may exceed that associated with the decrease in muscle mass. Thus, a combination of a decline in muscle mass and an intrinsic impairment in the contractile apparatus may contribute to the reduction in muscle strength with aging.

Whether muscular atrophy is secondary to a reduction in physical activity also contributes to weakness in the elderly is unclear, because contractile activity can produce muscular hypertrophy in even the oldest individuals. A reduced rate of protein synthesis is evident with aging, although this is not reflected by a reduction in myofibrillar mRNA. This suggests an alteration at the level of translation (88). Other mechanisms that may contribute to muscle atrophy include insulin resistance and decreased anabolic hormone concentrations (54,67,68).

Relatively little information exists concerning changes in muscle endurance and resistance to fatigue with aging. Findings are somewhat controversial, because some studies indicate no difference in fatigability, whereas others show an increased susceptibility to fatigue. The changes that occur in glycolytic and oxidative muscle enzyme activities with aging are unclear. Although a decrease in oxidative enzyme activities has been reported by some, others have reported no changes in these activities. Observations in muscle glycolytic capacity also vary (67,68,89,90). These variations may be explained in part by differences in the muscle groups studied. For example, citrate synthase activity decreases in the gastrocnemius and does not change in the vastus lateralis (91).

Although muscle atrophy is a consistent finding with aging, other alterations related to muscle functional capacity are somewhat more controversial. A conversion of type II to type I fibers has been seen, although many other studies suggest no changes in fiber type with aging (67,68,89–91). Lexell (89) reported a significant decline in muscle fiber number that begins at age 25 years but no preferential loss of either the type I or II fibers. The decline in fiber number has been attributed to a compromise at the level of the motor neuron, leading to neuronal loss with aging (67,68). The cause of this neuronal death, however, remains unknown (2).

Some fiber types may be more susceptible than others to the muscle atrophy of aging. Studies in men suggest that the cross-sectional area of the type I fibers are preserved whereas there is a decline in the area of the type IIa and IIb fibers (67,68,89,90). Thus, the reduction in type II fiber area with aging may account for the significant decline in muscle mass and force-generating ability. In women, however, a reduction in type I and

IIa fiber areas is evident in 70-year-old compared with 60-year-old women (92). Thus, there may be a gender-specific effect relative to fiber atrophy.

A final parameter important to muscle function and fatigability is capillary density. In human skeletal muscle, findings are again conflicting. Some work demonstrates no change in skeletal muscle capillarity (90), whereas others have reported a decline with aging (67,68,93).

## INTERACTION BETWEEN PHYSICAL CONDITIONING AND AGING

Repeated contractile activity, specifically resistance-oriented training, can be used to reverse the decrement in muscle strength and atrophy evident with aging. For such an intervention or treatment to be effective, however, the plasticity of skeletal muscle must be intact. Several studies have demonstrated that aged human skeletal muscle can respond robustly to resistance training in terms of muscle hypertrophy and other functional changes (94–97). Older men and women exhibit similar or even greater relative gains in strength compared with young individuals, provided that an adequate training program is used. If adequate training was not performed, only minimal gains are made.

Frontera et al. (97) trained 12 men (66 ± 2 years) three times per week for 12 weeks (Fig. 10). At the conclusion of training, knee extensor and flexor strength had increased by approximately 200% and 100%, respectively. This was accompanied by an 11% increase in quadricep cross-sectional area as determined from computed tomography. Specific histochemical analysis of muscle biopsy samples indicated a 30% hypertrophy of both type I and type II fibers. Increases in muscle citrate synthase activity and capillary density were also observed.

A similar program of resistance was performed for 8 weeks in institutionalized frail 90-year-old individuals (96). Initial strength levels were very low before training. The average increase in strength after 8 weeks of conditioning was 174%. This was accompanied by a mean increase in quadricep cross-sectional area of 15%. Even more im-

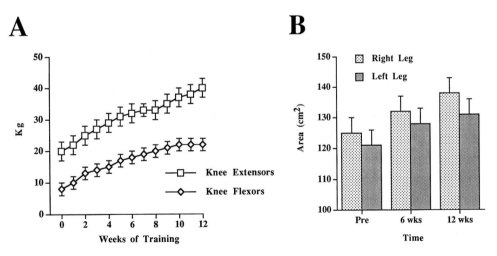

**FIG. 10.** Time course of improvements in strength (one repetition max) in the knee extensors and flexors of 66-year-old men (**A**). The increases in strength were accompanied by increases in thigh cross-sectional area, determined from computed tomography, at 6 and 12 weeks of the training (**B**). (From Ref. 90.)

portantly, there was an improvement in gait speed, suggesting an improved functional capacity.

It is not clear if the oxidative potential of human skeletal muscle decreases with the aging process. However, a reduction in cardiovascular fitness, as indicated by a decline in $Vo_2max$, is evident in both sedentary and trained individuals (Fig. 11). In sedentary individuals, this decline occurs at a rate of about 10% per decade (68,98,99).

Aged human skeletal muscle does respond to endurance training stimuli. $Vo_2max$ increased from 20% to 30% in individuals 60 to 80 years old with 3 months or more of endurance-oriented training (68). This increase in $Vo_2max$ is attributed, at least partially, to adaptations in skeletal muscle.

Significant increases in oxidative capacity and oxidative enzyme activities occur in the skeletal muscle of aged individuals with endurance training. Coggan et al. (100) examined 65-year-old men and women after 10 months of training four times a week for 45 minutes a session at 80% of maximal heart rate. With training, oxidative enzyme activities in skeletal muscle increased by approximately 25% to 50%, and $Vo_2max$ rose 28% with similar changes in the men and women. These changes were virtually equivalent to those in younger individuals (68). Meredith et al. (101) studied young (aged 24 years) and older (aged 65 years) men and women after 12 weeks of stationary cycling for 45 minutes a day 3 days a week at 70% of heart rate reserve. The increase in $Vo_2max$ was approximately 20% in each age group. The improvement in muscle oxidative capacity was much more pronounced, however, in the aged (128%) than in the young (28%) subjects.

Other adaptations occur in aged human skeletal muscle with endurance training. Muscle capillary density increases. There can be an increase in type IIa fibers accompanied by a decline in IIb fibers (100). However, these adaptations are only observed when the training stimulus is of a sufficient intensity over a period of 3 months or more (68). As in young subjects, a threshold stimulus is needed to induce positive adaptations.

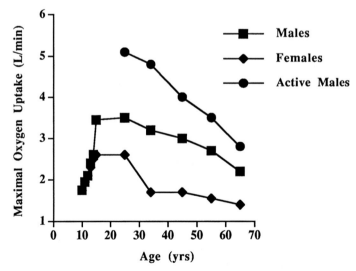

**FIG. 11.** Changes in maximal oxygen uptake with aging in men and women and active males. (From Refs. 98, 99). The data indicate similar rates of decline after approximately age 25 years but differing absolute values relative to gender and physical conditioning status.

This is particularly evident when examining cross-sectional studies comparing aged endurance athletes to their younger counterparts. Coggan et al. (102) compared skeletal muscle characteristics in aged (63 ± 6 years) and young (26 ± 3 years) endurance runners who were matched for performance and training volume. They found the activities of key oxidative enzymes were 25% to 30% higher in the aged runners. There were no differences in capillary density or in the percentages of type I, IIa, or IIb muscle fibers. These data indicate that training-induced adaptations in skeletal muscle can be maintained in aged individuals.

However, although the aged can exhibit positive adaptations with exercise, physical conditioning cannot totally reverse the impact of the aging process. Athletic performance in both power- and endurance-oriented events declines with age, even in the most highly motivated individuals (11,24). In relation to intervention, although the relative improvements with training are similar or even greater in aged and young subjects, the absolute values of many measures still remain depressed in the aged. This may be primarily due to the inherent fact that aged subjects enter such studies with a lower functional capacity of skeletal muscle. It cannot be denied, however, that physical conditioning improves muscle function robustly in aged subjects relative to their sedentary counterparts.

## REFERENCES

1. Edwards RHT. Human muscle function and fatigue. In: Porter R, Whelan J, eds. *Human muscle fatigue: physiological mechanisms*. London: Pitman Medical, 1981:1–18.
2. McComas AJ. *Skeletal muscle: form and function*. Champaign, IL: Human Kinetics, 1996.
3. Sejerstem OM, Vollestad WK, Hallén J, Bahr R. Acta Physiologica Scandinavica international symposia on muscle performance—fatigue, recovery and trainability. *Acta Physiol Scand* 1998;162:181–275.
4. Porter R, Whelan J, eds. *Human muscle fatigue: physiological mechanisms*. London: Pitman Medical, 1981.
5. Brooks GA, Fahey TD, White TP. *Exercise physiology: human bioenergetics and its applications*. Mountain View, CA: Mayfield Publishing Co., 1996:701–721.
6. Enoka RM, Stuart DG. Neurobiology of muscle fatigue. *J Appl Physiol* 1992;72:1631–1648.
7. Setchenov IM. Sur Frage nach der einsirkung sensitiver reize auf dre muskelarbeit des menschen. In: *Selected works*. Moscow: 1935:246–260.
8. Asmussen E, Mazin B. Recuperation after muscular fatigue by "diverting activities." *Eur J Appl Physiol* 1978;38:1–8.
9. Asmussen E, Mazin B. A central nervous component in local muscular fatigue. *Eur J Appl Physiol* 1978;38:9–15.
10. Newsholme EA, Blomstrand E, Ekblom B. Physical and mental fatigue: metabolic mechanisms and importance of plasma amino acids. *Br Med Bull* 1992;48:477–495.
11. Newsholme EA, Leech T, Duester G. *Keep on running: the science of training and performance*. Chichester, England: John Wiley and Sons, 1994:113–130, 238–239.
12. Bigland-Ritchie B, Jones DA, Hosking GP, Edwards RHT. Central and peripheral fatigue in sustained maximum voluntary contractions of human quadriceps muscle. *Clin Sci Mol Med* 1978;54:609–614.
13. Merton PA. Voluntary strength and fatigue. *J Physiol (Lond)* 1954;123:553–564.
14. Bergstrom J. Local changes of ATP and phosphylcreatine in human muscle tissue in connection with exercise. In: Chapman CB, ed. *Physiology of muscular exercise*. New York: American Heart Association, 1967:191–196.
15. Soderlund K, Greenhaff PL, Hultman E. Energy metabolism in type I and type II human muscle fibres during short term electrical stimulation at different frequencies. *Acta Physiol Scand* 1992;144:15–22.
16. Sahlin K, Tonkonogi M, Soderlund K. Energy supply and muscle fatigue in humans. *Acta Physiol Scand* 1998;162:261–266.
17. Greenhaff PL, Casey A, Short AH, Harris R, Soderlund K, Hultman E. Influence of oral creatine supplementation of muscle torque during repeated bouts of maximal voluntary exercise in humans. *Clin Sci* 1993;84:565–571.
18. Earnest CP, Snell PG, Rodriguez R, et al. The effect of monohydrate ingestion on anaerobic power indices, muscular strength, and body composition. *Acta Physiol Scand* 1995;153:207–209.
19. Thompson LV, Fitts RH. Muscle fatigue in the from semitendinosus: role of the high-energy phosphates and Pi. *Am J Physiol* 1992;263:C803–C809.
20. Wilkie DR. Muscular fatigue: effects of hydrogen ions and inorganic phosphate. *FASEB Proc* 1986;45:2921–2923.
21. Hultman E, Sjoholm H, Sahlin K, Edstrom L. Glycolytic and oxidative energy metabolism and contraction

characteristics of intact human muscle. In: Porter R, Whelan J, eds. *Human muscle fatigue: physiological mechanisms.* London: Pitman Medical, 1981:19–40.

22. Gevers W. Generation of protons by metabolic processes in heart cells. *J Mol Cell Cardiol* 1977;9:867–874.
23. Hargreaves M. Skeletal muscle carbohydrate metabolism during exercise. In: Hargreaves M, ed. *Exercise metabolism.* Champaign, IL: Human Kinetics, 1995:41–72.
24. Costill DL. *Inside running: basics of sports physiology.* Indianapolis, IN: Benchmark Press, 1986:85–122.
25. Jacobs I. Blood lactate: implications for training and sports performance. *Sports Med* 1986;3:10–28.
26. White TP, Brooks GA. [U-$^{14}$C]glucose, -alanine, and -leucine oxidation in rats at rest and two intensities of running. *Am J Physiol* 1981;240:E155–E165.
27. Romijn JA, Coyle EF, Sidossis LS, et al. Regulation of endogenous fat and carbohydrate metabolism in relation to exercise intensity and duration. *Am J Physiol* 1993;265:E380–E391.
28. Costill DL, Sherman M, Fink W, et al. The role of dietary carbohydrates in muscle glycogen resynthesis after strenuous running. *Am J Clin Nutr* 1981;34:1831–1836.
29. Kirwan JP, Costill DL, Mitchell JB, et al. Carbohydrate balance in competitive runners during successive days of intense training. *J Appl Physiol* 1988;65:2601–2606.
30. Ivy JL, Costill DL, Fink WJ, Lower RW. Influence of caffeine and carbohydrate feedings on endurance performance. *Med Sci Sports* 1979;11:6–11.
31. Spriet LL, MacLean DA, Dyck DJ, et al. Caffeine ingestion and muscle metabolism during prolonged exercise in humans. *Am J Physiol* 1992;262:E891–E898.
32. Kenney WL. Thermoregulation at rest and during exercise in healthy older adults. In: Holloszy JO, ed. *Exercise and sports sciences reviews.* Baltimore, MD: Williams & Wilkins, 1997:41–76.
33. Appell JH, Soares JMC, Duarte JAR. Exercise, muscle damage and fatigue. *Sports Med* 1992;13:108–112.
34. Mair J, Koller A, Artner-Dworzak E, et al. Effects of exercise on plasma myosin heavy chain fragments and MRI of skeletal muscle. *J Appl Physiol* 1992;72:656–661.
35. Salminen A. Lysosomal changes in skeletal muscle during the repair of exercise injuries in muscle fibers. *Acta Physiol Scand* 1985;539[Suppl]:1–31.
36. Newham DJ, McPhail G, Mills KR, Edwards RHT, Ultrastructural changes after concentric and eccentric contractions on human muscle. *J Neurol Sci* 1983;16:109–113.
37. Appell HJ, Forsberg S, Hollman W. Satellite cell activation in human skeletal-muscle after training evidence for muscle-fiber neoformation. *Int J Sports Med* 1988;9:297–302.
38. McCormick KM, Thomas DP. Exercise-induced satellite cell activation in senescent soleus muscle. *J Appl Physiol* 1992;72:888–892.
39. Kraus WE, Torgan CE, Taylor DA, Kenney WL. Thermoregulation at rest and during exercise in healthy older adults. In: Holloszy JO, ed. *Exercise and sports sciences reviews.* Baltimore, MD: Williams & Wilkins, 1994:313–360.
40. Brooke MH, Kaiser KK. Three myosin adenosine triphosphate systems: the nature of their pH lability and sulfhydryl dependence. *J Histochem Cytochem* 1970;18:670–672.
41. Hamalainen N, Pette D. Patterns of myosin isoforms in mammalian skeletal muscle fibers. *Microsc Res Tech* 1995;30:381–389.
42. Schiaffino S, Reggiani C. Molecular diversity of myofibrillar proteins: gene regulation and functional significance. *Physiol Rev* 1996;76:371–423.
43. Smerdu V, Karsch-Mizrachi I, Campione M, et al. Type IIx myosin heavy chain transcripts are expressed in type IIb fibers of human skeletal muscle. *Am J Physiol* 1994;267:C1723–C1728.
44. Simoneau JA, Bouchard C. Human variation in skeletal muscle fiber-type proportion and enzyme activities. *Am J Physiol* 1989;257:E567–E572.
45. Costill DL, Daniels J, Evans W, et al. Skeletal muscle enzymes and fiber composition in male and female track athletes. *J Appl Physiol* 1976;40:149–154.
46. Marin P, Andersen B, Krotkiewski M, Bjorntorp P. Muscle fiber composition and capillary density in women and men with NIDDM. *Diabetes Care* 1994;17:382–386.
47. Hickey MS, Carey JO, Azevedo JL, et al. Skeletal muscle fiber composition is related to adiposity and in vitro glucose transport rate in humans. *Am J Physiol* 1995;268:E453–E457.
48. Nyholm B, Qu Z, Kaal A, et al. Evidence of an increased number of type IIb muscle fibers in insulin-resistant first-degree relatives of patients with NIDDM. *Diabetes* 1997;46:1822–1828.
49. Bassett DR. Skeletal muscle characteristics: relationships to cardiovascular risk factors. *Med Sci Sports Exerc* 1994;26:957–966.
50. Kirschbaum BJ, Kucher HB, Termin A, et al. Antagonistic effect of chronic low frequency stimulation and thyroid hormone on myosin expression in rat fast-twitch muscle. *J Biol Chem* 1990;23:13974–13980.
51. Sullivan MJ, Duscha BD, Klitgaard H, et al. Altered expression of myosin heavy chain in human skeletal muscle in chronic heart failure. *Med Sci Sports Exerc* 1997;29:860–866.
52. Goldspink G, Scutt A, Martindale J, et al. Stretch and force generation induce rapid hypertrophy and myosin isoform gene switching in adult skeletal muscle. *Biochem Soc Trans* 1991;19:368–373.
53. Andersen P, Henriksson J. Training-induced changes in subgroups of human type II skeletal muscle fibers. *Acta Physiol Scand* 1977;99:123–125.
54. Kraemer WJ, Fleck SJ, Evans WJ. Strength and power training: physiological mechanisms of adaptation. In: Holloszy JO, ed. *Exercise and sports sciences reviews.* Baltimore, MD: Williams & Wilkins, 1996:363–397.

55. Tesch PA. Short- and long-term histochemical and biochemical adaptations in muscle. In: Komi P, ed. *Strength and power in sports. The encyclopedia of sports medicine.* England: Blackwell, 1992:239–248.

56. Roux W. *Gesammelte Abhandlugen uber Entwicklungsmechanik der Organismen.* Leipzig, Austria: Band I Funktionelle Anpassung, 1895.

57. Fox E, Bowers R, Foss M. *The physiological basis for exercise and sport.* Madison, WI: Brown and Benchmark, 1993:159–199.

58. Thistle H, Hislop H, Moffroid M, Lowman E. Isokinetic contraction: a new concept of resistance exercise. *Arch Phys Med Rehab* 1967;48:279–282.

59. Hortobagyi T, Hill JP, Houmard JA, et al. Adaptive responses to muscle lengthening and shortening in humans. *J Appl Physiol* 1996;80:765–772.

60. Dudley GA, Tesch PA, Miller BJ, Buchanan P. Importance of eccentric actions in performance to resistance training. *Aviat Space Environ Med* 1991;62:543–550.

61. Hather BM, Tesch PA, Buchanan P, Dudley GA. Influence of eccentric actions on skeletal muscle adaptations to resistance training. *Acta Physiol Scand* 1991;143:177–185.

62. Lesmes GR, Costill DL, Coyle EF, Fink WJ. Muscle strength and power changes during maximal isokinetic training. *Med Sci Sports* 1978;10:266–269.

63. Moffroid M, Whipple R, Hofkosh J, et al. A study of isokinetic exercise. *Phys Ther* 1968;49:735–746.

64. Tesch PA, Thorsson A, Coliander EB. Effects of eccentric and concentric resistance training on skeletal muscle substrates, enzyme activities and capillary supply. *Acta Physiol Scand* 1990;140:575–580.

65. Gonyea WJ, Ericson GC, Bonde-Peterson F. Skeletal muscle fiber splitting induced by weight-lifting exercise in cats. *Acta Physiol Scand* 1977;19:105–109.

66. Moritani T. Time course of adaptations during strength and power training. In: Komi P, ed. *Strength and power in sports. The encyclopedia of sports medicine.* Oxford, England: Blackwell, 1992:266–278.

67. Cartee GD. Aging skeletal muscle: response to exercise. In: Holloszy JO, ed. *Exercise and sports sciences reviews.* Baltimore, MD: Williams & Wilkins, 1994:91–120.

68. Rogers MA, Evans WJ. Changes in skeletal muscle with aging: effects of exercise training. In: Holloszy, JO, ed. *Exercise and sports sciences reviews.* Baltimore, MD: Williams & Wilkins, 1993:65–102.

69. Booth FW, Tseng BS, Fluck M, Carson JA. Molecular and cellular adaptation of muscle in response to physical training. *Acta Physiol Scand* 1998;162:343–350.

70. Pette D. Training effects on the contractile apparatus. *Acta Physiol Scand* 1998;162:367–376.

71. Coggan AR, Williams BD. Metabolic adaptations to endurance training: substrate metabolism during exercise. In: Hargreaves M, ed. *Exercise metabolism.* Champaign, IL: Human Kinetics, 1995:41–72.

72. Van der Vusse GJ, Reneman RS. Lipid metabolism in muscle. In: Rouell LB, Shepherd JT, eds. *Handbook of physiology. Exercise: regulation and interaction of Multiple systems.* Bethesda, MD: American Physiological Society, 1996:952–994.

73. Bouchard C, Dionne FT, Simoneau JA, Boulay MR. Genetics of aerobic and anaerobic performance. In: Holloszy JO, ed. *Exercise and sports sciences reviews.* Baltimore, MD: Williams & Wilkins, 1992:27–58.

74. Hickson RC. Interference of strength development by simultaneously training for strength and endurance. *Eur J Appl Physiol* 1980;45:255–263.

75. Dudley GA, Fleck SJ. Strength and endurance training: are they mutually exclusive? *Sports Med* 1987;4:79–85.

76. Coyle EF, Martin WH, Sinacore DR, et al. Time course of loss of adaptations after stopping prolonged intense endurance training. *J Appl Physiol* 1984;57:1858–1864.

77. Chi MMY, Hintz CS, Coyle EF, et al. Effects of detraining on enzymes of energy metabolism in individual human muscle fibers. *J Appl Physiol* 1983;244:C276–C287.

78. Hakkinen K, Komi PV. Electromyographic changes during strength training and detraining. *Med Sci Sports Exerc* 1983;15:455–460.

79. Hortobagyi T, Houmard JA, Stevenson JR, et al. The effects of detraining on power athletes. *Med Sci Sports Exerc* 1993;25:929–935.

80. Hickson RC, Foster C, Pollock ML, et al. Reduced training intensities and loss of aerobic power, endurance, and cardiac growth. *J Appl Physiol* 1985;58:492–499.

81. Houmard JA, Tyndall GL, Midyette JB, et al. Effect of reduced training and training cessation on insulin sensitivity and muscle GLUT-4. *J Appl Physiol* 1996;1:1162–1168.

82. Graves JE, Pollock ML, Leggett SH, et al. Effect of reduced training on muscular strength. *Int J Sports Med* 1988;9:316–319.

83. Jette AM, Branch LG. The Framingham disability study. II. Physical disability among the aging. *Am J Public Health* 1981;71:1211–1216.

84. Faulkner JA, Brooks SV, Zerba E. Skeletal muscle weakness and fatigue in old age: underlying mechanisms. In: Cristofalo XVJ, Lawton MP, eds. *Annual review of gerontology and geriatrics.* New York: Springer, 1990:147–166.

85. McCarter RJM. Age-related changes in skeletal muscle function. *Aging* 1990;2:27–38.

86. Larsson L, Grimby G, Karlsson J. Muscle strength and speed of movement in relation to age and muscle morphology. *J Appl Physiol* 1979;46:451–456.

87. Frontera WR, Hughes VA, Lutz KJ, Evans WJ. A cross-sectional study of muscle strength and mass in 45 to 78-year-old men and women. *J Appl Physiol* 1991;71:644–650.

88. Welle S, Bhatt K, Thornton. Polyadenylated RNA, actin mRNA, and myosin heavy chain mRNA in young and old skeletal muscle. *Am J Physiol* 1996;270:E224–229.

89. Lexell J. Human aging, muscle mass, and fiber type composition. *J Gerontol* 1995;50A:11–16.
90. Grimby G. Muscle performance and structure in the elderly as studied cross-sectionally and longitudinally. *J Gerontol* 1995;50A:17–22.
91. Houmard JA, Weidner ML, Gavigan KE, et al. Fiber type and citrate synthase activity in the human gastrocnemius and vastus lateralis with aging. *J Appl Physiol* 1988;85:1337–1341.
92. Essen-Guystavsson B, Borges O. Histochemical and metabolic characteristics of human skeletal muscle in relation to age. *Acta Physiol Scand* 1986;95:153–165.
93. Coggan AR, Spina RJ, King DS, et al. Histochemical and enzymatic comparison of the gastrocnemius muscle of young and elderly men and women. *J Gerontol Biol Sci* 1992;47:B71–76.
94. Brown AB, McCartney N, Sale DG. Positive adaptations to weight-lifting training in the elderly. *J Appl Physiol* 1990;69:1725–1733.
95. Charette SL, McEvoy L, Pyka G, et al. Muscle hypertrophy response to resistance training in older women. *J Appl Physiol* 1991;70:1912–1916.
96. Fiatarone MA, Marks EC, Ryan ND, et al. High intensity strength training in nonagenarians. Effects on skeletal muscle. *JAMA* 1990;263:3029–3034.
97. Frontera WR, Meredith CN, O'Reilly KP, et al. Strength conditioning in older men: skeletal muscle hypertrophy and improved function. *J Appl Physiol* 1988;64:1038–1044.
98. Hermansen L. Individual differences. In: Larson LA, ed. *Fitness, health, and work capacity. International standards for assessment.* New York: Macmillan, 1974.
99. Astrand PO, Rodahl KR. *Textbook of work physiology.* New York: McGraw-Hill, 1970.
100. Coggan AR, Spina RJ, King DS, et al. Skeletal muscle adaptations to endurance training in 60- to 70-year-old men and women. *J Appl Physiol* 1992;72:1780–1786.
101. Meredith C, Frontera W, Fisher E, et al. Peripheral effects of endurance training in young and old subjects. *J Appl Physiol* 1989;66:2844–2849.
102. Coggan AR, Spina RJ, Rogers MA, et al. Histochemical and enzymatic characteristics of skeletal muscle in master athletes. *J Appl Physiol* 1990;68:1896–1901.

# PART II

# Diseases of Muscle

*Diseases of Skeletal Muscle,*
edited by Robert L. Wortmann.
Lippincott Williams & Wilkins, Philadelphia © 2000

# 4

# Idiopathic Inflammatory Myopathies

## Chester V. Oddis

*Department of Medicine, University of Pittsburgh Medical Center and University of
Pittsburgh School of Medicine, Pittsburgh, Pennsylvania 15213*

The term inflammatory myopathy is often used interchangeably with the term myositis. The term idiopathic inflammatory myopathy is used to represent a group of diseases of unknown cause in which muscle injury results from inflammation. Today, the names polymyositis, dermatomyositis, inclusion body myositis, myositis associated with malignancy, myositis in overlap with another connective tissue disease, eosinophilic myositis, orbital myositis, myositis ossificans, and focal myositis are included among these disorders. The individual idiopathic inflammatory myopathies can be arbitrarily separated into "common" and "uncommon" (Table 1). The idiopathic inflammatory myopathies can affect individuals of all ages. Childhood forms, defined as myositis with onset before the age of 18, are discussed in Chapter 5.

## HISTORICAL OVERVIEW

Between 1886 and 1891, German clinicians were the first to publish clinical descriptions of polymyositis and dermatomyositis. The term polymyositis was coined by Wagner in 1886 (1), whereas Unverricht (2) introduced the term dermatomyositis in 1891. Nearly two thirds of the 19th century descriptions fit with polymyositis, whereas the remaining patients likely had dermatomyositis. In 1916, dermatomyositis associated with malignancy was initially reported (3), although a causal relationship between the two was not hypothesized until 1935 (4).

Inclusion body myositis was first pathologically described by Chou in 1967 (5), but the term was introduced by Yunis and Samaha (6) in 1971 when characteristic nuclear and cytoplasmic inclusions were seen in histopathologic sections of muscle tissue. The classification scheme generally applied to these diseases was published by Bohan and

**TABLE 1.** *Clinicopathologic classification of the idiopathic inflammatory myopathies*

| "Common" subtypes | "Uncommon" subtypes |
|---|---|
| Polymyositis | Eosinophilic myositis |
| Dermatomyositis | Orbital myositis |
| Inclusion body myositis | Myositis ossificans |
| Childhood myositis | Focal myositis |
| Malignancy-associated myositis | Giant cell myositis |
| Myositis in overlap with another connective tissue diseases | Granulomatous myositis |

Peter in 1975 (7). Before publication of their criteria, the literature was difficult to decipher because of the lack of standardization of disease definition.

## CLASSIFICATION AND DIAGNOSIS

The purpose of disease classification is to separate the disease of interest from others to determine incidence, prevalence, epidemiologic features, natural history, and response to therapies. This is necessary in situations where there are no specific diagnostic tests or unique disease markers. In such situations, classification allows the identification of homogeneous patient subsets that facilitate studies and analysis of disease-specific issues.

There are perhaps three general goals in establishing classification and diagnostic criteria in the inflammatory myopathies: to distinguish patients with myositis from patients with other connective tissue diseases or other conditions that cause weakness, to divide patients with idiopathic inflammatory myopathies into clinically meaningful subtypes (e.g. separating polymyositis from dermatomyositis or polymyositis from inclusion body myositis based on subclassification criteria), and to establish the diagnosis of myositis in patients with muscle injury secondary to inflammation. The distinction between classification and diagnostic criteria in the connective tissue diseases is often blurred, and considerable overlap exists when these terms are applied to criteria sets. Several classification schemes have been proposed, but to date none satisfactorily explains the marked heterogeneity inherent in these diseases.

Although earlier attempts at classification were made (8–11), the diagnostic criteria proposed in 1975 by Bohan and Peter (7) have been considered the gold standard for study of polymyositis and dermatomyositis (Table 2). These criteria were proposed pri-

**TABLE 2.** *Bohan and Peter (7) criteria for the diagnosis of polymyositis and dermatomyositis*

---

1. Symmetric proximal muscle weakness determined by physical examination
2. Elevation of serum skeletal muscle enzymes (particularly creatine phosphokinase and often aldolase), serum glutamate oxaloacetate and pyruvate transaminases, and lactate dehydrogenase
3. The electromyographic triad of short, small, polyphasic motor unit potentials; fibrillations, positive sharp waves, and insertional irritability; and bizarre high-frequency repetitive discharges
4. Muscle biopsy abnormalities of degeneration, regeneration, necrosis, phagocytosis, and an interstitial mononuclear infiltrate
5. Typical skin rash of dermatomyositis, including a heliotrope rash, Gottron's sign, and Gottron's papules

Definite disease requires four criteria (three plus rash) for dermatomyositis and four criteria without rash for polymyositis; probable disease must include three criteria (two plus rash) for dermatomyositis and three criteria without rash for polymyositis; and possible disease requires two criteria (one plus rash) for dermatomyositis and two criteria without rash for polymyositis.

For these criteria to be applied, the following disease had to be excluded:
  Central or peripheral neurologic disease
  Muscular dystrophy, especially Duchenne muscular dystrophy
  Granulomatous myositis such as sarcoidosis
  Infections, including trichinosis, schistosomiasis, trypanosomiasis, staphylococcosis, toxoplasmosis, influenza, or rubella
  Drugs and toxins, such as clofibrate, alcohol, and penicillamine
  Rhabdomyolysis
  Metabolic disorders such as McArdle's syndrome
  Endocrinopathies such as thyrotoxicosis, myxedema, hyperparathyroidism, diabetes mellitus, or Cushing's syndrome
  Myasthenia gravis
  Atheromatous microemboli
  Carcinomatous thromboembolization

---

**TABLE 3.** *Proposed criteria for diagnosis of inclusion body myositis*

Pathologic criteria
  Electron microscopy
  1. Microtubular filaments in the inclusions
  Light microscopy
  1. Lined vacuoles
  2. Intranuclear and/or intracytoplasmic inclusions
Clinical criteria
  1. Proximal muscle weakness (insidious onset)
  2. Distal muscle weakness
  3. Electromyographic evidence of a generalized myopathy (inflammatory myopathy)
  4. Elevation of muscle enzyme levels (creatine phosphokinase and/or aldolase)
  5. Failure of muscle weakness to improve on a high-dose corticosteroid regimen (at least 40 to 60
    mg/day for 3 to 4 months)

Definite inclusion body myositis (IBM) = pathologic electron microscopy criterion 1 and clinical criterion 1 plus one other clinical criterion. Probable IBM = pathologic light microscopy criterion 1 plus 3 other clinical criteria. Possible IBM = pathologic light microscopy criterion 2 plus any 3 clinical criteria.
  From Ref. 12, with permission.

marily for the purposes of clinical research and were developed to be specific rather than sensitive. Inclusion body myositis was almost never recognized at the time these criteria were developed. Criteria for the diagnosis of inclusion body myositis were proposed by Calabrese et al. in 1987 (Table 3) (12). The criteria proposed by Bohan and Peter have served remarkably well for over three decades.

In 1995, Tanimoto et al. (13) proposed a new criteria set for classification of polymyositis and dermatomyositis that represented a unique collaborative effort among rheumatologists, dermatologists, and neurologists (Table 4). This effort both broadened the spectrum of patients considered to have idiopathic inflammatory myopathies and allowed determination of criteria specificity by using comparative groups with noninflammatory neuromuscular diseases. These criteria included the five of Bohan and Peter plus four new ones. Individuals with inclusion body myositis, childhood myositis, and malig-

**TABLE 4.** *Tanimoto et al. (13) classification criteria for polymyositis and dermatomyositis*

1. Skin lesions
  a. Heliotrope rash (red-purple edematous erythema on the upper palpebra)
  b. Gottron's sign (red-purple keratotic, atrophic erythema, or macules on the extensor surface of
    finger joints)
  c. Erythema on the extensor surface of extremity joints; slightly raised red-purple erythema over
    elbows or knees
2. Proximal muscle weakness (upper or lower extremity and trunk)
3. Elevated serum creatine kinase or aldolase level
4. Muscle pain on grasping or spontaneous pain
5. Myogenic changes on electromyography (short-duration polyphasic motor unit potentials with
  spontaneous fibrillation potentials)
6. Positive anti-Jo-1 (histidyl-transfer RNA synthetase) antibody
7. Nondestructive arthritis or arthralgias
8. Systemic inflammatory signs (fever > 37°C at axilla, elevated serum C-reactive protein level, or
  accelerated erythrocyte sedimentation rate of more than 20 mm/h (Westergren method)
9. Pathologic findings compatible with inflammatory myositis (inflammatory infiltration of skeletal muscle
  with degeneration or necrosis of muscle fibers; active phagocytosis, central nuclei, or evidence of
  active regeneration may be seen)

Dermatomyositis = at least one item from criterion 1 and at least four from criteria items 2 through 9; polymyositis = at least four from criteria items 2 through 9.
  From Ref. 11, with permission.

**TABLE 5.** *Bohan and Peter (7) subtype classification*

Group 1: Primary idiopathic polymyositis
Group 2: Primary idiopathic dermatomyositis
Group 3: Dermatomyositis (or polymyositis) associated with neoplasia
Group 4: Childhood dermatomyositis (or polymyositis) associated with vasculitis
Group 5: Polymyositis or dermatomyositis associated with collagen-vascular disease (overlap group)

nancy-associated myositis are excluded. The latter exclusions and the inclusion of several nonspecific vaguely defined criteria limit the usefulness of this and previous criteria sets.

Bohan et al. (14) proposed a simple subclassification of five groups for the approach to myositis (Table 5), emphasizing that these did not have distinctive features but that future studies would likely elucidate differences. Another subclassification scheme based on clinical, immunopathologic, and morphologic features has been proposed by Dalakas et al. (15), dividing the idiopathic inflammatory myopathies among polymyositis, dermatomyositis, and inclusion body myositis. Accordingly, dermatomyositis is humorally mediated with the microvasculature targeted, and polymyositis and inclusion body myositis are characterized by an antigen-directed cytotoxic T-cell attack on myofibrils expressing class I major histocompatibility complex antigens. Although clinical heterogeneity among the three subgroups is recognized, the immunopathologic features are said to distinguish the myositis subsets from each other.

Each criteria set discussed above represents thoughtful approaches to the clinical evaluation of patients with suspected myositis. However, criteria sets require periodic reevaluation as concepts of disease pathogenesis evolve and new diagnostic modalities become available. The understanding of the immunology of the myositis syndromes has grown with the identification and characterization of autoantibodies associated with polymyositis and dermatomyositis (see Chapter 15). The anti-aminoacyl tRNA synthetases (anti-Jo-1 and others), anti-Mi-2, and anti-SRP occur almost exclusively in patients with myositis and thus have been termed myositis-specific autoantibodies. Each myositis-specific autoantibody is associated with characteristic clinical features in addition to myositis. However, a small number of patients with anti-synthetase autoantibodies have no evidence of myositis. Because of a low sensitivity of less than 50%, the absence of a myositis-specific autoantibody certainly does not exclude polymyositis or dermatomyositis, but their presence does have strong predictive value for the diagnosis of myositis.

Magnetic resonance imaging is a newer technique that has proven to be beneficial in assessing the presence and extent of muscle inflammation in the inflammatory myopathies (see Chapter 16). Magnetic resonance is not as specific or sensitive as a biopsy but is noninvasive and allows a much larger sampling.

A new classification system for myositis has been proposed by Targoff et al. (Table 6) (16,17) using myositis-specific autoantibodies status and magnetic resonance imaging data to modify the Bohan and Peter criteria (Table 2). In this criteria set, the high specificity of the myositis-specific autoantibodies would not compromise specificity, and abnormal magnetic resonance imaging results could substitute for the muscle weakness or enzyme elevation criteria. However, magnetic resonance imaging findings could not be used in addition to these criteria or in place of electromyography, biopsy, rash, or autoantibody criteria. This latter limitation is necessary because the specificity of edema on magnetic resonance imaging is not yet established.

Application of all criteria systems involve excluding all causes of myopathy. This relates to the insensitivity of all criteria developed to date. Bohan and Peter insisted on multiple exclusions (Table 2). Similarly, Targoff et al.'s criteria assumes that known infectious, toxic,

**TABLE 6.** *Proposed revised criteria for the diagnosis of idiopathic inflammatory myopathies*

1. Symmetric[a] proximal muscle weakness
2. Elevation of the serum levels of enzymes, including not only creatine kinase level but also aldolase, AST, ALT, and lactate dehydrogenase levels
3. Abnormal electromyogram with myopathic motor unit potentials, fibrillations, positive sharp waves, and increased insertional irritability
4. Muscle biopsy features of inflammatory infiltration and either degeneration/regeneration or perifascicular atrophy
5. Any of one of the myositis-specific autoantibodies (an antisynthetase, anti-Mi-2, or anti-SRP)
6. Typical skin rash of dermatomyositis that includes Gottron's sign, Gottron's papules, or heliotrope rash

[a]Symmetry is intended to denote bilateral but not necessarily equal involvement.
   Possible idiopathic inflammatory myopathy (IIM) = any two criteria; probable IIM = any three criteria; definite IIM = any four criteria. Results of magnetic resonance imaging that are consistent with muscle inflammation may be substituted for either criterion 1 or 2. Patients with IIM who satisfy criterion 6 may be subclassified as having dermatomyositis. Those who satisfy the proposed criteria for inclusion body myositis (17) may be subclassified as having inclusion body myositis. Criteria 1, 2, 3, 4 and 6 are the original Bohan and Peter criteria in similar form. ALT, alanine aminotransferase; AST, aspartate aminotransferase.
   From Ref. 16, with permission.

metabolic, dystrophic, or endocrine myopathies have been excluded. To date, all criteria proposed require physicians to make diagnoses by exclusion and will continue to do so until these diseases are more fully understood and better diagnostic tests developed.

## CLINICAL FEATURES

### Muscle Involvement

Although proximal muscle weakness is the most common symptom of an idiopathic inflammatory myopathy at disease onset, the clinical features at disease presentation vary considerably from patient to patient. In polymyositis and dermatomyositis the weakness is most frequently insidious, bilateral, symmetric, progressive, and painless over the course of months as opposed to weeks. The lower extremity is usually affected first, with individuals complaining of difficulty getting up out of a chair or walking up steps. Walking may become clumsy with a "waddling gait." People may fall and may be unable to get up without assistance. Upper extremity symptoms often follow with patients unable to raise their arms above their head or having difficulty combing their hair. Proximal weakness may be manifested by the inability to raise one's head from a pillow due to severe neck flexor involvement. Although less common, muscle pain may occur. This seems more common, particularly with exercise in patients with dermatomyositis.

Proximal dysphagia with nasal regurgitation of liquids and pulmonary aspiration is usually seen with severe disease and is a poor prognostic sign (18). Pharyngeal muscle weakness may also result in hoarseness or a change in voice, giving it a nasal quality. Muscle atrophy and joint contractures are very uncommon at disease presentation. Ocular and facial muscle weakness is very uncommon in any idiopathic inflammatory myopathy (19), and their presence should signal the likelihood of another diagnosis (Table 7).

Although weakness is the cardinal feature of an idiopathic inflammatory myopathy, it may not be the presenting feature. In 105 patients seen over a 12-year period, the earliest symptoms were polyarthritis, Raynaud's phenomenon, and sicca syndrome in half (20). These features often preceded the diagnosis of myositis by months or years. Similarly, proximal muscle weakness was the presenting symptom in only one third of a French Canadian cohort with myositis (21). A rare but increasingly recognized presentation of myositis (polymyositis more frequently than dermatomyositis) is a systemic symptom

**TABLE 7.** *Other causes of muscle weakness*

**Neurologic disorders**
  Spinal muscular atrophy
  Amyotrophic lateral sclerosis
  Myasthenia gravis
  Eaton-Lambert syndrome
  Guillain-Barré syndrome
  Chronic inflammatory demyelinating polyneuropathy
**Muscular dystrophies**
  Duchenne's
  Limb girdle
  Beckers
  Facioscapulohumeral
  Emery-Dreifuss
  Myotonic
**Metabolic myopathies**
  See Chapter 9
**Congenital myopathies**
  See Chapter 10
**Endocrine myopathies**
  Diabetic amyotrophy and/or neuropathy
  Hypothyroidism
  Hyperthyroidism
  Acromegaly
  Cushing's disease
  Addison's disease
  Vitamin D deficiency myopathy
**Toxic myopathies**
  Alcohol
  Drug-induced (cholesterol/lipid-lowering agents, colchicine, penicillamine,
    emetine, chloroquine, zidovudine, cocaine, heroine, corticosteroid)
**Carcinomatous neuromyopathy**
**Connective tissue and rheumatic diseases**
  Polymyalgia rheumatica
  Rheumatoid arthritis
  Systemic lupus erythematosus
  Sjögren's syndrome
  Systemic vasculitis (polyarteritis nodosa)
  Sarcoidosis
**Infectious**
  See Table 13 and Chapter 7

complex of fever, Raynaud's phenomenon, polyarthralgias or polyarthritis, muscle weakness, and dyspnea due to interstitial lung disease. This constellation of symptoms has been termed the "antisynthetase syndrome" due to an association with any one of several anti-aminoacyl-tRNA synthetase autoantibodies (see Chapter 15).

Fatigue is often the dominant complaint in patients with an inflammatory myopathy and may persist even after apparent adequate treatment with corticosteroids or other immunosuppressive agents. Fever is seen more commonly with childhood dermatomyositis than in adults. The antisynthetase syndrome provides the exception, where fever is common. Weight loss may occur as part of any systemic illness, but if severe may be a sign of concurrent malignancy. Weight loss may be associated with decreased oral caloric intake and attributed to pharyngeal dysfunction of striated muscle involvement or due to esophageal dysmotility commonly encountered in many connective tissue diseases.

### Cutaneous Involvement

The presence of skin involvement separates the patient with an inflammatory myopathy into the clinical classification of dermatomyositis, and there are a variety of rashes

**TABLE 8.** *Cutaneous features of the idiopathic inflammatory myopathies*

Specific signs in dermatomyositis
  Gottron's papules/sign (60% to 80% patients)
  Heliotrope rash (50% or less)
Less specific signs in dermatomyositis
  Photosensitivity (22)
  "V neck" sign
  "Shawl sign"
  Nailfold capillary changes or cuticular overgrowth
  Scalp involvement (23)
Other associated skin findings
  "Mechanics hands"
  Panniculitis
  Calcinosis (intradermal, subcutaneous, intramuscular)
  Vasculitis
  Vitiligo
  Cutaneous mucinosis (scleromyxedema)
  Multifocal lipoatrophy
  Poikiloderma (hyper/hypopigmented skin eruption)
  "Linear" lesions
  Acanthosis nigricans
  Bullous pemphigoid
  Acne fulminans

and cutaneous features that can be seen (Table 8). The specific rashes of dermatomyositis may precede, follow, or develop simultaneously with muscle symptoms. Although Gottron's papules are considered the only pathognomonic cutaneous feature of dermatomyositis, the presence of Gottron's sign and a heliotrope rash are specific enough to be included in criteria sets for the idiopathic inflammatory myopathies. Gottron's papules (Fig. 1A. See color plate 1 following page 85.) are scaly, erythematous, or violaceous plaques that are found over bony prominences, particularly the metacarpophalangeal and proximal and distal interphalangeal joints of the hands. Gottron's sign (Fig. 1B. See color plate 2 following page 85.) is a macular erythema that generally occurs in the same distribution as Gottron's papules but also is commonly seen over other extensor surfaces, such as the elbows, knees, hips, and ankles. Either or both of these rashes are found in approximately 60% to 80% of dermatomyositis patients. Later in the disease course, the affected skin lesions may become shiny, atrophic, and hypopigmented. The heliotrope rash, which is seen only in 50%, is purplish in color, may be edematous, and is typically located in the periorbital area (Fig. 2. See color plate 3 following page 85.). Photosensitivity is often manifested as a "V sign" over the anterior chest (22). Pruritus seems to distinguish the rash of dermatomyositis from that of systemic lupus erythematosus. The facial rash of dermatomyositis may in some patients also involve the nasolabial fold as opposed to the malar rash of systemic lupus erythematosus. The "shawl sign" is seen in dermatomyositis and is a rash located over the upper back and across the shoulders. Cuticular hypertrophy and hemorrhage with periungual erythema, telangiectasia, infarcts, and capillary dilatation are seen in some dermatomyositis patients and in those with myositis in overlap with another connective tissue disease. Severe calcinosis with subsequent skin ulceration, a potentially devastating complication seen in childhood dermatomyositis, is rare in adults. Rashes on the scalp are commonly seen in dermatomyositis and are often severe, misdiagnosed, and associated with patchy alopecia (23).

Cracking or fissuring of the lateral and palmar digital skin pads is termed "mechanic's hands" (Fig. 3). This is most frequently seen in patients with polymyositis and anti-tRNA synthetase or anti-PMScl autoantibody syndromes (24). Panniculitis, although rare in

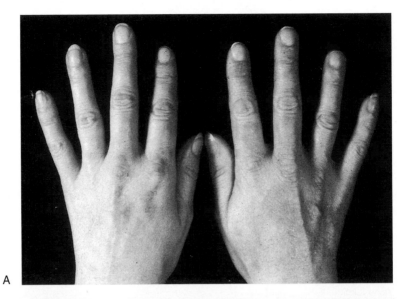

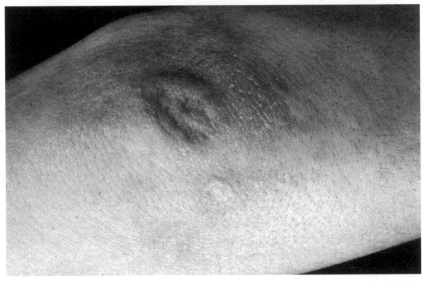

**FIG. 1. A:** Gottron's papules. Note the erythematous scaling rash over the knuckles (MCP, metacarpophalangeal joints) and dorsum of the hands in this patient with dermatomyositis. **B:** Gottron's sign. Note the similar appearing erythematous scaling rash over the elbow.

myositis, is increasingly reported and may be the presenting feature (25,26). Vasculitic skin changes occur in children and adults with dermatomyositis and have been associated in rare instances with the development of malignancy (27). Other much less common cutaneous features seen in the inflammatory myopathies are listed in Table 8.

Some patients may present with the classic rash of dermatomyositis and no demonstrable muscle weakness. In addition, muscle enzyme levels and electromyography are

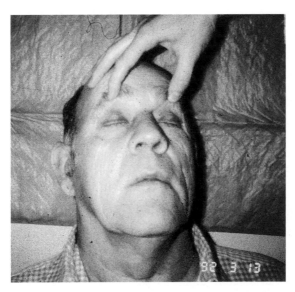

**FIG. 2.** Heliotrope rash of dermatomyositis. This erythematous and/or violaceous rash over the eyelids is characteristic of dermatomyositis in this middle-aged man.

normal. These patients are said to have "amyopathic dermatomyositis" or "dermatomyositis sine myositis" (28,29). Many of these patients will have a favorable outcome (30), but a poor prognosis and subsequent development of a malignancy have been reported (29,31,32). In some patients, partial or complete resolution of skin rash occurs. Others may develop muscle weakness requiring systemic corticosteroids. Several dermatologists have proposed that amyopathic dermatomyositis be added to the subclassification criteria proposed in Table 5 (26,30).

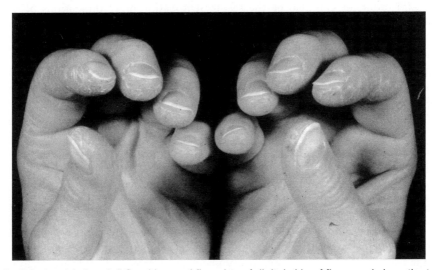

**FIG. 3.** "Mechanic's hands." Cracking and fissuring of digital skin of fingerpads in patients with anti-synthetase autoantibody. (Courtesy of Frederick W. Miller, M.D.)

## Articular Findings

Polyarthralgias and polyarthritis occur in roughly 25% to 50% of patients with inflammatory myopathy. The most common presentation is that of a mild nondeforming but inflammatory arthropathy affecting the small joints of the hands, wrists, and knees in a rheumatoid arthritis distribution. This type rarely develops into a chronic arthritis with joint deformity. Arthritis is more commonly seen in the subsets of myositis associated with another connective tissue disease or in patients with anti-tRNA synthetase autoantibodies.

A second form of more chronic deforming arthropathy has been reported. This may include arthritis of the hands with bony erosions, soft tissue calcification, and interphalangeal thumb joint instability ("floppy thumb sign") (33). Some patients with the anti-Jo-1 antibodies have a deforming but predominantly nonerosive arthritis with subluxations of the distal interphalangeal joints, especially the thumbs (34). This progression over time is seen radiographically in Fig. 4, and the photographs demonstrate the deforming pseudorheumatoid appearance of the hand. This arthropathy may be refractory to conventional treatment and may be complicated by widespread calcification resulting from hydroxyapatite deposition (35).

## Pulmonary Involvement

Pulmonary involvement is common in idiopathic inflammatory myopathy, occurring in as many as 40% to 50% of patients (Table 9). When present, dyspnea is a serious symptom and warrants an aggressive diagnostic approach (36). Dyspnea may result from nonparenchymal pulmonary problems, including respiratory (diaphragm and intercostal) muscle weakness or associated cardiac dysfunction. Respiratory muscle weakness leads to ventilatory failure in only a small percentage of patients (37). However, hypercapnia is likely when respiratory muscle strength drops below 30% of normal and when vital capacity is less than 55% predicted (38).

Aspiration pneumonia is often secondary to pharyngeal striated muscle involvement. Pulmonary problems can also be the result of infection or complications of therapy. Fulminant *Pneumocystis carinii* pneumonia has been reported in lymphopenic, but human immunodeficiency virus-negative, patients after relatively short periods of prednisone therapy (39). This has a very poor prognosis. Methotrexate may lead to pneumonitis that presents acutely with fever, dyspnea, and pulmonary infiltrates. This complication resolves with drug discontinuation and institution of high-dose corticosteroid therapy.

Pulmonary parenchymal disease can also develop. Dyspnea with diffuse alveolitis is an ominous feature. Although sometimes progressing rapidly, dyspnea in this setting typically develops insidiously along with a nonproductive cough and occasional fever. Respiratory crackles and tachypnea are found on physical examination. Chest radiographs may demonstrate predominantly bibasilar infiltrates or a more diffuse reticulonodular pattern. High-resolution computed tomography reveals varying degrees of alveolitis with a "ground glass" appearance or fibrosis. The presence of alveolitis indicates a more favorable potentially treatment-responsive condition. Arterial hypoxemia with exercise desaturation is common, and pulmonary function testing reveals restrictive physiology and a decrease in diffusion capacity. This form of pulmonary involvement may be fatal in weeks to months or rapidly decompensate to adult respiratory distress syndrome (40). Alveolitis has been re-

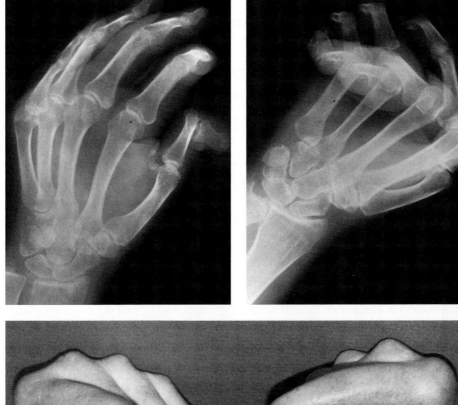

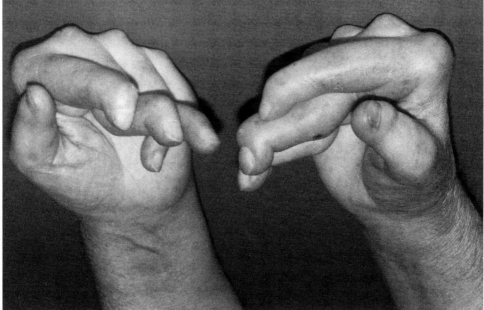

**FIG. 4. A:** Radiograph of the hand of a patient with the anti-Jo-1 autoantibody demonstrating subluxation of interphalangeal joint of the thumb ("floppy thumb sign"). **B:** Radiograph of same hand as in A taken 4 years later showing progressive deformity with several metacarpophalangeal (MCP), proximal interphalangeal (PIP), and distal interphalangeal (DIP) joint subluxations. **C:** Photograph of patient's hands taken at the same time as in B showing deformity of multiple joints and pseudorheumatoid appearance.

**TABLE 9.** *Causes of dyspnea in the inflammatory myopathies*

Nonpulmonary causes
   Respiratory muscle weakness (diaphragmatic, intercostal)
   Cardiac dysfunction (myocarditis, congestive heart failure, arrhythmia from
      conduction system disease)
Pulmonary causes
   Aspiration pneumonia (pharyngeal myopathy)
   Methotrexate pneumonitis
   Active severe alveolitis (often anti-synthetase antibody positive)
   Slowly progressive (fibrotic) interstitial lung disease
   Asymptomatic (radiographic) bibasilar fibrosis (mild restrictive PFTs)
   Pulmonary hypertension (primary or secondary)
   Alveolar hemorrhage (capillaritis)
   Pneumomediastinum

PFTs, pulmonary function tests.

ported in patients association with circulating anti-aminoacyl-tRNA synthetase autoantibodies (41). In some cases, the dyspnea dominates the clinical presentation to the point that the myositis is overlooked. Interstitial lung disease with anti-synthetase autoantibodies is observed in patients with no clinical evidence of myositis (42).

A more slowly progressive form of interstitial lung disease and pulmonary fibrosis may also occur in polymyositis, dermatomyositis, or overlap myositis. This may be seen in the presence or absence of an anti-synthetase autoantibody, and the course is clearly different from that described above, even though pulmonary fibrosis may become severe (43). Some patients with myositis and pulmonary fibrosis may be completely asymptomatic from the pulmonary perspective, demonstrating only radiographic bibasilar fibrosis and no functional compromise. Bronchoalveolar lavage, radionuclide scans, and high-resolution computed tomograph have been used to follow the progress of pulmonary involvement in selected cases (44–46).

In an attempt to correlate histologic features with clinical, radiographic, and prognostic variables, lung tissue from 15 patients with polymyositis or dermatomyositis was studied (47). Three histologic patterns emerged: bronchiolitis obliterans organizing pneumonia, interstitial pneumonia, and diffuse alveolar damage. Patients with bronchiolitis obliterans organizing pneumonia had a more favorable progression than those with interstitial pneumonia, but all three patients with diffuse alveolar damage died. The histologic subclassification was a better predictor of survival than the radiographic or clinical features.

Many patients with myositis-associated interstitial lung disease with progressive fibrosis develop pulmonary hypertension, often secondary to chronic hypoxemia, leading to pulmonary vasoconstriction. However, some patients develop a primary pulmonary hypertension syndrome with decompensation and death (48). Other less common pulmonary manifestations of myositis include pulmonary capillaritis with diffuse alveolar hemorrhage (49) and spontaneous pneumomediastinum (50,51).

## Cardiac Abnormalities

Cardiac involvement is common in the idiopathic inflammatory myopathies but seldom symptomatic until far advanced. The frequency of cardiac dysfunction is dependent on the diagnostic method used to assess disease activity. A persistently elevated creatine kinase-MB fraction is believed to predict or indicate extensive cardiac disease

(52,53), but a rising MB fraction to total creatine kinase ratio may be more specific for cardiac involvement (54). However, an elevated creatine kinase-MB isoenzyme fraction does not necessarily signify involvement. This fraction may be elevated because it is present in regenerating skeletal muscle fibers, a large number of which may be found in myositis. Measurements of cardiac troponin I are reportedly more useful in distinguishing whether creatine kinase-MB elevations are due to myocardial or skeletal muscle injury (55).

The precise relationship of electrocardiographic abnormalities to myositis-associated cardiac disease is unclear. Noninvasive modalities such as electrocardiography, Holter monitoring, and echocardiography may detect a high frequency of asymptomatic nonspecific abnormalities. Electrocardiographic abnormalities occur in about one third of patients with polymyositis, but heart block causing sudden death is very rare (56). Extensive noninvasive studies reveal that left ventricular diastolic dysfunction is frequently detectable but subclinical (57). Radioisotopic assessment of cardiac muscle dysfunction in myositis, using $^{99m}$Tc-pyrophosphate uptake, detected a correlation between increased myocardial uptake and poor outcome with inflammatory and degenerative myocardial changes at autopsy (58). Myocardial disease may also be detected by anti-myosin antibody scintigraphy (59).

Less common but serious features of cardiac involvement include myocarditis leading to congestive heart failure (60), endomyocardial fibrosis (61), or pericardial effusion with tamponade (62). The effect of treatment with corticosteroids leading to atherosclerosis and premature cardiovascular mortality is poorly studied but undoubtedly significant.

### Gastrointestinal Involvement

Dysphagia, or difficulty swallowing, is found in up to 50% to 60% of patients at some point in their disease course and is common during the active phase of myositis (63). Generally, dysphagia is considered a poor prognostic sign (14,18). The swallowing mechanism may be affected at a variety of sites, ranging from the tongue and facial muscles to the smooth and striated muscle of the esophagus (64). Cervical or pharyngeal (termed proximal) dysphagia leads to difficulty initiating the swallowing process with nasal regurgitation of liquids, dysphonia, and, if severe, aspiration of oral contents into the tracheobronchial tree, leading to chemical or bacterial pneumonitis. Patients with pharyngeal dysphagia clinically are more likely to demonstrate neck flexor weakness and have difficulty lifting their head off a pillow. The pharyngeal musculature is striated in nature and thus can become inflamed, weak, and dysfunctional, like striated muscle in other locations. Cricopharyngeal muscle dysfunction resulting from inflammation must be considered in the evaluation of any myositis patient with proximal dysphagia. The symptoms of cricopharyngeal dysfunction are slightly different than those seen with the pharyngeal dysphagia of active myositis. In this setting, patients cough with swallowing and often complain of a blocking sensation. Swallowing is unaffected by body position and is easier with liquids (65). The cricopharyngeal muscle involvement may result in fibrosis, hypertrophy, and achalasia (66). Dysphagia from cricopharyngeal dysfunction is quite common and increasingly recognized in patients with inclusion body myositis and is due to the same inflammatory fibrosing pathologic process that occurs in polymyositis or dermatomyositis (67). The correct diagnosis is made by videofluoroscopy optimally performed with a speech therapist.

Distal dysphagia implicates dysfunction of the smooth rather than skeletal muscle. Symptoms include the sensation of food sticking in the retrosternal area and pyrosis that tend to be worse on reclining. Such symptoms are often of greater concern in patients with myositis and an associated connective tissue disease, especially systemic sclerosis. However, many patients with inflammatory myopathy not associated with another connective tissue disease have clinical, radiographic, or manometric evidence of distal esophageal dysmotility (68,69). Very rarely, megaesophagus or motor dysfunction of the entire gastrointestinal tract may occur (70). All forms of distal dysphagia may allow chronic reflux symptoms and predispose to stricture formation or Barret's esophagus.

The gastrointestinal manifestations common in children with dermatomyositis (i.e., mucosal ulceration with perforation and hemorrhage due to vasculitis) are rarely seen in adults. However, adults with coexistent myositis and inflammatory bowel disease are reported (71–73). Other uncommon gastrointestinal features in idiopathic inflammatory myopathy include malabsorption, primary biliary cirrhosis (74), adult celiac disease (75), and pneumatosis cystoides intestinalis (76).

### Vascular Disease

Raynaud's phenomenon is frequently observed in all subsets of idiopathic inflammatory myopathy except perhaps those with malignancy-associated myositis. Raynaud's is a common feature of the anti-synthetase syndrome and of myositis associated with other connective tissue diseases. Vascular thrombosis is rarely observed in adults. However, the coexistence of childhood dermatomyositis with fulminant disseminated large vein thrombosis and a circulating lupus anticoagulant has been reported in an 8-year-old child (77). Systemic vasculitis is common in children. In contrast, systemic vasculitis is an uncommon association with myositis in adults even though cutaneous vasculitis may be a prominent feature of dermatomyositis in this age group (27). The inflammatory vascular lesions include tender dermal and/or subcutaneous nodules, periungual infarcts, digital ulcerations, and retinal vasculitis. Retinal vasculitis causing irreversible visual loss has been reported in dermatomyositis (78).

### Renal Manifestations

Renal involvement in idiopathic inflammatory myositis is quite uncommon except in the setting of overlap syndromes with systemic lupus erythematosus or with systemic sclerosis. Very rarely, patients with polymyositis develop acute renal failure secondary to rhabdomyolysis with myoglobinemia and myoglobinuria, leading to acute tubular necrosis. These presentations are characterized by the triad of a high serum creatine kinase myoglobulinuria and pigmented casts in the urine (79). Renal histology in this instance generally reveals normal glomeruli, but "myoglobin" casts are found in necrotic tubules (see Chapter 13).

Very occasionally, patients with an idiopathic inflammatory myopathy develop proteinuria. This may occur in isolation or be associated with urinary sediment abnormalities (80). Renal biopsies have showed focal mesangial proliferative glomerulonephritis with immunoglobulin and complement deposition. Although immune complex-mediated injury has been postulated, evidence for that mechanism is lacking. Serum complement levels are normal, and cryoglobulins have not been found. Membranous nephropathy is exceedingly rare unless there is an associated malignancy or evidence of systemic lupus erythematosus (81). Hematuria and hemaglobinuria may be seen in myositis patients, with the latter possibly a reflection of myoglobinuria because both cause a "positive hemoglobin" reaction on dipstick testing of urine. "Apparent hematuria" may therefore be more apparent than real in myositis and is present when rhabdomyolysis develops, even if subclinical (82). Progression to any form of chronic renal failure is very unusual regardless of the cause of urinary sediment abnormalities.

## Associated Conditions

Hypothyroid myopathy is well known to masquerade as polymyositis (83), but thyroid diseases are associated with immune-mediated disorders, including the idiopathic inflammatory myopathies. In fact, in a large cohort, 11 of 315 patients with idiopathic inflammatory myopathies had Hashimoto's thyroiditis (84). Myositis may coexist in patients with Graves' disease and antithyroglobulin antibodies (85,86). Autoimmune hematologic complications in myositis are uncommon, but Evans' syndrome (autoimmune hemolytic anemia with thrombocytopenia) and idiopathic thrombocytopenia have been reported with dermatomyositis (87,88).

## INCLUSION BODY MYOSITIS

Inclusion body myositis was first reported in 1967 (5), but awareness of the entity remained limited until the late 1980s when criteria for its classification were proposed (12). Although precise figures on the incidence and prevalence of inclusion body myositis are not known, this entity is certainly more common than previously thought and is being increasingly diagnosed as its features are better recognized. Some reports indicate that this entity composes 15% to 28% of all inflammatory myopathies (89). Inclusion body myositis has both a sporadic and hereditary form, with the latter transmitted in both autosomal recessive and autosomal dominant patterns (90–92). Inflammatory infiltrates are less commonly detected in familial inclusion body myositis (93).

Inclusion body myositis is a disorder of predominantly middle-aged and older individuals and, unlike the other idiopathic inflammatory myopathies, has a male predominance (2:1). Over 80% of cases in one series were over the age of 50 years (94), and the mean age in another cohort was 61 years (95). In its fully developed form, inclusion body myositis has distinctive clinical features, but its slow progression often delays the diagnosis. It is not uncommon for inclusion body myositis to be misdiagnosed or to present as treatment-resistant polymyositis (12). Although the presenting features of inclusion body myositis may be identical to those of polymyositis, the presentation is more typically characterized by painless proximal (early) and distal (later) muscle weakness of insidious onset (Table 10). Patients often have considerable difficulty in determining the

**TABLE 10.** *Clinical features of inclusion body myositis*

1. Insidious yet progressive proximal (early) and distal (late) muscle atrophy and weakness
2. Affects predominantly middle-aged and elderly population (M/F = 2:1)
3. Rare association with malignancy or other connective tissue disease
4. Creatine kinase normal or only low-level elevation (usually <5–6 times normal)
5. Mixed myopathic and neuropathic electromyographic features
6. Resistance to corticosteroids and immunosuppressive drugs

onset of their symptoms and usually report a functional deficit as the initial disease feature.

Muscle weakness and atrophy may be more asymmetric than in polymyositis or dermatomyositis, with selective disease affecting the iliopsoas, quadriceps, biceps, or triceps muscle groups. The intrinsic muscles of the hand may be affected with finger flexor weakness, forearm atrophy (Fig. 5), and the progressive inability to grasp or pinch. Foot drop is observed and its presence in a middle-aged "refractory" myositis patient is strongly suggestive of inclusion body myositis. Falling episodes occur more frequently as the disease progresses and as distal muscle involvement complicates established proximal deficits. Dysphagia secondary to cricopharyngeus muscle involvement is seen in approximately one third of patients and may be severe (95,96). Dysphagia is a presenting symptom of disease in some (97). Inclusion body myositis may also involve respiratory muscles and may lead to respiratory failure (98).

The serum creatine kinase level is only moderately elevated in most patients with inclusion body myositis and may be normal in a percentage. Autoantibodies, including the myositis-specific autoantibodies, are typically absent except for the occasional nonspecific or age-dependent antinuclear antibody or the rare patient with inclusion body myositis and another connective tissue disease. The association of other connective tissue or immunologic diseases with inclusion body myositis, although sporadic and perhaps epidemiologically flawed by ascertainment bias, raises the possibility of a unifying underlying autoimmune mechanism. Dermatomyositis (99), scleroderma (100), Sjögren's syndrome (101), systemic lupus erythematosus (102), rheumatoid arthritis (103), sar-

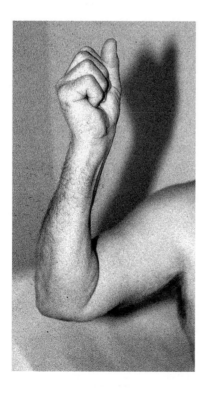

**FIG. 5.** Characteristic forearm muscle atrophy ("scooped out" appearance) in male patient with inclusion body myositis.

coidosis (104), and common variable immunodeficiency (105) have all been reported concurrently with inclusion body myositis.

Electromyography is helpful in diagnosis because a mixed myopathic and neuropathic picture is frequently observed. Electrophysiologic evaluation of patients with inclusion body myositis reveals features not commonly seen in patients with other inflammatory myopathies in about a third of cases (106).

The histopathologic features of inclusion body myositis include myofiber necrosis with regeneration and a chronic inflammatory infiltrate in addition to three distinctive features: rimmed vacuoles, intranuclear and cytoplasmic inclusion bodies, and deposits of amyloidogenic proteins in rimmed vacuoles (107).

The relationship between malignancy and inclusion body myositis is weaker than other inflammatory myopathies. However, coexistence of those conditions has been reported. Male patients with inclusion body myositis and either prostate or bladder cancer have been reported, and the relationship between inclusion body myositis and genitourinary malignancy is potentially intriguing. At least 11 cases of inclusion body myositis and malignancy have been reported (108). The response of the muscle disease to treatment of the neoplasm has varied from no improvement to significant response (108,109).

## MALIGNANCY-ASSOCIATED MYOSITIS

An increase in incidence of cancer in patients with polymyositis was first noted in 1916 (110). Although the relationship between inflammatory myopathy and malignancy is controversial, circumstantial evidence suggests a pathologic relationship between the two disease processes. Such evidence includes the recrudescence of muscle symptoms with tumor recurrence after complete resolution of myositis with initial cancer resection or chemotherapy-induced remission and cases of new onset dermatomyositis occurring with tumor recurrence.

Myositis with cancer is unusual in children and is more common in people over 50 years old. The male to female ratio in patients with malignancy and myositis is approximately 1:1. The true incidence of malignancy is difficult to determine because many studies involve small numbers of patients and many populations are quite select. For example, community studies report a much lower occurrence of malignancy compared with larger medical center and university populations.

The issue is further complicated by variations in the temporal relationship between development of the muscle disease and the malignancy. In over 80% of instances, the diagnosis of myositis and cancer were made within 1 year of each other, with the myositis preceding the malignancy slightly more commonly (111). Longitudinal observations of patients with myositis after diagnosis have not identified a long-term increased frequency of malignancy (111,112), but this is also controversial (113).

Although each subgroup of inflammatory myopathy has been reported to occur with malignancy, data for an association with dermatomyositis are most compelling (Table 11) (14,20,111–130). A Swedish population-based study demonstrated a significantly increased risk of cancer and mortality in the dermatomyositis subset (111). In a retrospective study of adult myositis in the United States, a statistically higher frequency of malignancy was found in dermatomyositis compared with polymyositis (7/27 versus 1/31) (131). Similarly, a population-based investigation in Finland observed a strong association of dermatomyositis but not polymyositis with cancer, especially within 1 year after

**TABLE 11.** *Frequency of malignancy in several case*
*series of polymyositis and dermatomyositis*

| Study (reference) | Dermatomyositis, n/n (%) | Polymyositis, n/n (%) |
|---|---|---|
| Bohan et al. (14) | 8/60 (13) | 5/50 (10) |
| Callen (114) | 7/27 (26) | 1/31 (3) |
| Vesterager et al. (115) | 9/18 (50) | — |
| Mola et al. (116) | 2/12 (20) | 0/7 (0) |
| Holden et al. (117) | 4/24 (17) | 0/12 (0) |
| Henriksson and Sandstedt (118) | 3/45 (7) | 4/62 (6) |
| Hoffman et al. (119) | 1/12 (8) | 1/15 (7) |
| Goh and Rajan (120) | 6/10 (60) | — |
| Tymms and Webb (20) | 7/36 (19) | 9/69 (13) |
| Baron and Small (121) | 5/11 (45) | 2/11 (18) |
| Benbassat et al. (122) | 10/39 (26) | 3/21 (14) |
| Manchul et al. (112) | 10/31 (32) | 7/40 (18) |
| Hidano et al. (123) | 112/569 (20) | — |
| Lakhanpal et al. (124) | 11/50 (22) | 18/65 (28) |
| Duncan et al. (125) | 10/39 (26) | — |
| Cox et al. (126) | 20/49 (41) | — |
| Bonnetblanc et al. (127) | 13/32 (41) | — |
| Oddis et al. (128) | 12/122 (10) | 13/200 (7) |
| Sigurgeirsson et al. (111) | 59/392 (15) | 37/396 (9) |
| Love et al. (129) | 10/89 (11.2) | 2/60 (3.3) |
| Airio et al. (130) | 19/71 (27) | 12/175 (7) |
| Maoz et al. (113) | 9/20 (45) | 4/15 (27) |

From Ref. 114, with permission.

the onset of dermatomyositis (130). Although one case-control study showed an increased risk of cancer before or concurrent with the diagnosis of inflammatory myopathy (112), another failed to detect any association (124). Finally, a recent report from Israel that followed patients for an 11-year period found malignancy occurring in 27% with polymyositis and 45% with dermatomyositis, a frequency 12.6 times that expected in the general population (113).

Cutaneous necrosis or vasculitis (132) and dermatomyositis sine myositis (32) may be predictors of malignancy. In contrast, the presence of pulmonary fibrosis, myositis-associated or specific autoantibodies, or an associated connective tissue disease decreases the likelihood of cancer (129).

The types of cancers that occur coincidentally with myositis are usually those expected based on the patient's age and sex. Many types of cancers are seen in myositis, including Hodgkin's and non-Hodgkin's lymphomas, hematopoietic malignancies, melanoma, genitourinary, gastrointestinal (particularly gastric), breast, and thymic tumors. However, nasopharyngeal malignancy and ovarian carcinoma deserve special mention. Asian and Chinese patients may have an overrepresentation of nasopharyngeal carcinoma with dermatomyositis (120,133,134). Gynecologic malignancies, in particular ovarian cancer, are increased in many case series. Cherin et al. (135) observed ovarian cancer in 7 of 45 women with dermatomyositis and malignancy, a much greater frequency than the 1% expected. Four of 15 women with dermatomyositis developed metastatic ovarian carcinoma a mean of 20 months after the diagnosis of dermatomyositis (136).

Another compounding factor in determining the true relationship between myositis and malignancy today includes the therapeutic agents often used to treat the muscle disease. The use of methotrexate, azathioprine, and chlorambucil have been associated with increased risk of developing malignancies. This has been reported when these agents were used to treat myositis or other rheumatic diseases (137–139). The use of cytotoxic drugs in the treatment of dermatomyositis has not been shown to increase the risk of subsequent malignancy (130).

## MYOSITIS IN OVERLAP WITH ANOTHER CONNECTIVE TISSUE DISEASE

Another connective tissue disorder can be diagnosed in approximately 20% of individuals with idiopathic inflammatory myopathies (14). These overlap syndromes include myositis in association with scleroderma, systemic lupus erythematosus, rheumatoid arthritis, Sjögren's syndrome and other immune-mediated entities. In general, the overlap myositis syndromes are characterized by higher frequencies of Raynaud's phenomenon and polyarthritis, a higher titer antinuclear antibody, and milder myositis with a favorable response to corticosteroids (129).

Patients with scleroderma may have a bland noninflammatory fibrotic myopathy with normal or slightly elevated creatine kinase levels or, less commonly, scleroderma with all the features of polymyositis, including high enzyme levels, inflammatory electromyographic changes, and abnormal muscle biopsy with lymphocytic infiltrates (140). Necrotizing myopathy associated with localized scleroderma has been reported (141). Polymyositis-systemic sclerosis overlap syndromes may be identified by the presence of the anti-PM-Scl (24) or anti-Ku (142) autoantibodies (see Chapter 15).

Muscle weakness is a common complaint in systemic lupus erythematosus (143). Myositis may account for this symptom in approximately 10% of patients. There is the increased frequency of abnormal muscle biopsies in systemic lupus erythematosus with changes varying among myositis, vasculitis, and a vacuolar myopathy (144,145). Myositis may be the initial manifestation of systemic lupus erythematosus. In many cases, the muscle disease responds promptly to corticosteroids (143). Eleven patients with lupus myositis (those fulfilling criteria for each diagnosis) were retrospectively compared with 19 polymyositis or dermatomyositis patients. At presentation, both groups showed similar significant increases in serum creatine kinase levels and comparable reductions in muscle strength. Using uniform methods of clinical and functional assessment over a mean of 7.4 years, both groups followed either a relapsing and remitting or a chronic persistent course. At last follow-up, quadriceps strength remained significantly depressed. These results show that lupus myositis can be as severe as pure polymyositis or dermatomyositis and should be treated aggressively.

Muscular involvement in rheumatoid arthritis is rare even though rheumatoid arthritis patients complain of significant muscle weakness and limited endurance. Although muscle biopsies in rheumatoid arthritis more commonly demonstrate type II fiber atrophy, some patients have myositis with necrosis and mononuclear cell infiltration. Twenty-one (6%) of 350 rheumatoid arthritis patients from a single center who developed muscle symptoms (most commonly weakness and atrophy) and/or an elevated creatine kinase (8/21) were studied by electromyography and biopsy (146). In 13 cases a treatable disease was identified such as inflammatory or toxic myopathy, and in all but 1 patient the treatment response was satisfactory.

In 1972, Sharp et al. (147) described an overlap syndrome, termed mixed connective tissue disease, with variable features of systemic sclerosis, systemic lupus erythematosus, rheumatoid arthritis, and myositis and the circulating anti-ribonucleoprotein antibodies. Since its description, mixed connective tissue disease has been the subject of considerable debate. The original claims that the syndrome was clinically identifiable by a unique group of features (i.e., that the presence of high titers of antibodies to ribonucleoprotein was a unique serologic feature; that cerebral, pulmonary, and renal involvement and vasculitis did not occur; and that mixed connective tissue disease was benign and responsive to low-dose corticosteroid therapy) have not stood the test of time. A subsequent evaluation of 22 of the original 25 patients 8 years later noted that 17 patients had sufficient data to make another diagnosis. Ten had scleroderma and five had coexistent myositis (148). High-dose corticosteroids were required in many patients, and many sclerodermatous manifestations were unresponsive to steroids. In addition, the association of anti-ribonucleoprotein with clinical mixed connective tissue disease was proven not to be specific (148). The contention of a benign prognosis was further belied when a review of five series of mixed connective tissue disease patients demonstrated a 13% mortality within 12 years (149). Some believe it best to classify the combination of features previously termed mixed connective tissue disease as an undifferentiated connective tissue disease (or syndrome) of which myositis is frequently a benign more corticosteroid-responsive feature.

Myositis has been reported in patients with primary Sjögren's syndrome, although the association is probably present in less than 5% of patients (150). In general, patients respond to corticosteroids alone or to the addition of immunosuppressive drugs. Other immune-mediated disorders with a reported myositis component include the polymyalgia rheumatica, seronegative spondyloarthropathies, primary biliary cirrhosis, psoriatic arthritis, inflammatory bowel disease, myasthenia gravis, Behçet's disease, Wegener's granulomatosis, Churg-Straus syndrome, polyarteritis nodosa, adult Still's disease, amyloidosis, and graft-versus-host disease (151–153).

## UNCOMMON CLINICAL SUBTYPES OF IDIOPATHIC INFLAMMATORY MYOPATHIES

### Eosinophilic Myositis

Myositis with an eosinophilic inflammatory infiltrate can take many forms (154,155). Muscle involvement frequently occurs as part of the spectrum of hypereosinophilic syndrome but is the presenting symptom in only 15% of patients. Eosinophilic myopathy may also occur with parasitic and other infections, drug or toxic myopathies, sarcoidosis, and rarely other connective tissue diseases. For example, the ingestion of contaminated L-tryptophan has led to eosinophilia-myalgia syndrome, a multisystem disease with severe myalgias, muscle weakness, neuropathy, sclerodermatous skin changes, and occasionally eosinophilic perimyositis (156).

The term eosinophilic myositis represents a distinct syndrome of idiopathic eosinophilic inflammatory myopathy. Histopathology can show a localized or diffuse process ranging from isolated perimyositis to frank infiltration with eosinophils. Clinically, eosinophilic myositis may be associated with a variety of systemic features resembling those seen in immunologically mediated disorders (154,155), but laboratory findings are variable. A significant number of patients (25% to 35%) have a normal peripheral eosinophil count and/or serum creatine kinase level. The diagnosis is generally made by exclusion after ruling out an infectious process, drug or toxin ingestion, or an associated autoimmune disease.

Eosinophilic fasciitis can be distinguished from eosinophilic myositis by eosinophilia in association with thickening of the skin and subcutaneous tissue resembling scleroderma. In contrast to scleroderma, patients lack Raynaud's phenomenon, and the diagnosis is made by a full thickness biopsy from skin down to muscle tissue, revealing fascial

**TABLE 12.** *Clinical and pathologic classifications of idiopathic eosinophilic myositis*

|  | Focal eosinophilic myositis | Eosinophilic polymyositis | Eosinophilic perimyositis |
|---|---|---|---|
| Systemic symptoms | No | Yes | Prodromal (gastrointestinal arthralgias, fever) |
| Muscle involvement | Lower extremity | Proximal muscles myocardium | Lower extremity |
| Histology | Deep eosinophilic infiltration with fiber invasion and necrosis | Perivascular eosinophilic cuffing, diffuse infiltration | Fascial and perimysial infiltrate |
| Prognosis | Spontaneous or steroid-induced recovery, can relapse | Steroid-induced recovery, can relapse | Spontaneous recovery |

thickening with eosinophil and mononuclear cell infiltration. A recently proposed classification of idiopathic eosinophilic myositis divides the syndrome into three distinct entities: focal eosinophilic myositis, eosinophilic polymyositis, and eosinophilic perimyositis (Table 12) (157). A cutaneous manifestation resembling cellulitis and skin vasculitis has also been reported in association with eosinophilic myositis (158,159).

## Orbital Myositis

Idiopathic orbital myositis is an inflammatory process affecting the extraocular muscles of the eye in the absence of thyroid ophthalmopathy. It occurs most commonly in young to middle-aged adults and has a female predilection. Patients classically present with pain exacerbated by any eye movement. Vision remains normal, but patients complain of diplopia and have proptosis with eyelid swelling, conjunctival injection, and, rarely, a palpable mass. The severity of eye movement restriction varies with the duration of symptoms and the degree of extraocular muscle inflammation and edema. The medial rectus is most commonly involved, although any or all muscles may be affected (160). The differential diagnosis includes orbital cellulitis, tumor, Wegener's granulomatosis, arterial venous malformation, and cavernous sinus thrombosis, but thyroid eye disease is most commonly confused with idiopathic orbital myositis. Thyroid ophthalmopathy, seen with Graves' disease or other autoimmune thyroid disorders, is more insidious in onset, associated with lid lag and most frequently involves the inferior rectus, the least commonly involved extraocular muscle in idiopathic orbital myositis.

Although idiopathic orbital myositis has been seen with many different diseases, an immune-mediated pathogenesis is suggested by the association with a variety of autoimmune disorders such as Crohn's disease, systemic lupus erythematosus, giant cell polymyositis, giant cell myocarditis, asthma, and rheumatoid arthritis (161,162). The treatment of choice is systemic corticosteroids, and response is usually prompt. Risk factors for recurrent disease include male gender, lack of proptosis, eyelid retraction, horizontal recti inflammation, involvement of multiple or bilateral extraocular muscles, and muscle tendon sparing (163).

## Myositis Ossificans

Myositis ossificans is a condition of heterotopic nonneoplastic ossification of striated muscle and connective tissue. The most common variant is posttraumatic. Curiously, an identifiable trauma can be confirmed in only 60% to 70% of cases (164). Typically, heterotopic bone remains confined to a single muscle or muscle group (165,166). Less commonly, myositis ossificans may follow repetitive injury such as is sustained in horseback riding or rifle shooting. Another variant of localized myositis ossificans is seen in paraplegic patients in the muscles below the level of spinal cord injury. The cause of myositis ossificans in immobilized muscles is unknown, but the histopathology in that form and the posttraumatic form are similar. Localized myositis ossificans is generally benign even though the lesions can be very painful and functionally disabling. In localized variants, excision may be curative.

Fibrodysplasia (myositis) ossificans progressiva is a rare but disabling hereditary form of myositis ossificans. This form is believed to initially result from a spontaneous genetic mutation and is then inherited in an autosomal dominant pattern with complete penetrance and variable expressivity. Heterotopic calcification occurs in many muscle groups associated with several skeletal abnormalities, including congenitally shortened first metatarsal bones, short thumbs, and other digital abnormalities. Mental retardation and deafness can occur. Clinical presentation is variable, and trauma may or may not be associated with the subsequent development of a painful inflammatory mass that calcifies. Early fibrodysplasia ossificans progressiva lesions demonstrate primitive cartilage and fibroblastic proliferation with inflammation. Soft tissue calcifications result from proteoglycans and glycoprotein accumulations and bind calcium. Most patients have established soft tissue calcification by age 10 years. Spinal involvement may develop, appearing clinically and radiographically similar to ankylosing spondylitis (167). Although the diaphragm, cardiac, and smooth muscles are generally spared, death may result from restrictive respiratory failure or aspiration pneumonia. Unfortunately, resection of ossified tissue leads to further "traumatic" ossification. The differential diagnosis includes calcification after soft tissue injury from trauma, infection, or malignancy.

Calcification of skeletal muscle can also occur as myositis ossificans circumscripta, a more localized process beginning as a hematoma with calcifications developing parallel to the axis of a long bone and muscle and in dermatomyositis, scleroderma, multiple exostoses (Ollier's disease), periostitis, and chronic renal failure. Heterotopic ossification of muscle has been described in the setting of adult respiratory distress syndrome after neuromuscular blockade (168).

## Focal Myositis

In 1977, Heffner et al. (169) described the clinical and pathologic features of 16 patients with focal myositis. Since the original description, other patients with focal myositis at different locations and with varying presentations have been reported. This rare disorder generally presents with a painful mass in the lower extremity with a history of acute or subacute onset (169). It usually resolves without treatment, is associated with a normal serum creatine kinase level, and has no systemic effects. Over 50% of patients have a painful calf or thigh mass that may be misdiagnosed as thrombophlebitis or soft tissue tumor. Focal myositis has also been observed affecting the sternocleidomastoid muscles; temporalis muscle and psoas muscle; and muscles of the tongue and floor of the mouth, abdominal wall, upper arms, and forearms. Magnetic resonance imaging is helpful initially in diagnosis and useful in follow-up. The differential diagnosis of focal myositis includes trauma, thrombophlebitis, abscess, cellulitis, sarcoma, metastatic muscle tumors, pyomyositis, myositis ossificans, diabetic muscle infarction, and pseudotumor. Other localized pseudotumoral forms of myositis include localized nodular myositis, nodular fascitis, and proliferative myositis. The histopathology of these differ from that of focal myositis but have similar clinical presentations. The histopathology of focal myositis includes varying degrees of muscle fiber necrosis and regeneration, variations in fiber size, occasional lymphocytic infiltrates, and abundant interstitial fibrosis limited to the muscle (169). In contrast, nodular fasciitis and proliferative myositis involve adjacent muscular fascia, although often there are self-limited reports of focal myositis evolving into polymyositis within a year or more. In some cases, focal myositis can be recurrent (170).

Diabetic muscle infarction presents similarly with a palpable muscle mass (often in the thigh) with localized pain, swelling, and limited range of motion (171). Patients generally have longstanding insulin-dependent diabetes with many end-organ vascular complications. The onset is acute and rarely includes systemic features.

## EPIDEMIOLOGY

The annual incidence of polymyositis and dermatomyositis ranges from two to ten new cases per million depending on the population studied. A trend toward increasing incidence over time has been observed and may be explained by improved diagnostic techniques and increased physician awareness (172). Most epidemiologic studies report incidence peaks in childhood and adult patients, although inflammatory myopathy may occur in any age group (173–175). This disparity in incidence along with other distinguishing clinical and histologic features (see Chapters 5 and 6) among adults and children supports the concept of diagnostic and pathogenetic differences between childhood and adult forms of myositis. Myositis associated with malignancy and inclusion body myositis are more common in individuals over 50 years.

Overall, the average female to male incidence ratio exceeds 2:1, with women predominating in disease occurring between ages 15 and 44 years. The ratio is near unity in myositis associated with malignancy. In myositis associated with another connective tissue disease, females predominate 10:1 and the African American to white incidence ratio is 3 to 4:1. Males, however, predominate with a 2:1 ratio in inclusion body myositis. These figures do not apply to the more uncommon variants of idiopathic inflammatory myopathy (Table 1), which are much more rare and difficult to describe epidemiologically.

## GENETIC AND ENVIRONMENTAL FACTORS

The occurrence of dermatomyositis in monozygotic twins (176) and the association of myositis with certain HLA-DRB1 and DQA1 alleles (177) support a genetic predisposition to disease in some families. The strongest genetic risk factor for idiopathic inflammatory myopathy is the haplotype A1-B8-DR3 (DRB1*0301)-DQA1*0501 (178). This human leukocyte antigen haplotype is seen commonly with other connective tissue diseases. Individuals with an idiopathic inflammatory myopathy have an increased frequency of an autoimmune disease in other family members (179). The prevalence of autoimmune diseases is approximately fourfold increased in first-degree relatives of idiopathic inflammatory myopathy patients compared with a prevalence rate in relatives of control subjects (21.9% versus 4.9%, respectively). Genetic modeling analyses sup-

**TABLE 13.** *Potential environmental triggers for idiopathic inflammatory myopathies*

Infectious
  Viral (hepatitis B and C, influenza A and B, human immunodeficiency virus, human T-cell
    leukemia virus type I, echovirus, coxsackie)
  Parasites (lyme, toxoplasmosis)
  Bacterial (staphylococcus, streptococcus, clostridial)
Noninfectious
  Drugs (D-penicillamine, cimetidine, L-tryptophan, cholesterol-lowering agents)
  Biologics (human growth hormone therapy, interleukin-2 therapy, vaccines)
  Surgical implants (silicone, collagen)
  Occupational (silica, polyvinyl chloride, dyes and organic solvents)
  Ultraviolet light

ported a non-Mendelian polygenic inheritance pattern for these families, supporting the concept that many autoimmune disorders share genes that synergistically act to increase the risk of disease.

Striking associations of environmental factors with myositis onset have not been identified (Table 13) (151). However, occupational exposure to silica (180), ingestion of contaminated L-tryptophan preparations, and collagen and silicone implants may be implicated in the development of inflammatory myopathy (181,182). Seasonal and geographic clustering of myositis has been reported (183), indicating that a common environmental factor such as a bacterial or viral infection could trigger disease onset (Table 13) (151). Excessive physical activity and emotional stress have also been proported as significant risk factors for disease onset, but these associations have not been confirmed (184).

## TREATMENT

An accurate assessment of prognosis and therapeutic responses is difficult in idiopathic inflammatory myopathies. First, myositis is rare, and most studies involve single referral centers reporting retrospectively on small numbers of patients followed for relatively brief periods of time. Second, these cross-sectional studies combine patients with early and late disease, limiting the ability to identify prognostic factors. Third is the lack of a pathophysiologically meaningful classification system. None of the proposed classification schemes have been validated. Finally, no objective criteria for improvement and deterioration in myositis have been standardized. To begin to address these questions will require long-term prospective follow-up of well-defined incident cohorts of myositis patients using validated outcome measures.

The management of patients with idiopathic inflammatory myopathies is therefore challenging because of the low prevalence and heterogeneous presentations. It is difficult for most clinicians to accumulate sufficient experience to feel comfortable managing patients with myositis. This situation is further complicated by the lack of well-controlled clinical trials comparing various methods of treatment. Nevertheless, a combination of several disease assessment tools are generally used to evaluate and design treatment regimens for the individual patient with myositis. These multifaceted assessment schemes are similarly used to assess treatment response in published studies. Rider (185) recently proposed several elements to consider in a composite index of disease activity and damage in inflammatory myopathies. Finally, our ability to evaluate therapies is hindered by the marked heterogeneity inherent in the diagnosis and classification of these diseases.

As the various subgroups of idiopathic inflammatory myopathies are better defined, future treatment will include a more effective delineation of subjects. This may come from more discriminating analysis using magnetic resonance imaging and serologic markers such as myositis-specific autoantibodies, classification of specific lymphocyte subsets, or identifying the presence of certain cytokines. Until then, treatments remain largely empiric (151,152,186–188). Accordingly, the treatment of each patient must be individualized, and the monitoring of disease activity must be customized.

## Initial Therapeutic Considerations

Corticosteroids are the agents of choice for the initial treatment of myositis. Doses vary depending on the patient and the prescribing physician's preferences. Options include a single morning dose or divided doses. A single daily dose will limit steroid-related toxicity, but divided doses are believed to be more potent. Daily doses of 60 mg of prednisone (or 1 to 2 mg/kg) are usually chosen. A delay in diagnosis, for whatever reason, may unfavorably impact on disease prognosis, and patients with a long delay between the onset of muscle weakness and diagnosis of myositis are less likely to respond completely to prednisone than patients with shorter delays (187). In patients with severe disease (e.g., bedridden, swallowing dysfunction) or extramacular manifestations such as interstitial lung disease or myocarditis, intravenous pulse methylprednisolone may be used to gain more rapid disease control.

Once initiated, the high daily dose of prednisone is continued until a definite treatment response is attained. Ideally, this means strength has normalized and the serum creatine kinase level has returned to the normal range. This usually takes at least 4 to 8 weeks. Thereafter, prednisone is consolidated to a single morning dose, if it was given initially in divided doses, and a tapering of the dosage begins. The prednisone taper is continued at approximately 20% to 25% of the existing dose each month (187). Patients are evaluated regularly by assessing manual muscle strength and measuring serum creatine kinase levels. A conversion to alternate day prednisone dosing may be attempted when the disease is judged to be in remission. Many will maintain prednisone therapy at a dose of 5 to 10 mg/day until the disease has been suppressed for approximately 1 year.

An alternative corticosteroid regimen more rapidly converts a high single daily dose of prednisone (80 to 100 mg/day) to a lower alternate day dosage schedule (188). Successful disease control has been achieved with an initial 80- to 100-mg daily single dose for 3 to 4 weeks followed by an approximate 12-week taper to an alternate day dose schedule of 80 to 100 mg. In this regimen, the alternate "off-day" dose is gradually reduced by about 10 mg/week.

The regimen chosen must be individualized depending on the severity of the disease and rate of response. With disease relapse, defined by worsening weakness and an increase in serum creatine kinase level, prednisone dosage is increased or another immunosuppressive agent may be added. It may or may not be necessary to raise the prednisone dose to the level at which treatment was initiated to regain control of the disease. Many treatment failures or relapses are the result of not using enough corticosteroid for a long enough interval.

In some individuals, improvement in muscle strength will lag behind creatine kinase normalization by weeks and sometimes months. Patients should be reassured that abnormal creatine kinase often predicts future improvement in muscle strength. In others, strength may improve despite creatine kinase levels remaining elevated. Occasionally, an excellent clinical response is seen with the patient reporting normal muscle strength, but the creatine kinase never returns to normal. Therefore, although useful and predictive

(187), the creatine kinase should not be used exclusively or in lieu of other disease activity parameters.

Although prednisone may be curative for some patients, its overzealous use may lead to unwanted corticosteroid-related side effects (189). Corticosteroid myopathy, which causes selective atrophy of type II muscle fibers, is of particular concern. This is suggested by continued or worsening proximal muscle weakness after an interval of improvement or when the serum creatine kinase level has improved, stabilized, or even normalized. The dilemma is whether the weakness represents a disease flare or steroid myopathy. There is no specific diagnostic test that can effectively answer the question other than a trial of rapidly reducing the dose and seeing weakness resolve in the setting of drug-induced myopathy or raising the dose and seeing improvement in the setting of active inflammation.

It is worth considering using a second immunosuppressive agent at the time of diagnosis. This rationale stems from a retrospective analysis assessing the predictors of response to several treatment regimens in the idiopathic inflammatory myopathies. Up to 40% of patients with myositis have corticosteroid-resistant disease, and patients with muscle symptoms greater than 9 months are less likely to respond completely to initial treatment and may benefit from early second-line therapy (190). Another retrospective analysis demonstrated a favorable outcome in patients receiving initial combined treatment compared with corticosteroids alone (191). In addition, corticosteroids are clearly toxic, and many believe morbidity and perhaps mortality resulting from their use is underappreciated (192). These data provide rationale supporting the early introduction of corticosteroid-sparing agents.

The designation of myositis as "refractory" has not been adequately defined or uniformly agreed on. However, persistent disease activity despite adequate initial corticosteroids beyond 6 weeks to 3 months should lead one to consider adding a second agent, if that has not already been done, and question the accuracy of diagnosis. A careful reassessment may be in order. Other diseases, such as inclusion body myositis, a metabolic myopathy, toxic myopathy, or muscular dystrophy, should be excluded (Table 7).

### Additional Immunosuppressive Therapy

Although most patients with inflammatory myopathy have at least a partial response to corticosteroid therapy, many require additional immunosuppressive agents. These can be used as steroid-sparing agents in the case of serious steroid-induced complications, disease relapse after repeated tapering attempts, rapidly progressive disease with serious extramuscular manifestations, or simply the ineffectiveness of prednisone as a single agent.

Methotrexate is perhaps the most commonly recommended immunosuppressive agent for myositis, despite there being no controlled trial attesting to its efficacy (193). Methotrexate was first reported effective in 1971 when five of seven patients with steroid-resistant polymyositis responded favorably to its intravenous use (194). Many subsequent reports have demonstrated the efficacy of methotrexate in routine and refractory myositis, and one retrospective review suggested that weekly doses of 25 mg or less led to lower corticosteroid requirements (195). Methotrexate can be administered orally, subcutaneously, intravenously, or intramuscularly. The subcutaneous route is recommended when doses exceed 20 mg/week. Intramuscular injection is not routinely recommended because administration by that route does not improve blood levels and may falsely raise serum creatine kinase levels. Parenteral methotrexate may be increased to 30 to 50 mg/week, and leucovorin can be administered 12 hours after dosing if flu-like symptoms, mucositis, or gastrointestinal side effects have developed. Daily doses of folic acid (1 to 2 mg) may also help patients tolerate methotrexate treatments.

Azathioprine is another agent that may be used if treatment with prednisone as a single agent has been less than effective. In one of the few controlled, prospective, double-blind trials of an immunosuppressive agent in myositis, no difference was found between azathioprine and prednisone versus prednisone alone at 3 months (196). However, during the unblinded phase of the trial, patients taking the combination of azathioprine and prednisone functioned better and required less maintenance than those using prednisone alone at 1 and 3 years (197). Azathioprine typically has a slower onset of action than methotrexate (4 to 10 weeks) and should not be considered a failure until continued for at least 6 months. Recommended daily doses are in the range of 100 to 200 mg or 2 to 3 mg/kg.

A recently reported randomized crossover study from the National Institutes of Health compared two aggressive regimens to treat 30 patients with refractory myositis (Table 14) (198). Although the study lacked the power to effectively compare both treatment regimens, data analysis suggested that the oral methotrexate and azathioprine were superior to intravenous methotrexate. In fact, the oral combination was effective in patients who failed to respond to either drug alone, suggesting this combination should be used in patients with treatment-resistant myositis before choosing other potentially toxic regimens.

The use of cyclophosphamide in myositis is controversial. It was ineffective in 11 patients with refractory idiopathic inflammatory myopathy when administered in monthly intravenous pulses (199). However, nearly all patients had long-standing disease, two had inclusion body myositis and eight had interstitial lung disease. Each of these is considered a very poor prognostic feature. Conversely, several authors reported efficacy with monthly pulse cyclophosphamide in lupus myositis, myositis with Sjögren's syndrome, and the interstitial lung disease in patients with polymyositis and dermatomyositis (200–203). Cyclophosphamide can be given orally starting at 50 mg/day and the dose raised to approximately 2 mg/kg/day to achieve disease control or until leukopenia or other side effects develop.

Chlorambucil was used in five patients with dermatomyositis refractory to prednisone, azathioprine, and methotrexate (204). Three patients continued on prednisone with a chlorambucil dose of 4 mg/day. Improvement occurred in 4 to 6 weeks in all five patients, and steroids were eventually discontinued in four patients. Four patients stopped the chlorambucil after 13 to 30 months due to disease remission. Toxicity was minimal with transient leukopenia in two patients.

**TABLE 14.** *Two cytotoxic regimens in randomized trial of refractory myositis*

1. Combination oral methotrexate (MTX) and azathioprine (AZA)
   Month 1: MTX 7.5 mg/wk + AZA 50 mg/day
   Month 2: MTX 15 mg/wk + AZA 100 mg/day
   Months 3–6: MTX 22.5–25 mg/wk + AZA 150 mg/day
2. Intravenous MTX with leucovorin rescue every 2 weeks for 6 months
   MTX 500 mg/m$^2$, followed 24 h later by oral leucovorin 50 mg/m$^2$ every 6 h for four doses

Prednisone dosage was maintained constant for 1 month and then was tapered to 0.25 mg/kg every other day over the next 5 months.
From Ref. 198, with permission.

Others have treated refractory cases of myositis with combinations that include prednisone and methotrexate with either chlorambucil (6 mg daily) or cyclophosphamide (25 to 50 mg daily). These regimens contain alkylating agents that have been associated with the development of late malignancy (138,139).

Cyclosporine is an immunosuppressive agent that acts by inhibiting the calcium-dependent pathway of T-cell activation. It blocks the transcription of genes coding for cytokines, specifically the interleukin-2 genes, and thus blocks development of cytotoxic lymphocyte and T-helper cell proliferation. There have been no controlled studies in the adult myositis population, and nearly all reports of cyclosporine efficacy are based on case reports or small series of patients (205–211). The effective dose generally ranges from 2.5 to 7.5 mg/kg/day. Improvement may begin between 2 and 6 weeks. Cyclosporine was used as initial therapy in ten patients with dermatomyositis and compared to 45 historic control subjects treated with combination prednisone and azathioprine (208). Cyclosporine was at least as effective, more rapid in onset, and associated with only one major side effect (nonoliguric renal dysfunction with the serum creatinine rising to 1.9 mg/dL). In addition, cyclosporine was effective in a patient with refractory anti-Jo-1 antibody-positive polymyositis (210) and in combination with high-dose intravenous immune globulin (IVIg) in two patients with dermatomyositis (211). The side-effect profile of cyclosporine includes nephrotoxicity, hypertension, hypertrichosis, gingival hypertrophy, anemia, and rarely lymphoproliferative malignancy.

Tacrolimus (FK 506) is another agent that inhibits the activation of CD4+ T-helper cells through several calcium-associated events involved in lymphokine gene transcription. This novel immunosuppressive agent is currently used to prevent allograft rejection in transplant recipients. Tacrolimus use was assessed in eight patients with refractory myositis, six of whom had the anti-Jo-1 antibody and two with the anti-SRP autoantibody. The creatine kinase level dropped significantly in all patients, functional status improved, and corticosteroid requirements were lowered in all eight patients. Extramuscular manifestations, including arthropathy, mechanic's hands, and interstitial lung disease, also improved (212).

## Intravenous Immune Globulin and Other Therapies

IVIg has been reported as efficacious in a variety of immunologically mediated diseases, including the idiopathic inflammatory myopathies. Although the mechanism of action remains speculative, IVIg may block Fc receptors on vascular walls, eliminate circulating immune complexes, or neutralize a yet unidentified causative agent. In a randomized, double-blind, placebo-controlled trial, 15 patients with refractory dermatomyositis were given high-dose IVIg while continuing maintenance prednisone (mean dose, 25 mg/day) (213). Patients received either placebo or a single monthly 2-g/kg infusion for 3 consecutive months. Patients receiving IVIg had significant improvement in muscle strength and a composite functional status measure. After crossover, 12 patients with severe disability improved to near normal function. Five responders were rebiopsied and showed marked histologic improvement.

IVIg has not been studied in a controlled fashion in polymyositis, although significant clinical improvement was noted in 15 of 20 patients with refractory polymyositis or dermatomyositis. In a separate study (214), improvement was noted in only 3 of 11 patients with myositis given IVIg as first-line therapy (215). The assessment of IVIg in many studies is limited by inconsistent measures of disease activity, varying regimens of administration, differences in gamma globulin preparations, and the heterogeneous nature of the patients studied. Because IVIg is prepared from pooled plasma, different preparations may have different activities. Furthermore, the long-term efficacy of IVIg remains questionable because tachyphylaxis has been reported (216). Although generally well tolerated with minimal side effects, flushing, headache, myalgias, and aseptic meningitis have been observed (217). IVIg remains a very expensive treatment option and it may, at best, be most indicated for use in dermatomyositis or as a "bridge" while waiting for other agents to take effect.

Plasmapheresis and plasma exchange potentially reduce the amount of circulating antibody and cytokines, thereby limiting tissue deposition of immunoglobulins and altering humoral and cellular immune responses. Older uncontrolled trials reported plasmapheresis to be efficacious in patients with polymyositis (218). However, in a prospective study, 39 patients with myositis were randomly assigned to receive plasma exchange, leukapheresis, or sham apheresis in a double-blind trial (219). Only 3 of 13 patients in each group had improvement in muscle strength or functional capacity. Although leukapheresis and plasma exchange were deemed ineffective, the study was limited in duration (1 month) and 26 of 39 patients had circulating anti-Jo-1 or anti-SRP antibodies, which are known to be associated with a poor prognosis. In another report, two patients with refractory polymyositis responded dramatically to a combination of plasma exchange and IVIg despite the failure in one patient when each treatment was used separately (220).

Total body irradiation has been reported in a small number of patients with severe life-threatening refractory disease (221–224). Of the seven patients in these reports all responded, but one died after developing bone marrow suppression. Three additional patients with intractable polymyositis failed to respond to total body irradiation (225). Other unproved but potentially helpful modalities include thymectomy (226) and photopheresis (227).

Routine and opportunistic infectious complications can occur, particularly when immunosuppressive therapy is administered. Unusual infections include Ludwig's angina (228), disseminated histoplasmosis (229), and progressive multifocal leukoencephalopathy secondary to Jacob-Creutzfeld virus infection (230).

## Inclusion Body Myositis

Although recognition of inclusion body myositis is improving, this disease is often diagnosed long after its onset or at times when atrophy and weakness are profound. At the present, the likelihood of a beneficial treatment response from any therapy is quite low. There are numerous reports of treatment failure in patients with inclusion body myositis (12,231,232). In one prospective trial, muscle biopsies were performed before and after corticosteroid treatment in eight patients (232). Although inflammation decreased in the muscle biopsy specimens and the serum creatine kinase levels fell to normal, muscle strength worsened in these patients, suggesting that the inflammatory response in inclusion body myositis plays a secondary role in disease pathogenesis. An initial uncontrolled study using IVIg showed that three of four patients improved (233), leading to a subsequent randomized crossover trial of IVIg in 19 patients (234). One third of the 19 patients objectively improved with an increase in functional status and a significant improvement in swallowing function. However, of nine patients with inclusion body myositis treated in a separate open IVIg trial, two showed subjective improvement but all experienced declines in muscle strength (235).

It has been suggested that slowing the progression of weakness is an acceptable goal in treating inclusion body myositis. A retrospective review combined with a randomized prospective immunosuppressive therapeutic trial showed that azathioprine and methotrexate halted disease progression in 23% of retrospectively analyzed patients, whereas 74% prospectively studied patients had disease improvement or stabilization with oral azathioprine and methotrexate combined with biweekly IVIg for 3 to 6 months (236). Because of the inability to accurately assess slow inexorable deterioration in inclusion body myositis, Calabrese and Chou (107) suggested the following therapeutic approach:

1. A trial of 40 to 60 mg/day of prednisone for 3 months in newly diagnosed inclusion body myositis patients. A favorable response includes a clear increase in strength and reduction of the serum creatine kinase level.
2. If improvement occurs, azathioprine or methotrexate is added and the corticosteroid dosage is tapered.
3. In patients with very high levels of muscle enzymes, marked inflammatory infiltrates on muscle biopsy, or an associated autoimmune disease, another immunosuppressive agent is added after the initial steroid trial for 3 additional months even in the absence of a clear initial clinical response to steroids.
4. For those showing no demonstrable improvement after 3 months of corticosteroids, particularly in the presence of marked muscle atrophy, treatment with immunosuppressive agents should be discontinued.

These general guidelines require some individualization but nevertheless serve to potentially prevent treatment-related morbidity in patients with a poorly responsive but slowly progressive and relatively non–life-threatening disease.

Adjunctive nonpharmacologic measures are important in inclusion body myositis. Because patients have both proximal and distal muscle weakness, the ability to perform activities of daily living are significantly compromised. Adaptive devices and the use of leg braces or orthotic devices may prolong the ability to ambulate, prevent falling episodes, and delay the need for a wheelchair. Physical therapy with strength training may also be useful (237).

### Extramuscular Manifestations

Constitutional symptoms, including fatigue and fever, generally respond to corticosteroids, whereas Raynaud's phenomenon is best managed with common sense measures such as dressing warmly, avoiding cold exposure, and discontinuing the use of tobacco. Biofeedback is helpful in some cases, as is drug therapy with a calcium channel blocker (for example, nifedipine at a dose equivalent to 30 to 60 mg daily).

The rash of dermatomyositis may be particularly refractory to treatment and proceed in an independent discordant fashion from the muscular manifestations (237). Sunscreens are essential. Topical and oral corticosteroids may lessen erythema and pruritus but often do not eradicate the rash. Immunosuppressive agents have been used with inconsistent results. Methotrexate use may lead to improvement. In an open study, hydroxychloroquine in a dosage of 200 to 400 mg/day was added to corticosteroids in seven patients (238). The rash improved in all patients, and three had total resolution of skin disease. Hydroxychloroquine may not affect muscle inflammation, however. Quinacrine (100 mg daily) and isotretinoin (0.5 to 1.0 mg/kg/day) have been used in patients with refractory rash with some good results. The latter drug is teratogenic and must not be used by females who are or can become pregnant.

Subcutaneous calcification is an unusual manifestation in adult myositis but can occur in overlap syndromes and in the rare adult with dermatomyositis (239). Calcinosis is very resistant to treatment. The secondary soft tissue inflammation from calcinosis will rarely respond to oral colchicine (0.5 to 1.2 mg daily for 7 to 10 days) (240,241). Other proposed, but generally ineffective, therapies include low-dose warfarin (242), aluminum hydroxide (243), and probenecid (244). Diltiazem (240 to 480 mg/day) was given to four patients with calcinosis and limited systemic sclerosis. Each patient had a reduction or disappearance of calcific lesions (245). In some cases, surgical excision of calcium may be necessary if the deposits interfere with function.

Polyarthralgias and arthritis usually resolve promptly with corticosteroid therapy. The chronic rheumatoid-like arthropathy may require the same remittive agents used to treat other forms of inflammatory polyarthritis.

A variety of conditions may result in dyspnea in patients with myositis (Table 9). The most worrisome intrinsic pulmonary problem is a rapidly progressive diffuse alveolitis. In a report of 14 Japanese patients with myositis, including nine with dermatomyositis and interstitial lung disease (246), response to corticosteroids was poor, and six patients died from respiratory failure. Another report described three cases of idiopathic inflammatory myopathy with interstitial lung disease in which the addition of intravenous pulse cyclophosphamide therapy within 6 months of the development or exacerbation of pulmonary dysfunction led to a favorable outcome (203). Over a 10-year period, 104 Spanish patients with idiopathic inflammatory myopathy were prospectively evaluated (247). Eight patients had interstitial lung disease, six of eight had the anti-Jo-1 antibody, and six of seven had anti-endothelial cell antibodies. In contrast to many other reports (37,246,248), where interstitial lung disease is associated with a poor prognosis, those patients with dermatomyositis and interstitial lung disease had a similar survival to patients without lung disease. Aggressive therapy with immunosuppressive drugs was generally begun early in these patients. Prednisone alone was effective in only three of eight. The remaining five received varying immunosuppressive combinations of prednisone, cyclophosphamide, azathioprine, and/or cyclosporine (247).

Using cyclophosphamide by the intravenous route may help avoid substantial toxicity, including myelosuppression, hemorrhagic cystitis, and increased risk of malignancy. Six patients with rapidly progressive interstitial lung disease associated with a connective tissue disease were treated with intravenous pulse cyclophosphamide (238). Patients received six to nine cycles of therapy at 0.5 g/m$^2$ body surface area together with 50 mg of prednisolone that was tapered to 5 to 7.5 mg/day. All patients showed improvement in exercise tolerance and lung function. Elevated bronchoalveolar lavage neutrophils dropped substantially, and high-resolution computed tomography changes regressed in four. Intravenous pulse cyclophosphamide has been well tolerated in many but may be associated with substantial toxicity. Intravenous cyclophosphamide therapy should probably be reserved for patients with high inflammatory indices of interstitial lung disease activity (249).

The prevalence of cardiac involvement in myositis is difficult to estimate, but congestive heart failure is uncommon. Abnormalities detected by the various methods of assessment discussed earlier may resolve after treatment with high doses of prednisone for 6 to 8 weeks (250). There are little data on the use of other immunosuppressive agents to treat cardiac complications. Pericardial disease should response to corticosteroid therapy.

Various esophageal, gastric, and intestinal problems complicate the management of myositis. Proximal dysphagia due to pharyngeal weakness may require supplemental feedings or parenteral hyperalimentation. Distal dysphagia and pyrosis secondary to esophageal dysmotility and reflux esophagitis require aggressive therapy to relieve symptoms and prevent stricture formation. Preventive measures include elevation of the head of the bed and not reclining after meals, whereas medications such as antacids, H2-receptor antagonists, and proton-pump inhibitors are useful as well. Stricture formation may require esophageal dilatation. Malabsorption, although less common than that seen in systemic sclerosis, should be managed with frequent small meals, fat-soluble vitamin supplementation, prokinetic agents (metaclopramide, cisapride), and rotating antibiotics such as ampicillin, tetracycline, and metranidazole to decrease bowel bacterial overgrowth. Cricopharyngeal achalasia can be treated effectively with cricopharyngeal myotomy (66,67). Vasculitic gastrointestinal involvement requires high-dose corticosteroids and often the addition of another immunosuppressive agent such as cyclophosphamide.

Cancer in myositis patients is usually obvious rather than occult (112,124). Thus, the workup for malignancy should consist of a meticulous history and physical examination and routine laboratory evaluation with directed individualized follow-up of any abnormality detected that cannot be explained by myositis (e.g., iron-deficiency anemia, blood in the stool, microscopic hematuria, or an abnormal mammogram). Callen (114) recommended a complete blood count, multiphasic chemistry screen, urinalysis, stool hematest, chest radiograph routinely, and a mammogram and perhaps a pelvic ultrasound or computed tomography in women. Young men should have a careful testicular examination and older men a serum prostate-specific antigen. Because of the difficulty and delay in diagnosis of ovarian cancer and its poor prognosis, some recommend that women of any age with dermatomyositis undergo frequent gynecologic evaluations, including pelvic examinations, transvaginal ultrasound and/or pelvic computed tomography, and serial serum CA-125 testing. A search for nasopharyngeal cancer should be performed in dermatomyositis patients from areas prevalent for this tumor (120,133,134).

### Rehabilitation and Physical Therapy Issues

Rehabilitation and physical therapy may play a critical role in the management of patients with idiopathic inflammatory myopathy (251,252). The remarkable heterogeneity among patients with the same inflammatory myopathy underscores the importance of an individualized approach. A patient with acute severe polymyositis with respiratory involvement requires a different approach than the polymyositis patient managed in the outpatient setting who continues to work full time. Similarly, patients with myositis in overlap with another connective tissue disease often have specific functional problems unique to the underlying rheumatic process. Inclusion body myositis has its own particular management needs (236). The timing and intensity of physical therapy has been controversial. The goals of any rehabilitative program include preserving existing muscle function, preventing disuse atrophy that can occur with the inactivity seen with acute disease, and avoiding joint contractures that result from limited joint mobility and fibrotic healing of inflamed muscles (see Chapter 19).

During active myositis, when muscles are weak and creatine kinase levels are elevated, therapy should be aimed at passive range of motion exercises with prescribed periods of bed rest. Patients in this acute phase may also require a collar for neck support, periodic speech therapy evaluation to assess swallowing dysfunction, and breathing exercises with serial measurement of forced vital capacity. Deep heat therapy to joint and muscle areas may be helpful in combination with stretching exercises. During the recovery phase when strength is better and the muscle enzymes are improving or normal, a more aggressive isometric (static) exercise program for major muscle groups with continued range of motion and vigorous stretching can be instituted.

More aggressive rehabilitative approaches have been suggested in patients with stable disease despite elevated creatine kinase levels. Five patients with active myositis began an alternating program of resistive and nonresistive exercise during rehabilitation and routine pharmacologic treatment. Four of five patients demonstrated increased strength, and no patient had clinically significant increases in creatine kinase levels (253). Another patient with active stable polymyositis received a 4-week isometric strengthening program demonstrating increased strength without a sustained rise in serum creatine kinase levels (254). Thus, even in the setting of active myositis, more aggressive rehabilitative techniques have not led to a clinical or biochemical disease flare.

During disease remission in the chronic phase of myositis, patients should perform active isotonic and resistive exercises with low weight to improve muscle tone and strength. In addition, due to general deconditioning, an aerobic exercise program should be encouraged (e.g., a stationary bike without resistance or lap swimming in a pool) (251).

## PROGNOSIS

Corticosteroids have had a clear positive impact on survival. In the presteroid era, up to 50% of patients died (255). Recent reports indicate a 90% survival among patients with polymyositis and dermatomyositis 5 years after initial diagnosis (128). Improved survival is likely due to earlier diagnosis, improvement in general medical care, and more judicious use of immunosuppressive drugs for refractory disease and extramuscular organ involvement. The best survival rates are for inclusion body myositis and myositis associated with another connective tissue disease. Concerning circulating autoantibodies, the presence of anti-SRP has the worst prognosis, with a 30% 5-year survival, followed by the anti-synthetase subset 65%. The best antibody-associated 5-year survival is among those with anti-PM-Scl and anti Mi-2 patients at 95% (129). Factors known to be associated with poor survival include older age at disease onset, delayed initiation of therapy (173), pharyngeal dysphagia with pulmonary aspiration, interstitial lung disease (248), myocardial involvement, and complications of immunosuppressive therapy.

The determinants of disability are different from those associated with death. Patients with inclusion body myositis, for example, have the worse functional outcome but a very good survival rate due to limited systemic complications. In one 20-year study of 118 patients with polymyositis, dermatomyositis, and connective tissue disease overlap, two thirds of the 82 survivors had no functional disability (256). Another study reported 87% of 107 patients with minimal or no disability after a mean follow-up of 5 years if they initially improved with medical treatment (257). In a prospective longitudinal study of a national cohort of 257 patients with polymyositis and dermatomyositis, the Health Assessment Questionnaire was used to analyze change in functional status between years 3 through 7 after diagnosis of myositis (192). Disability increased with disease duration and corticosteroid-related morbidity. Osteonecrosis and osteoporotic fracture contributed significantly to functional disability. Other sequelae leading to disability include calcinosis, arthropathy, pulmonary fibrosis, and congestive cardiomyopathy.

## REFERENCES

1. Wagner E. Ein Fall von akuter polymyositis. *Deutsch Arch Klin Med* 1886;40:241–266.
2. Unverricht H. Dermatomyositis acuta. *Deutsch Med Wochnscher* 1891;17:41–44.
3. Kankeleit H. Uber primare nichteitrige polymyositis. *Deutsch Arch Klin Med* 1916;120:335–348.
4. Bazecny R. Dermatomyositis. *Arch Dermatol Syph* 1935;171:242–251.
5. Chou SM. Myxovirus like structures in a case of human chronic polymyositis. *Science* 1967;158:1453–1455.
6. Yunis EJ, Samaha FJ. Inclusion body myositis. *Lab Invest* 1971;25:240–248.
7. Bohan A, Peter JB. Polymyositis and dermatomyositis. *N Eng J Med* 1975;292:344–347, 403–407.
8. Walton JN, Adams RD. *Polymyositis.* Baltimore: Williams & Wilkins, 1958.
9. Rowland LP, Clark C, Olarte M. Therapy for dermatomyositis and polymyositis. *Adv Neurol* 1977;17:63–70.
10. Research Group on Neuromuscular Diseases of the World Federation of Neurology. Classification of the neuromuscular disorders. *J Neurol Sci* 1968;6:165–175.
11. Gardner-Medwin D, Walton JN. The clinical examination of the voluntary muscles. In: Walton JN, ed. *Disorders of voluntary muscle.* New York: Churchill Livingstone, 1974.
12. Calabrese LH, Mitsumoto H, Chou SM. Inclusion body myositis presenting as treatment-resistant polymyositis. *Arthritis Rheum* 1987;30:397–403.
13. Tanimoto K, Nakano K, Kano S, et al. Classification criteria for polymyositis and dermatomyositis. *J Rheumatol* 1995;22:668–674.
14. Bohan A, Peter JB, Bowman R, Pearson CM. A computer-assisted analysis of 153 patients with polymyositis and dermatomyositis. *Medicine* 1976;55:89–104.
15. Dalakas MC. Clinical, immunopathologic and therapeutic considerations of inflammatory myopathies. *Clin Neuropharmacol* 1992;15:327–351.
16. Targoff IN, Miller FW, Medsger TA Jr, Oddis CV. Classification criteria for the idiopathic inflammatory myopathies. *Curr Opin Rheum* 1997;9:527–535.
17. Griggs RC, Askanas VA, DiMauro S, et al. Inclusion body myositis and myopathies. *Ann Neurol* 1995;38:705–713.
18. Medsger TA, Robinson H, Masi AT. Factors affecting survivorship in polymyositis. A life-table study of 124 patients. *Arthritis Rheum* 1971;14:249–258.
19. Bogousslavsky J, Perentes E, Regli F, Deruaz JP. Polymyositis with severe facial involvement. *J Neurol* 1982;228:277–281.
20. Tymms KE, Webb J. Dermatopolymyositis and other connective tissue diseases. A review of 105 cases. *J Rheumatol* 1996;12:1140–1148.
21. Uthman I, Vazquez-Abad D, Senecal J-L. Distinctive features of idiopathic inflammatory myopathies in French Canadians. *Semin Arthritis Rheum* 1996;26:447–458.
22. Cheong W-K, Hughes GRV, Norris PG, Hawk JLM. Cutaneous photosensitivity in dermatomyositis. *Br J Dermatol* 1994;131:205–208.
23. Kasteler JS, Callen JP. Scalp involvement in dermatomyositis. *JAMA* 1994;272:1939–1941.
24. Oddis CV, Okano Y, Rudert WA, et al. Serum autoantibody to the nucleolar antigen PM-Scl. *Arthritis Rheum* 1992;35:1211–1217.
25. Sabroe RA, Wallington TB, Kennedy CTC. Dermatomyositis treated with high-dose intravenous immunoglobulins and associated with panniculitis. *Clin Exp Dermatol* 1995;20:164–167.
26. Ishikawa O, Tamura A, Ryuzaki K, et al. Membranocystic changes in the panniculitis of dermatomyositis. *Br J Dermatol* 1996;134:773–776.
27. Feldman D, Hochberg MC, Zizic TM, Stevens MB. Cutaneous vasculitis in adult polymyositis/dermatomyositis. *J Rheumatol* 1983;10:85–89.
28. Euwer RL, Sontheimer RD. Amyopathic dermatomyositis: a review. *J Invest Dermatol* 1993;100:S124–127.
29. Fudman EJ, Schnitzer TJ. Dermatomyositis without creatine kinase elevation. A poor prognostic sign. *Am J Med* 1986;80:329–332.
30. Cosnes A, Amaudric F, Gheradi R, et al. Dermatomyositis without muscle weakness: long term followup of 12 patients without systemic corticosteroids. *Arch Dermatol* 1995;131:1381–1385.
31. Osman Y, Narita M, Kishi K, et al. Case report: amyopathic dermatomyositis associated with transformed malignant lymphoma. *Am J Med Sci* 1996;311:240–242.
32. Whitmore SE, Watson R, Rosenshein NB, Provost TT. Dermatomyositis sine myositis: association with malignancy. *J Rheumatol* 1996;23:1010–105.
33. Bunch TW, O Duffy JD, McLeod RA. Deforming arthritis of the hands in polymyositis. *Arthritis Rheum* 1976;19:243–247.
34. Oddis CV, Medsger TA Jr, Cooperstein LA. A subluxing arthropathy associated with the anti-Jo-1 antibody in polymyositis/dermatomyositis. *Arthritis Rheum* 1990;33:1640–1645.
35. Citera G, Lazaro MA, Cocco JAM, et al. Apatite deposition in polymyositis subluxing arthropathy. *J Rheumatol* 1996;23:551–553.
36. Marie I, Harton P-Y, Hachulla E, et al. Pulmonary involvement in polymyositis and in dermatomyositis. *J Rheumatol* 1998;25:1336–1343.
37. Dickey BF, Myers AR. Pulmonary disease in polymyositis/dermatomyositis. *Semin Arthritis Rheum* 1984;14:60–76.

38. Braun NMT, AroyanS, Rochester DF. Respiratory muscle and pulmonary function in polymyositis and other proximal myopathies. *Thorax* 1983;38:616–623.
39. Bachelz H, Schremmer B, Cadranel J, et al. Fulminant *Pneumocystis carinii* pneumonia in 4 patients with dermatomyositis. *Arch Intern Med* 1997;157:1501–1503.
40. Clawson KC, Oddis CV. Adult respiratory distress syndrome in polymyositis patients with the anti-Jo-1 antibody. *Arthritis Rheum* 1995;38:1519–1523.
41. Marguerie C, Bunn CC, Beynon HLC, et al. Polymyositis, pulmonary fibrosis and autoantibodies to aminoacyl-tRNA synthetase enzymes. *Q J Med* 1990;77:1019–1038.
42. Friedman AW, Targoff IN, Arnett FC. Interstitial lung disease with autoantibodies against aminoacyl-tRNA synthetases in the absence of clinically apparent myositis. *Semin Arthritis Rheum* 1996;26:459–467.
43. Takizawa H, Suzukin, Yangawa T, et al. Outcome in patients with interstitial lung disease and polymyositis-dermatomyositis, a subgroup with poor prognosis. *Jpn J Thorac Dis* 1996;34:1093–1097.
44. Hill C, Romas E, Kirkham B. Use of sequential DTPA clearance and high resolution computerized tomography in monitoring interstitial lung disease in dermatomyositis. *Br J Rheumatol* 1996 35:164–166.
45. Ramsey SC, Yeates MG, Burke WMJ, et al. Quantitative pulmonary gallium scanning in interstitial lung diseases. *Eur J Nucl Med* 1992;19:80–85.
46. Wells AIJ, Hansell DM, Harraison NK. Clearance of inhaled 99mTc-DTPA predicts the clinical course of fibrosing alveolitis. *Eur Respir J* 1993;6:797–802.
47. Tazelaar HD, Viggiano W, Pickersgill J, Colby TV. Interstitial lung disease in polymyositis and dermatomyositis. Clinical features and prognosis as correlated with histologic findings. *Am Rev Respir Dis* 1990;141:727–733.
48. Grateau G, Roux M-E, Franck N, et al. Pulmonary hypertension in a case of dermatomyositis. *J Rheumatol* 1993;20:1452–1453.
49. Schwarz MI, Sutarik JM, Nick JA, et al. Pulmonary capillaritis and diffuse alveolar hemorrhage. A primary manifestation of polymyositis. *Am J Respir Crit Care Med* 1995;151:2037–2040.
50. Bradley JD. Spontaneous pneumomediastinum in adult dermatomyositis. *Ann Rheum Dis* 1986;45:780–782.
51. Cicuttini FM, Fraser KJ. Recurrent pneumomediastinum in adult dermatomyositis. *J Rheumatol* 1989;16:384–386.
52. Askari AD, Huettner TL. Cardiac abnormalities in polymyositis/dermatomyositis. *Semin Arthritis Rheum* 1982;12:208–219.
53. Strongwater SL, Annesely T, Schnitzer TJ. Myocardial involvement in polymyositis. *J Rheumatol* 1983;10:459–463.
54. El Allaf M, Chapelle J-P, El Allaf D, et al. Differentiating muscle damage from myocardial injury by means of the serum creatine kinase (CK) isoenzyme MB mass measurement/total CK activity ratio. *Clin Chem* 1986;32:291–295.
55. Adams JE, Bodor GS, Davila-Roman VG, et al. Cardiac troponin I. A marker with high specificity for cardiac injury. *Circulation* 1993;88:101–106.
56. Stern R, Goodbold JH, Chess Q, Kagan LJ. ECG abnormalities in polymyositis. *Arch Intern Med* 1984;44:2185–2189.
57. Gonzalez-Lopez L, Gamez-Nava JI, Sanchez L, et al. Cardiac manifestations in dermato-polymyositis. *Clin Exp Rheumatol* 1996;14:373–379.
58. Buchpiguel CA, Roizenblatt S, Lucena-Fernandes MF, et al. Radioisotopic assessment of peripheral and cardial muscle involvement and dysfunction in polymyositis/dermatomyositis. *J Rheumatol* 1991;18:1359–1363.
59. Le Guludec D, Lhote F, Weinmann P, et al. New application of myocardial antimycin scintigraphy: diagnosis of myocardial disease in polymyositis. *Ann Rheum Dis* 1993;52:235–238.
60. Bhan A, Baithun SI, Kopelman P, Swash M. Fatal myocarditis with acute polymyositis in a young adult. *Postgrad Med J* 1990;66:229–231.
61. Rossi MA. Endomyocardial fibrosis in dermatomyositis. *Int J Cardiol* 1990;28:119–122.
62. Yale SH, Adlakha A, Stanton MS. Dermatomyositis with pericardial tamponade and polymyositis with pericardial effusion. *Am Heart J* 1993;126:997–999.
63. Willig TN, Paulus J, Guily JLS, et al. Swallowing problems in neuromuscular disorders. *Arch Phys Med Rehabil* 1994;75:1175–1181.
64. Sonies BC. Evaluation and treatment of speech and swallowing disorders associated with myopathies. *Curr Opin Rheumatol* 1997;9:486–495.
65. Dietz F, Logeman JA, Sahgal V, Schmid FR. Cricopharyngeal muscle dysfunction in the differential diagnosis of dysphagia in polymyositis. *Arthritis Rheum* 1980;23:491–495.
66. Kagen LJ, Hochman RB, Strong EW. Cricopharyngeal obstruction in inflammatory myopathy (polymyositis/dermatomyositis). Report of three cases and review of the literature. *Arthritis Rheum* 1985;28:630–636.
67. Darrow DH, Hoffman HT, Barnes GJ, Wiley CA. Management of dysphagia in inclusion body myositis. *Arch Otolaryngol Head Neck Surg* 1992;118:313–317.
68. deMerieuz P, Verity A, Clements PJ, Paulus HE. Esophageal abnormalities and dysphagia in polymyositis and dermatomyositis. Clinical, radiographic, and pathologic features. *Arthritis Rheum* 1983;26:961–968.
69. Jacob H, Berkowitz D, McDonald E, et al. The esophageal motility disorder of polymyositis. A prospective study. *Arch Intern Med* 1983;143:2262–2264.

70. Caramaschi P, Biasi D, Carletto A, et al. Megaesophagus in a patient affected by dermatomyositis. *Clin Rheumatol* 1997;16:106–110.

71. Kaneoka H, Iyadomi I, Hiida M, et al. An overlapping case of ulcerative colitis and polymyositis. *J Rheumatol* 1990;17:274–276.

72. Leibowitz G, Eliakim R, Amir G, Rachmilewitz D. Dermatomyositis associated with Crohn's disease. *J Clin Gastroenterol* 1984;18:48–52.

73. Heub D, Hauser I, Riess R. Atypical inflammatory myopathy associated with Crohn's disease. *Clin Neuropathol* 1996;15:150–154.

74. Boki KA, Dourakis SP. Polymyositis associated with primary biliary cirrhosis. *Clin Rheumatol* 1995;14: 375–378.

75. Evron E, Abarbanel JM, Branski D, Sthoeger ZM. Polymyositis, arthritis, and proteinuria in a patient with adult celiac disease. *J Rheumatol* 1996;23:782–783.

76. Pasquier E, Wattiaux MJ, Peigney N. First case of pneumatosis cystoides intestinalis in adult dermatomyositis. *J Rheumatol* 1993;20:499–503.

77. Huemer C, Duesse M, Seerainer W, Lubec G. Juvenile dermatomyositis with major thrombosis—an unusual course. *Clin Exp Rheumatol* 1995;13:795.

78. Yeo LMW, Swaby DSA, Situnayake RD, Murray PI. Irreversible visual loss in dermatomyositis. *Br J Rheumatol* 1995;34:1179–1181.

79. Thakur VC, DeSalvo J, McGrath H, Jr, et al. Case report: polymyositis-induced myoglobinuric acute renal failure. *Am J Med Sci* 1996;312:85–87.

80. Dyck RF, Katz A, Gordon DA, et al. Glomerulonephritis associated with polymyositis. *J Rheumatol* 1979;6: 336–344.

81. Makino H, Hirata K, Matsuda M, et al. Membranous nephropathy developing during the course of dermatomyositis. *J Rheumatol* 1994;21:1377–1378.

82. Lim R, Parker JLW. Apparent haematuria: an early sign in polymyositis. *Br Med J* 1988;296:1725–1726.

83. Hochberg MC, Koppes GM, Edwards CQ, et al. Hypothyroidism presenting as a polymyositis-like syndrome. *Arthritis Rheum* 1976;19:1363–1366.

84. Plotz PH, Dalakas M, Leff RL, et al. Current concepts in the idiopathic inflammatory myopathies: polymyositis, dermatomyositis, and related disorders. *Ann Intern Med* 1989;111:143–157.

85. Zingrillo M, Errico M, Simone P, et al. A case of dermatomyositis associated with hypothyroidism and hypoparathyroidism after surgery for Graves' disease. *J Endocrinol Invest* 1990;13:949–950.

86. Hardiman O, Molloy F, Brett F, Farrell M. Inflammatory myopathy in thyrotoxicosis. *Neurology* 1997;48: 339–341.

87. Cooper C, Fairris G, Cotton DWK, et al. Dermatomyositis associated with idiopathic thrombocytopenia. *Dermatologica* 1986;172:173–176.

88. Hay EM, Makris M, Winfield J, Winfield DA. Evans' syndrome associated with dermatomyositis. *Ann Rheum Dis* 1990;40:793–794.

89. Askanas V, Engel WN. Sporadic inclusion-body myositis and hereditary inclusion body myopathies: current concepts of diagnosis and pathogenesis. *Curr Opin Rheumatol* 1998;10:530–542.

90. Massa R, Weller B, Karpati G, et al. Familial inclusion body myositis among Kurdish-Iranian Jews. *Arch Neurol* 1991;48:519–522.

91. Neville HE, Baumbach LL, Ringel SP, et al. Familial inclusion body myositis: evidence for autosomal dominant inheritance. *Neurology* 1992;42:897–902.

92. Argov Z, Eisenberg I, Mitrani-Rosenbaum S. Genetics of inclusion body myopathies. *Curr Opin Rheumatol* 1998;10:543–547.

93. Griggs RC, Askanas V, DiMauro S, et al. Inclusion body myositis and myopathies. *Ann Neurol* 1995;38: 705–713.

94. Lotz BP, Engel AG, Nishino H, et al. Inclusion body myositis: observations in 40 patients. *Brain* 1989;112: 727–747.

95. Mayers ME, Chou SM, Calabrese LH. Inclusion body myositis: analysis of 32 cases. *J Rheumatol* 1992;19: 1385–1389.

96. Verma A, Bradley WG, Adesina AM, et al. Inclusion body myositis with cricopharyngeus muscle involvement and severe dysphagia. *Muscle Nerve* 1991;14:470–473.

97. Riminton DS, Chambers ST, Parkin PJ, et al. Inclusion body myositis presenting solely as dysphagia. *Neurology* 1993;43:1241–1243.

98. Cohen R, Lipper S, Dantzker DR. Inclusion body myositis as a cause of respiratory failure. *Chest* 1993; 104:975–977.

99. Lane RJM, Fulthorpe JJ, Hudgson P. Inclusion body myositis: a case with associated collagen vascular disease responding to treatment. *J Neurol Neurosurg Psychiatry* 1985;48:270–273.

100. Salama J, Tome FMS, Lebon P, et al. Myositie a inclusions: ettude clinique, morphologique et virologique concernant une nouvelle observation associ 6e A une sclerodermie generallise 6 et A un syndrome de Klinefelter. *Rev Neurol (Paris)* 1980;136:863.

101. Khraishi MM, Jay V, Keystone EC. Inclusion body myositis in association with vitamin B12 deficiency and Sjögren's syndrome. *J Rheumatol* 1992;19:306–309.

102. Yood RA, Smith TW. Inclusion body myositis and systemic lupus erythematosus. *J Rheumatol* 1985;12:568–570.

103. Soden M, Boundy K, Burrow D, et al. Inclusion body myositis in association with rheumatoid arthritis. *J Rheumatol* 1994;21:344–346.
104. Danon MJ, Perurena OH, Ronan S, et al. Inclusion body myositis associated with systemic sarcoidosis. *Can J Neurol Sci* 1986;13:334–336.
105. Dalakas MC, Illa I. Common variable immunodeficiency and inclusion body myositis: a distinct myopathy mediated by natural killer cells. *Ann Neurol* 1995;37:806–810.
106. Shields RW, Wilborn AJ, Levin KH, et al. Inclusion body myositis: the EMG features. *Neurology* 1989;39:233.
107. Calabrese LH, Chou SM. Inclusion body myositis. *Rheum Dis Clin North Am* 1994;20:955–972.
108. Jensen ML, Wieting JM, Andary MT, et al. Inclusion body myositis and transitional cell carcinoma of the bladder: significant resolution of symptoms after tumor excision. *Arch Phys Med Rehabil* 1997;78:327–329.
109. Ytterberg SR, Roelofs RI, Mahowald ML. Inclusion body myositis and renal cell carcinoma. *Arthritis Rheum* 1993;36:416–421.
110. Stertz G. Polymyositis. *Berl Klin Wochenschr* 1916;53:489.
111. Sigurgeirsson B, Lindelof B, Edhag O, Allander E. Risk of cancer in patients with dermatomyositis or polymyositis. *N Engl J Med* 1992;326:363–367.
112. Manchul LA, Jin A, Pritchard KI, et al. The frequency of malignant neoplasms in patients with polymyositis-dermatomyositis. *Arch Intern Med* 1985;145:1835–1839.
113. Maoz CR, Langevitz P, Livneh A, et al. High incidence of malignancies in patients with dermatomyositis and polymyositis: an 11 year analysis. *Semin Arthritis Rheum* 1998;27:319–324.
114. Callen JP: Relationship of cancer to inflammatory muscle diseases: dermatomyositis, polymyositis, and inclusion body myositis. *Rheum Dis Clin North Am* 1994;20:943–953.
115. Vesterager L, Worm AM, Thomsen K. Dermatomyositis and malignancy. *Clin Exp Dermatol* 1980;5:31–35.
116. Mola Em, Bernardo IM, Banos JG, et al. Dermatomiositis y polimiositis. Revision de 17 casos. *Rev Clin Esp* 1980;159:251–255.
117. Holden DJ, Brownell AK, Fritzler MJ. Clinical and serologic features of patients with polymyositis or dermatomyositis. *Can Med Assoc J* 1985;132:649–653.
118. Henriksson KG, Sandstedt P. Polymyositis—treatment and prognosis. *Acta Neurol Scand* 1982;65:280–300.
119. Hoffman GS, Franck WA, Raddatz DA, et al. Presentation, treatment and prognosis of idiopathic inflammatory muscle disease in a rural hospital. *Am J Med* 1983;75:433–438.
120. Goh CL, Rajan VS. Dermatomyositis in a skin clinic. *Ann Acad Med Singapore* 1983;12:6–12.
121. Baron M, Small P. Polymyositis/dermatomyositis: clinical features and outcome in 22 patients. *J Rheumatol* 1985;12:283–286.
122. Benbassat J, Gefel D, Larholt K, et al. Prognostic factors in polymyositis/dermatomyositis. *Arthritis Rheum* 1985;28:249–255.
123. Hidano A, Kaneko K, Arai Y, et al. Survey of the prognosis for dermatomyositis with special reference to its association with malignancy and pulmonary fibrosis. *J Dermatol* 1986;113:233–241.
124. Lakhanpal S, Bunch TW, Ilstrup DM, Melton LJ, III. Polymyositis-dermatomyositis and malignant lesions: does an association exist? *Mayo Clin Proc* 1986;61:645–653.
125. Duncan AG, Richardson KB, Klein JB, et al. Clinical, serologic and immunogenetic studies in patients with dermatomyositis. *Acta Dermatol Venereol* 1990;71:312–316.
126. Cox NH, Lawrence CM, Langtry JAA, et al. Dermatomyositis. *Arch Dermatol* 1990;126:61–65.
127. Bonnetblanc JM, Bernard P, Fayol J, et al. Dermatomyositis and malignancy. *Dermatologica* 1990;180:212–216.
128. Oddis C, Medsger TA Jr, Hill P. Followup of a national cohort of 322 polymyositis-dermatomyositis (polymyositis-dermatomyositis) patients. *Arthritis Rheum* 1991;34:S148.
129. Love LA, Leff RL, Fraser DD, et al. A new approach to the classification of idiopathic inflammatory myopathy: myositis-specific autoantibodies define useful homogeneous patient groups. *Medicine* 1991;70:360–374.
130. Airio A, Pukkala E, Isomaki H. Elevated cancer incidence in patients with dermatomyositis: a population based study. *J Rheumatol* 1995;22:1300–1303.
131. Callen JP, Hyla JF, Bole GG Jr, Kay DR. The relationship of dermatomyositis and polymyositis to internal malignancy. *Arch Dermatol* 1980;116:295–298.
132. Basset-Seguin N, Roujeau J-C, Gheradi R, et al. Prognostic factors and predictive signs of malignancy in adult dermatomyositis. *Arch Dermatol* 1990;126:633–637.
133. Peng J-C, Sheen T-S, Hsu M-M. Nasopharyngeal carcinoma with dermatomyositis. *Arch Otolaryngol Head Neck Surg* 1995;121:1298–1301.
134. Hu W, Chen D, Min H. Study of 45 cases of nasopharyngeal carcinoma with dermatomyositis. *Am J Clin Oncol* 1996;19:35–38.
135. Cherin P, Piette J-C, Herson S, et al. Dermatomyositis and ovarian cancer: a report of 7 cases and literature review. *J Rheumatol* 1993;20:1897–1899.
136. Whitmore SE, Rosenshein NB, Provost TT. Ovarian cancer in patients with dermatomyositis. *Medicine* 1994;73:153–160.
137. Bittar BF, Rose CD. Early development of Hodgkin's lymphoma in association with the use of methotrexate for the treatment of dermatomyositis. *Ann Rheum Dis* 1995;54:607–608.
138. Wallace DJ, Metzger AL, White KK. Combination immunosuppressive treatment of steroid-resistant dermatomyositis/polymyositis. *Arthritis Rheum* 1985;28:590–592.

139. Cagnoli M, Marchesoni A, Tosi S. Combined steroid, methotrexate and chlorambucil therapy for steroid-resistant dermatomyositis. *Clin Exp Rheumatol* 1991;9:658–659.
140. Olsen NJ, King LE Jr, Park JH. Muscle abnormalities in scleroderma. *Rheum Dis Clin North Am* 1996;22:783–796.
141. Dunne JW, Heye N, Edis RH, Kakulas BA. Necrotizing inflammatory myopathy associated with localized scleroderma. *Muscle Nerve* 1996;19:1040–1042.
142. Yamanishi Y, Maeda H, Katayama S, et al. Scleroderma-polymyositis overlap syndrome associated with anti-Ku antibody and rimmed vacuole formation. *J Rheumatol* 1996;23:1991–1994.
143. Garton MJ, Isenberg DA. Clinical features of lupus myositis versus idiopathic myositis: a review of 30 cases. *Br J Rheumatol* 1997;36:1067–1074.
144. Finol HJ, Montagnanis, Marquez A, et al. Ultrastructural pathology of skeletal muscle in systemic lupus erythematosus. *J Rheumatol* 1990;17:210–219.
145. Lim KL, Abdul-Wahab R, Lowe J, Powell RJ. Muscle biopsy abnormalities in systemic lupus erythematosus: correlation with clinical and laboratory parameters. *Ann Rheum Dis* 1994;53:178–182.
146. Miro O, Pedrol E, Casademont J, et al. Muscle involvement in rheumatoid arthritis: clinicopathological study of 21 symptomatic cases. *Semin Arthritis Rheum* 1996;25:421–428.
147. Sharp GC, Irwin WS, Tan EM, et al. Mixed connective tissue disease—an apparently distinct rheumatic disease syndrome associated with a specific antibody to an extractable nuclear antigen. *Am J Med* 1972;52:148–159.
148. Nimelstein SH, Brody S, McShane D, Holman HR. Mixed connective tissue disease: a subsequent evaluation of the original 25 patients. *Medicine* 1980;59:239–248.
149. Black C, Isenberg DA. Mixed connective tissue disease—goodbye to all that. *Br J Rheumatol* 1992;31:695–700.
150. Kraus A, Cifuentes M, Villa AR, et al. Myositis in primary Sjögren's syndrome: report of 3 cases. *J Rheumatol* 1994;21:649–653.
151. Miller FW. Inflammatory myopathies: polymyositis, dermatomyositis, and related conditions. In: Koopman WJ, ed. *Arthritis and allied conditions*. Baltimore: William & Wilkins, 1997:1422.
152. Wortmann RL. Inflammatory diseases of muscle and other myopathies. In: Kelley WN, Harris ED Jr, Ruddy S, Sledge CB, eds. *Textbook of rheumatology*, 5th ed. Philadelphia: W.B. Saunders, 1997:1177–1206.
153. Parker PM, Openshaw H, Forman SJ. Myositis associated with graft-versus-host disease. *Curr Opin Rheumatol* 1997;9:513–519.
154. Kaufman LD, Kephart GM, Seiderman RJ, et al. The spectrum of eosinophilic myositis. *Arthritis Rheum* 1993;36:1014–1024.
155. Pickering MC, Walport MJ. Eosinophilic myopathic syndromes. *Curr Opin Rheumatol* 1998;10:504–510.
156. Kaufman LD, Seidern RJ, Gruber BL. L-Tryptophan associated eosinophilic perimyositis, neuritis, and fasciitis: a clinicopathologic and laboratory study of 25 patients. *Medicine* 1990;69:187–199.
157. Hall FC, Krausz T, Walport MJ. Idiopathic eosinophilic myositis. *Q J Med* 1995;88:581–586.
158. Espino-Montoro A, Medina M, Marin-Martin J, et al. Idiopathic eosinophilic myositis associated with vasculitis and symmetrical polyneuropathy. *Br J Rheumatol* 1997;36:276–279.
159. Trueb RM, Lubbe J, Torricelli R, et al. Eosinophilic myositis with eosinophilic cellulitis like skin lesions. *Arch Dermatol* 1997;133:203–206.
160. Siatkowski RM, Capo H, Bryne SF, et al. Clinical and echographic findings in idiopathic orbital myositis. *Am J Ophthalmol* 1994;118:343–350.
161. Serop S, Vianna RNG, Claeys M, DeLaey JJ. Orbital myositis secondary to systemic lupus erythematosus. *Acta Ophthalmol* 1994;72:520–523.
162. Scott IU, Siatkowski RM. Idiopathic orbital myositis. *Curr Opin Rheumatol* 1997;9:504–512.
163. Mannor GE, Rose GE, Moseley IF, Wright JE. Outcome of orbital myositis. *Ophthalmology* 1997;104:409–414.
164. Siegert JJ, Wortmann RL. Myositis ossificans simulating acute monoarticular arthritis. *J Rheumatol* 1986;13:652–654.
165. Cushner FD, Morwessel RM. Myositis ossificans traumatic. *Orthop Rev* 1992;21:1319–1323.
166. Nuovo MA, Norman A, Chumas J, et al. Myositis ossificans with atypical clinical, radiographic, or pathologic findings: a review of 23 cases. *Skeletal Radiol* 1992;21:87–95.
167. Bridges AJ, Hsu K-C, Singh A, et al. Fibrodysplasia (myositis) ossificans progressiva. *Semin Arthritis Rheum* 1994;24:155–164.
168. Goodman TA, Merkel PA, Perlmutter G, et al. Heterotopic ossification in the setting of neuromuscular blockage. *Arthritis Rheum* 1997;40:1619–1627.
169. Hefner RR, Jr, Armbrustmacher VW, Earle KM. Focal myositis. *Cancer* 1977;40:301–306.
170. Sieb JP, Ries F, Traber F, et al. Recurrent focal myositis. *Muscle Nerve* 1997;20:1205–1206.
171. Umpierrez GE, Stiles RG, Kleinbart J, et al. Diabetic muscle infarction. *Am J Med* 1996;101:245–250.
172. Oddis CV, Conte CG, Steen VD, et al. Incidence of polymyositis-dermatomyositis: a 20-year study of hospital diagnosed cases in Allegheny County, PA 1963–1982. *J Rheumatol* 1990;17:1329–1334.
173. Hochberg MC. Epidemiology of polymyositis/dermatomyositis. *Mt Sinai J Med* 1988;55:447–449.
174. Cronin ME, Plotz PH. Idiopathic inflammatory myopathies. *Rheum Dis Clin North Am* 1990;16;655–665.
175. Pachman LM. Inflammatory myopathy in childhood. *Rheum Dis Clin North Am* 1994;20:919–926.
176. Harati Y, Niakan E, Bergman EW. Childhood dermatomyositis in monozygotic twins. *Neurology* 1986;36:721–723.

177. Arnett FC, Targoff IN, Mimori T, et al. Interrelationship of major histocompatibility complex class II alleles and autoantibodies in four ethnic groups with various forms of myositis. *Arthritis Rheum* 1996;39:1507–1518.
178. Garlepp MJ. Immunogenetics of inflammatory myopathies. *Baillieres Clin Neurol* 1993;2:579–597.
179. Ginn LR, Llin J-P, Plotz PH, et al. Familial autoimmunity in pedigrees of idiopathic inflammatory myopathy patients suggests common genetic risk factors for many autoimmune diseases. *Arthritis Rheum* 1998;41: 400–405.
180. Koeger AC, Alcaix D, Rozenberg S, et al. Occupational exposure to silicon and dermato-polymyositis: 3 cases. *Ann Med Intern (Paris)* 1991;142:409–413.
181. Cukier J, Beauchamp RA, Spindler JS, et al. Association between bovine collagen dermal implants and a dermatomyositis or a polymyositis-like syndrome. *Ann Intern Med* 1993;118:920–928.
182. Bridges AJ, Conley C, Wang G, et al. A clinical and immunologic evaluation of women with silicone breast implants and symptoms of rheumatic disease. *Ann Intern Med* 1993;118:929–936.
183. Leff RL, Burgess SH, Miller FW, et al. Distinct seasonal patterns in the onset of adult idiopathic inflammatory myopathy in patients with anti-Jo-1 and anti-signal recognition particle autoantibodies. *Arthritis Rheum* 1991; 34:1391–1396.
184. Lyon ME, Bloch DA, Hollak B, et al. Predisposing factors in polymyositis-dermatomyositis: results of a nationwide survey. *J Rheumatol* 1989;16:1218–1224.
185. Rider GL. Assessment of disease activity and its sequelae in children and adults with myositis. *Curr Opin Rheumatol* 1996;8:495–506.
186. Mastaglia FL, Phillips BA, Zilko P. Treatment of inflammatory myopathies. *Muscle Nerve* 1997;20: 651–644.
187. Oddis CV, Medsger TA Jr. Relationship between serum creatine kinase level and corticosteroid therapy in polymyositis-dermatomyositis. *J Rheumatol* 1988;15:807–811.
188. Dalakas M. Treatment of polymyositis and dermatomyositis. *Curr Opin Rheumatol* 1989;1:443–449.
189. Morand EF. Corticosteroids in the treatment of rheumatologic diseases. *Curr Opin Rheumatol* 1998;10: 179–183.
190. Joffe MM, Love LA, Leff RL, et al. Drug therapy of the idiopathic inflammatory myopathies: predictors of response to prednisone, azathioprine, and methotrexate and a comparison of their efficacy. *Am J Med* 1993;94: 379–387.
191. Lilley H, Dennett X, Byrne E. Biopsy proven polymyositis in Victoria 1982–1987: analysis of prognostic factors. *J R Soc Med* 1994;87:323–326.
192. Clarke AE, Bloch DA, Medsger TA Jr, Oddis CV. A longitudinal study of functional disability in a national cohort of patients with polymyositis/dermatomyositis. *Arthritis Rheum* 1995;38:1218–1224.
193. Wilke WE. Methotrexate uses in miscellaneous inflammatory diseases. *Rheum Dis Clin North Am* 1997;23: 855–882.
194. Sokoloff MC, Goldberg LS, Pearson CM. Treatment of corticosteroid-resistant polymyositis with methotrexate. *Lancet* 1971;1:14–16.
195. Newman ED, Scott DW. The use of low-dose methotrexate in the treatment of polymyositis and dermatomyositis. *J Clin Rheumatol* 1995;1:99–102.
196. Bunch TW, Worthington JW, Combs JJ, et al. Azathioprine with prednisone for polymyositis. *Ann Intern Med* 1980;92:365–369.
197. Bunch TW. Prednisone and azathioprine for polymyositis. *Arthritis Rheum* 1981;24:45–48.
198. Villalba L, Hicks JE, Adams EM, et al. Treatment of refractory myositis. *Arthritis Rheum* 1998;41:392–399.
199. Cronin ME, Miller FW, Hicks JE, et al. The failure of intravenous cyclophosphamide therapy in refractory idiopathic inflammatory myopathy. *J Rheumatol* 1989;16:1225–1228.
200. Boulware DW, Makkena R. Monthly cyclophosphamide in lupus pneumonitis and myositis. *J Rheumatol* 1991; 18:153.
201. LeRoy JP, Drosos AA, Yiannapoulos DI, et al. Intravenous pulse cyclophosphamide therapy in myositis and Sjögren's syndrome. *Arthritis Rheum* 1990;33:1579–1581.
202. Kono WH, Klashman DJ, Gilbert RC. Successful IV pulse cyclophosphamide in refractory polymyositis in 3 patients with systemic lupus erythematosus. *J Rheumatol* 1990;17:982–983.
203. Al-Janadi M, Smith CD, Karsh J. Cyclophosphamide treatment of interstitial pulmonary fibrosis in polymyositis/dermatomyositis. *J Rheumatol* 1989;16:1592–1596.
204. Sinoway PA, Callen JP. Chlorambucil: an effective corticosteroid-sparing agent for patients with recalcitrant dermatomyositis. *Arthritis Rheum* 1993;36:319–324.
205. Casato M, Bonomo I, Caccavo C, Giorgi A. Clinical effects of cyclosporin in dermatomyositis. *Clin Exp Dermatol* 1990;15:121–123.
206. Lueck CJ, Trend P, Swash M. Cyclosporin in the management of polymyositis and dermatomyositis. *J Neurol Neurosurg Psychiatry* 1991;54:1007–1008.
207. Mehregan DR, Su D. Cyclosporine treatment for dermatomyositis/polymyositis. *Cutis* 1993;51:59–61.
208. Grau JM, Herrero C, Casademont J, et al. Cyclosporine A as first choice therapy for dermatomyositis. *J Rheumatol* 1994;21:381–382.
209. Langford CA, Klippel JH, Barlow JE, et al. Use of cytotoxic agents and cyclosporine in the treatment of autoimmune disease. Part 1. Rheumatologic and renal diseases. *Ann Intern Med* 1998;128:1021–1028.

210. Tellus MM, Buchanan RRC. Effective treatment of anti-Jo-1 antibody-positive polymyositis with cyclosporin. *Br J Rheumatol* 1995;34:1187–1188.

211. Saddeh C, Bridges W, Burwick F. Dermatomyositis: remission induced with combined oral cyclosporine and high-dose intravenous immune globulin. *South Med J* 1995;88:866–870.

212. Oddis CV, Sciurba FC, Elmagd KA, Stard TE. Tacrolimus in refractory polymyositis with interstitial lung disease. *Lancet* 1999;353:1762–1763.

213. Dalakas MC, Illa I, Dambrosia JM, et al. A controlled trial of high-dose intravenous immune globulin infusions as treatment for dermatomyositis. *N Engl J Med* 1993;329:1993–2000.

214. Cherin P, Herson S, Wechsler B, et al. Efficacy of intravenous gammaglobulin therapy in chronic refractory polymyositis and dermatomyositis: an open study with 20 adult patients. *Am J Med* 1991;91:162–168.

215. Cherin P, Piette JC, Wechsler B, et al. Intravenous gamma globulin as first line therapy in polymyositis and dermatomyositis: an open study in 11 adult patients. *J Rheumatol* 1994;21:1092–1097.

216. Reimhold AAM, Weinblatt ME. Tachyphylaxis of intravenous immunoglobulin in refractory inflammatory myopathy. *J Rheumatol* 1994;21:1144–1146.

217. Sekul EA, Cupler EJ, Dalakas MC. Aseptic meningitis associated with high-dose intravenous immunoglobulin therapy: frequency and risk factors. *Ann Intern Med* 1994;121:259–262.

218. Dau PC. Plasmapheresis in idiopathic inflammatory myopathy. *Arch Neurol* 1981;38:544–552.

219. Miller FW, Leitman SF, Cronin ME, et al. Controlled trial of plasma exchange and leukapheresis in polymyositis and dermatomyositis. *N Engl J Med* 1992;326:1380–1384.

220. Herson S, Cherin P, Coutellier A. The association of plasma exchange synchronized with intravenous gamma globulin therapy in severe intractable polymyositis. *J Rheumatol* 1992;19:828–829.

221. Engel WK, Lichter AS, Galdi AP. Polymyositis: remarkable response to total body irradiation. *Lancet* 1981;1:658.

222. Hubbard WN, Walport MJ, Halnan KE, et al. Remission from polymyositis after total body irradiation. *Br Med J* 1982;284:1915–1916.

223. Morgan SH, Bernstein RM, Coppen J, et al. Total body irradiation and the course of polymyositis. *Arthritis Rheum* 1985;28:831–835.

224. Kelly JJ, Madoc-Jones Y, Adelman LS, et al. Response to total body irradiation in dermatomyositis. *Muscle Nerve* 1988;11:120–123.

225. Cherin P, Herson S, Coutellier A, et al. Failure of total body irradiation in polymyositis: report of three cases. *Br J Rheum* 1992;31:282–283.

226. Cumming WJK. Thymectomy in refractory dermatomyositis. *Muscle Nerve* 1989;12:424.

227. DeWilde A, Geller A, Szer IS, et al. Extracorporeal photochemotherapy as adjunctive treatment in juvenile dermatomyositis: a case report. *Arch Dermatol* 1002;128:1656–1657.

228. Fridrich KL, Taylor RW, Olson RAJ. Dermatomyositis presenting with Ludwig's angina. *Oral Surg Oral Med Oral Pathol* 1987;63:21–24.

229. Voloshin DK, Lacomis D, McMahon D. Disseminated histoplasmosis presenting as myositis and fasciitis in a patient with dermatomyositis. *Muscle Nerve* 1995;18:531–535.

230. Rankin E, Scaravilli F. Progressive multifocal leukoencephalopathy in a patient with rheumatoid arthritis and polymyositis. *J Rheumatol* 1995;22:777–779.

231. Lotz BMP, Engel AG, Nishino H, et al. Inclusion myositis: observation in 40 patients. *Brain* 1989;112:727–747.

232. Barohn RJ, Amato AA, Sabenk Z, et al. Inclusion body myositis: explanation for poor response to immunosuppressive therapy. *Neurology* 1995;45:1302–1304.

233. Soiueidan SA, Dalakas MC. Treatment of inclusion-body myositis with high-dose intravenous immunoglobulin. *Neurology* 1993;43:876–879.

234. Dalakas MC, Dambrosia JM, Sekul EA, et al. The efficacy of high-dose intravenous immunoglobulin in patients with inclusion-body myositis. *Neurology* 1995;45:S208.

235. Amato AA, Barohn RJ, Jackson CE, et al. Inclusion body myositis: treatment with intravenous immunoglobulin. *Neurology* 1994;44:1516–1518.

236. Leff RL, Miller FW, Hicks J, et al. The treatment of inclusion body myositis: a retrospective review and a randomized, prospective trial of immunosuppressive therapy. *Medicine* 1993;72:225–235.

237. Drake LA, Dinehart SM, Farmer ER, et al. Guidelines for care for dermatomyositis. *J Am Acad Dermatol* 1996;34:824–829.

238. Woo TY, Callen JP, Voorhees JJ, et al. Cutaneous lesions of dermatomyositis are improved by hydroxychloroquine. *J Am Acad Dermatol* 1984;10:592–600.

239. Cohen MG, Nash P, Webb J. Calcification is rare in adult-onset dermatopolymyositis. *Clin Rheum* 1986;5:512–516.

240. Taborn J, Bole GG, Thompson GR. Colchicine suppression of local and systemic inflammation due to calcinosis universalis in chronic dermatomyositis. *Ann Intern Med* 1978;89:648–649.

241. Fuchs D, Fruchter L, Fishel B, et al. Colchicine suppression of local inflammation due to calcinosis in dermatomyositis and progressive systemic sclerosis. *Clin Rheumatol* 1986;5:527–530.

242. Berger RG, Featherstone GL, Raasch RH, et al. Treatment of calcinosis universalis with low-dose warfarin. *Am J Med* 1987;83:72–76.

243. Wang W-J, Lo W-L, Wong CK. Calcinosis cutis in juvenile dermatomyositis: remarkable response to aluminum hydroxide therapy. *Arch Dermatol* 1988;124:1721–1722.

244. Skuterud E, Sydnes OA, Haavik TK. Calcinosis in dermatomyositis treated with probenecid. *Scand J Rheumatol* 1981;10:92–94.
245. Palmieri GMA, Sebes JJ, Aelion JA, et al. Treatment of calcinosis with diltiazem. *Arthritis Rheum* 1995;38: 1646–1654.
246. Takizawa H, Shiga J, Moroi Y, et al. Interstitial lung disease in dermatomyositis: clinicopathological study. *J Rheumatol* 1987;14:102–107.
247. Grau JM, Miro O, Pedrol E, et al. Interstitial lung disease related to dermatomyositis. Comparative study with patients without lung involvement. *J Rheumatol* 1996;23:1921–1926.
248. Arsura EL, Greenberg AS. Adverse impact of interstitial pulmonary fibrosis on prognosis in polymyositis and dermatomyositis. *Semin Arthritis Rheum* 1988;18:29–37.
249. Schnabel A, Reuter M, Gross WL. Intravenous pulse cyclophosphamide in the treatment of interstitial lung disease due to collagen vascular diseases. *Arthritis Rheum* 1998;41:1215–1220.
250. Askari AD. The heart in polymyositis and dermatomyositis. *Mt Sinai J Med* 1988;55:479–482.
251. Hicks JE. Rehabilitating patients with idiopathic inflammatory myopathy. *J Musculoskel Med* 1995;12:41–54.
252. Hicks JE. Role of rehabilitation in the management of myopathies. *Curr Opin Rheumatol* 1998;10:548–555.
253. Hicks JE, Miller FW, Plotz P, et al. Isometric exercise increases strength and does not produce sustained creatinine phosphokinase increases in a patient with polymyositis. *J Rheumatol* 1993;20:1399–1401.
254. Escalante A, Miller L, Beardmore TD. Resistive exercise in the rehabilitation of polymyositis/dermatomyositis. *J Rheumatol* 1993;20:1340–1344.
255. Oddis CV, Medsger TA Jr. Prognosis in polymyositis-dermatomyositis. In: Bellamy N, ed. *Prognosis in the rheumatic diseases*. London: Kluwer Academic Publisher, 1991:233–250.
256. DeVere R, Bradley WG. Polymyositis: its presentation, morbidity and mortality. *Brain* 1975;98:637–666.
257. Henriksson KG, Sandstedt P. Polymyositis-treatment and prognosis. *Acta Neurol Scand* 1982;65:280–300.

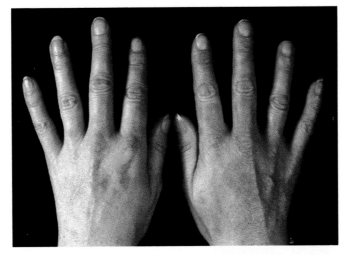

**COLOR PLATE 1.** Gottron's papules. Note the erythematous scaling rash over the knuckles (metacarpal phalangeal joints) and dorsum of the hands in this patient with dermatomyositis.

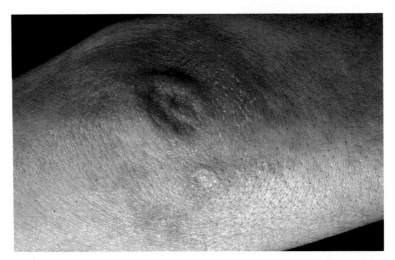

**COLOR PLATE 2.** Gottron's sign. Note the similar appearing erythematous scaling rash over the elbow.

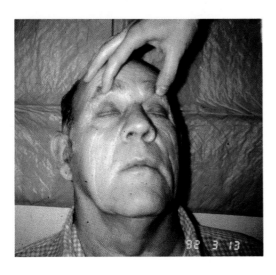

**COLOR PLATE 3.** Heliotrope rash of dermatomyositis. This erythematous and/or violaceous rash over the eyelids is characteristic of dermatomyositis in this middle-aged man.

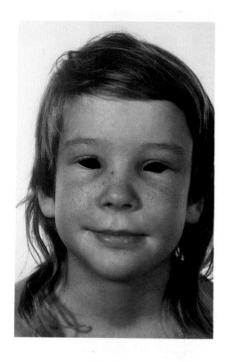

**COLOR PLATE 4.** The rash of juvenile dermato-myositis crosses the nasal bridge and could be confused with mild sunburn. However, there is edema of the upper eyelids and prominence of vascular markings at the upper eyelid margins.

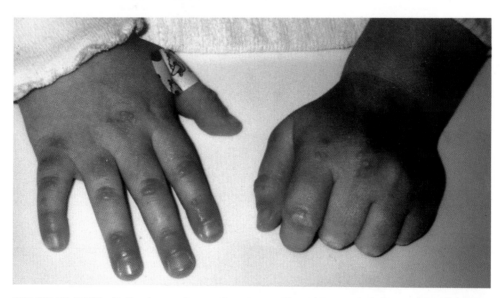

**COLOR PLATE 5.** Gottron's papules, erythema, over the metacarpal phalangeal and interphalangeal joints, and periungual erythema that accompanies abnormal nailfold capillary studies.

*Diseases of Skeletal Muscle,*
edited by Robert L. Wortmann.
Lippincott Williams & Wilkins, Philadelphia © 2000

# 5

# Inflammatory Myopathies in Children

Lauren M. Pachman

*Department of Pediatrics, Northwestern University Medical School, Chicago, Illinois;*
*Division of Pediatric Immunology and Rheumatology,*
*The Children's Memorial Hospital, Chicago, Illinois 60614*

The primary clinical feature of both juvenile dermatomyositis and polymyositis in children is chronic and progressive weakness of proximal muscles. In juvenile dermatomyositis, vasculopathy and distinctive skin manifestations are commonly associated with muscle involvement; in polymyositis, the skin is spared. The criteria proposed by Bohan and Peter in 1975 (1) are used to classify children with idiopathic inflammatory myopathies (see Chapter 4). In children, the distribution of the inflammatory change in muscle is often focal. This may confound the process of obtaining sufficient evidence to fulfill these criteria. In practice, using these criteria for diagnosis, although moderately useful, is imperfect and depends on selection of the appropriately involved muscle for electromyography and muscle biopsy. Therefore, in early or mild disease, diagnosis and institution of therapy may be delayed, with less than fortunate consequences (2).

Because myositis is often a component of other autoimmune or connective tissue diseases, exclusion of conditions such as systemic lupus erythematosus, mixed connective tissue disease (3), chronic arthritis in children (especially of systemic onset) (4), the spondyloarthropathies, Sjögren's syndrome and infection (5) is essential. Inclusion body myositis, which often runs a steroid-resistant course, has also been described in children (6). Other forms of inflammatory myopathy in children can be found to be concentrated in one specific area, such as orbital (7), nodular, or proliferative myositis (8), or involve an eosinophilic infiltration of the fascia (9). Association with malignancy is frequent in adults with dermatomyositis (10) but not children (11). Only sporadic cases of both an inflammatory myopathy and malignancy have been cited (12). Furthermore, a population-based canvass did not find malignancy in children aged 16 years or under (13).

## CLINICAL PRESENTATION

In children, juvenile dermatomyositis predominates, with juvenile polymyositis accounting for about 8% or less of cases of inflammatory myopathy (14). The most common physical findings of juvenile dermatomyositis children at diagnosis are rash, weakness, muscle pain, and fever. Dysphagia, hoarseness, abdominal pain, arthritis, calcifications, and melena may also be present (Table 1). In addition, hepatosplenomegaly and generalized lymphadenopathy are present at onset or before initiation of therapy in about 5% of children. When present, splenomegaly can persist for several months (2,15).

**TABLE 1.** *Symptoms present in 70 newly diagnosed children with juvenile dermatomyositis*

| Symptom | Number | Percent |
|---|---|---|
| Rash | 79 | 100 |
| Weakness | 79 | 100 |
| Muscle pain | 58 | 73 |
| Fever | 51 | 65 |
| Dysphagia | 35 | 44 |
| Hoarseness | 34 | 43 |
| Abdominal pain | 29 | 37 |
| Arthritis | 28 | 35 |
| Calcifications | 18 | 23 |
| Melena | 10 | 13 |

From Ref. 2, with permission.

## Cutaneous Manifestations

In half of the children with juvenile dermatomyositis, the rash predates the onset of muscle weakness. In contrast, proximal weakness is the first symptom in about a quarter of the cases, with the onset of rash and weakness coinciding in the remainder. The distribution comparing minority and nonminority children and the interval between the first and second symptom are shown in Table 2. Typically, the rash has a violaceous or heliotrope hue and is often most prominent on the eyelid. Small infarctions, often over the medial canthus, may be seen in those children who have a prominent component of vasculopathy. Many children with juvenile dermatomyositis are photosensitive and may sunburn easily. Sun exposure can precipitate the rash and exacerbate the symptoms either initially or once the disease has been diagnosed and treated. One of the first symptoms may be intermittent periorbital edema. Periorbital erythema and edema with or without eyelid telangiectasia, which may persist long after other signs and symptoms of other disease activity have resolved, are seen in 50% to 90% of affected children.

As in children with systemic lupus, the erythema may cross the bridge of the nose (Fig. 1A. See color plate 4 following page 85.). Other areas of erythema involving the upper torso, the extensor surfaces of the arms and legs, the medial malleoli of the ankles, and the buttocks may occur even in the absence of raised serum concentrations of muscle-derived enzymes. Partial baldness may result as a consequence of chronic scalp inflammation (16), which is particularly distressing to the adolescent. The skin over the knuckles is often either hypertrophic or pale red (Gottron's sign), evolving into colorless bands of atrophic skin, which, during active disease, may have a papular "alligator skin" appear-

**TABLE 2.** *First symptom (rash and/or weakness) of juvenile dermatomyositis and interval of time (median in months) before second symptom*

| | N | Rash first | Rash–weakness interval[a] | Weakness first | Weakness–rash interval[a] | Rash and weakness occurred at the same time |
|---|---|---|---|---|---|---|
| White | 59 | 30 | 2.0 (0.2–12.9) | 15 | 2.0 (0.7–9.6) | 14 |
| Minority | 20 | 12 | 3.5 (1.0–9.4) | 4 | 6.0 (4.6–20.0) | 4 |
| All | 79 | 42 | 2.0 (0.2–12.9) | 19 | 3.2 (0.7–20.0) | 18 |

[a]Values are medians, with range in parentheses.
From Ref. 2, with permission.

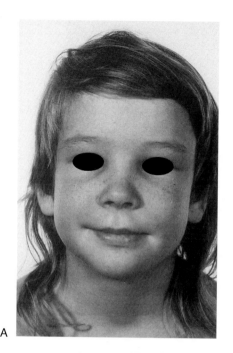

A

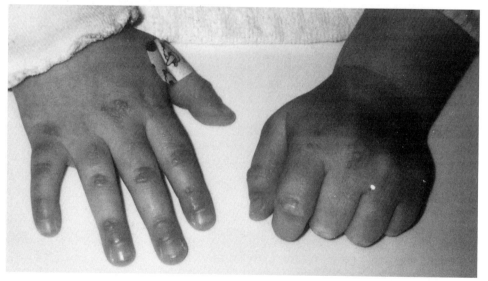

B

**FIG. 1. A:** The rash of juvenile dermatomyositis crosses the nasal bridge and could be confused with mild sunburn. However, there is edema of the upper eyelids and prominence of vascular markings at the upper eyelid margins. **B:** Gottron's papules, erythema, over the metacarpal phalangeal and interphalangeal joints, and periungual erythema that accompanies abnormal nailfold capillary studies.

ance (Gottron's papules) (Fig. 1B. See color plate 5 following page 85.). These hypertrophic lesions (which fade as the disease resolves), occur primarily over the metacarpal phalangeal joints, the extensor aspect of the elbows or the knees. Some children develop the cutaneous manifestations of juvenile dermatomyositis with no evidence of muscle involvement (dermatomyositis sine myositis). Some believe that children with the amyopathic form of juvenile dermatomyositis will eventually develop myositis often with calcinosis (17), but others disagree (18).

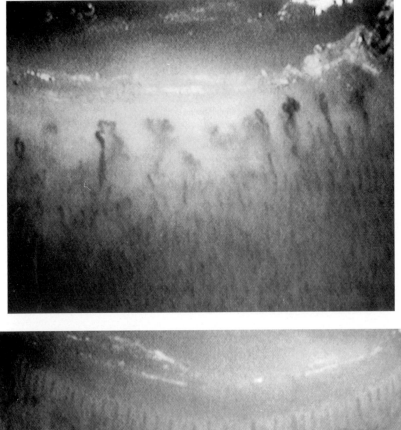

C

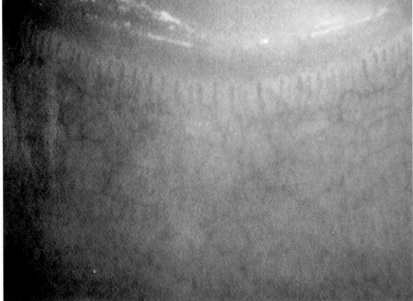

D

**FIG. 1.** *Continued.* **C:** Abnormal nailfold capillaries in a child with chronic symptoms of juvenile dermatomyositis showing avascularity at the edge of the fingernail with decreased end-row capillary loops. Those that remain are dilated and tortuous and demonstrate terminal bush formation typical of this disease. **D:** Nailfold capillaries after healing, showing a residual prominent subcapillary venous plexus but resolution of avascularity and terminal bush formation.

Manifestations of diffuse vasculopathy include dilated and abnormal nailbed capillaries (Fig. 1C), infarction of oral epithelium and skin folds, or digital ulceration. Diffuse vasculopathy is clearly associated with more severe disease, is correlated with the child's clinical course (19), and repairs with resolution of disease (Fig. 1D). The progression and regression of the vasculopathy can be quantitated by freeze-frame video nailfold microscopy (20,21). Increased disease duration is associated with an increased number of bushy loops and prominence of the subcapillary venous plexus. Elevated serum levels of creatine kinase are also associated with increased numbers of bushy loops (22).

Other cutaneous signs in juvenile dermatomyositis include florid erythematous gum hypertrophy and paronychia, often on the great toes. The paronychia may improve with symptomatic care, which may require parenteral antibiotics and return of sufficient peripheral vascular blood flow. The lacy patterning on the skin of livedo reticularis is frequent in children who present with Raynaud's phenomenon. The findings of livedo reticularis may rarely indicate the presence of a hypercoagulable state associated with circulating anticardiolipin antibodies.

If the symptoms of juvenile dermatomyositis have been present for a period of time, there is a greater likelihood that the cutaneous findings of partial lipodystrophy may be evident on physical examination (23,24). These signs may be quite subtle when they first appear. The subcutaneous tissue loss is pronounced in the buccal fat and may be progressive in the extremities. Involved areas are not tender despite the presence of a lymphohistiocytic panniculitis (25). In this uncommon disorder there is symmetric absence of subcutaneous fat with accentuation of muscularity, triglyceridemia, glucose intolerance-associated acanthosis nigricans, hirsutism, and hepatomegaly (26–28). If the onset is before menarche in females, sterility may follow. Partial lipodystrophy has been described in children with juvenile rheumatoid arthritis, insulin-dependent diabetes mellitus, Hashimoto's thyroiditis (29), membranoproliferative glomerulonephritis (30), systemic lupus erythematosus (31), and coeliac disease (32) as well as in juvenile dermatomyositis (23,33). However, in patients with juvenile dermatomyositis, partial lipodystrophy appears to be more common than previously appreciated (24).

## Musculoskeletal Symptoms

Proximal muscle weakness as seen by difficulty in climbing stairs, getting up from a chair, combing hair, or Gower's sign (using the hands to push off from the body in an attempt to stand) is common. Weakness of neck flexors is a particularly sensitive indicator of muscular impairment. Muscle strength testing in children is different from that in adults. For example, a child under the age of 4 years will not be able to do a situp (clear the scapula from the floor when lying on their back), even when normal.

The functional disability from muscle involvement can be measured reliably by the Child Health Assessment Questionnaire (34). Over 60% of children complain of pain on muscle compression, but it is less severe than the muscle pain observed in the infectious myopathies. Usually the child is more comfortable when the limbs are held in the flexed position, promoting the development of flexion contractures, which can be ameliorated in the early phase of the illness by gentle passive stretching of the affected areas.

Active myosis can often be confirmed by electromyography or muscle biopsy and can often be present despite normal serum levels of muscle-derived enzymes (35). The use of magnetic resonance imaging-directed biopsies (see Chapter 16) minimizes error in sam-

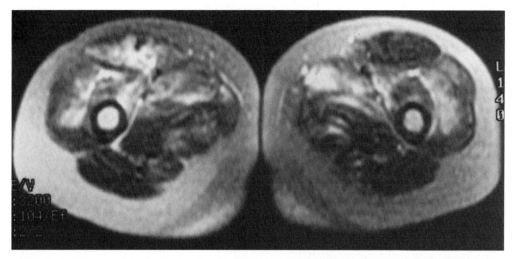

**FIG. 2.** An abnormal magnetic resonance image in a child with active juvenile dermatomyositis. The T2-weighted image with fat suppression shows a focal distribution of muscle involvement. The black areas are more normal muscles, whereas the white areas reflect edema and local inflammation.

pling of uninvolved areas in this focal disease (Fig. 2) (36) and can, under special circumstances, provide an excellent method to monitor a child's response to therapy (37–39). The magnetic resonance image may normalize several months after the muscle enzymes have stabilized in the normal range (40). $^{32}$P-magnetic resonance spectroscopy has been used for the past few years and gives useful information about muscle strength and performance in children (41). Decreased bone density is frequent in untreated patients with juvenile dermatomyositis. This places the child at risk of bony fracture (42,43), a risk further increased by steroid administration.

### Calcinosis Associated with a Depressed Serum Osteocalcin

The appearance of nonbony calcium deposits in soft tissue can be present at the time of diagnosis in 26% to 28% of patients with juvenile dermatomyositis (2,15). Calcinosis appears to be a correlate of disease chronicity that may be a consequence of delay in diagnosis and the resulting insufficient therapy (2). The calcifications may occur at pressure points such as the elbows or buttocks but also can be found in fascia surrounding muscle (Fig. 3). The calcifications may change in appearance from massive accumulations to become thinner more pancake-like collections that then may resolve spontaneously. Others may drain as a white cheesy or serosanguinous exudate and leave dry pitted scars. In persistent active myositis, the calcifications may progress to form a sheath that impairs motion or breaks the barrier of the skin, forming a site of entry for infection. Septicemia after disruption of the skin barrier by calcium deposits is not uncommon and contributes heavily to morbidity and mortality from this disease. The calcifications are not correlated with the presence of antinuclear antibodies, immune complexes, or class II human leukocyte antigens (HLA) (44). Calcinosis is associated with an increased urinary excretion of γ-carboxyglutamic acid, a component of the vitamin K-dependent coagulation pathway (45). The etiology of the calcinosis must be determined and clearly

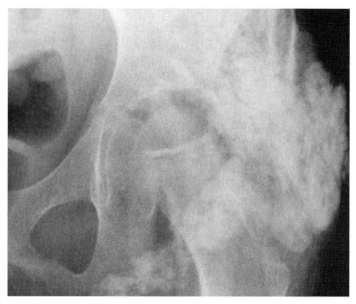

**FIG. 3.** Calcinosis in a child with chronic symptoms of juvenile dermatomyositis, seen on radiograph of the proximal part of the lower extremity. The dense white deposits are clearly seen but are only slightly palpable on physical examination.

differentiated from other syndromes in which calcinosis occurs, such as in heterotopic calcinosis or that after trauma.

## Cardiorespiratory Abnormalities

Electrocardiographic abnormalities are present at the time of disease onset in over half the children with definite juvenile dermatomyositis. Asymptomatic conduction abnormalities predominate, with an occasional complete right bundle branch block (46). These abnormalities usually resolve with decrease in disease activity. Dilated cardiomyopathy can be a presenting complaint (47,48), and tachycardia during the disease course reflects cardiac compromise.

Pulmonary fibrosis is more commonly found in individuals who have circulatory antibodies to tRNA synthetases (see Chapter 15). However, a decrease in ventilatory capacity with a normal diffusion of carbon dioxide was found in 78% of patients with juvenile dermatomyositis who were negative for anti-Jo-1, an anti-tRNA synthetase antibody. This decrease in ventilatory capacity can be associated with diminished speech volume. Vocal cord nodules have been documented in about 3% of children. These presumably result from forcing speech in an attempt to be heard and cause a persistently husky voice.

## Gastrointestinal Involvement

Significant gastrointestinal complications indicate a poor prognosis. Decreased esophageal motility can be documented by a radiographic cookie swallow, which may show airway penetration and retained barium in a widened atonic pyriform sinus (49).

The swallowing of liquids may be severely impaired. Esophageal reflux may result in aspiration pneumonia. Smooth muscle dysfunction can also result in decreased lower gastrointestinal muscle motility, making constipation an annoying symptom. Involvement of the masseter muscles may result in difficulty in chewing.

Vasculopathy may affect any part of the gastrointestinal tract. In severe disease, weight loss and mucosal ulceration with melena and the possibility of life-threatening perforation, peritoneal infection, and massive blood loss can occur. In the young child, development of normal speech patterns can be disturbed. Soft palate involvement is often revealed by nasal high-pitched speech. This usually resolves with a decrease in the inflammatory component of the myositis.

### Genitourinary Function

Rhabdomyolysis and primary compromise of the renal parenchyma itself may occur in children with an active myopathic process, requiring prompt hydration and monitoring of renal function (see Chapter 13). Necrosis of the ureter has been reported. This occurs in the middle one-third (iliac) segment, presumably because of the relatively sparse blood supply to this region compared with the upper (lumbar) and lower (pelvic) segments (50).

Menses may cease during severe disease, only to resume once the active inflammation is controlled. Anticardiolipin antibodies have been identified in some patients with juvenile dermatomyositis (51) and can be associated with increased fetal wastage (52,53). Birth control measures should take into account the possible presence of anticardiolipin antibodies to avoid the risk of increased intravascular thrombosis, but a successful pregnancy can be maintained in young women with active illness.

### Ophthalmologic Findings

Infarctions of eye-related tissue most often occur over the medial canthus and result in a depressed scar. In active disease, transient retinal exudates and "cotton wool" spots may occur after the occlusion of small vessels. These occlusions can cause intraretinal edema with injury to retinal nerve fibers, optic atrophy, and sustained visual loss. Neovascularization of the retina with spontaneous regression has also been reported (54). Disease of conjunctival vessels can also lead to an avascular zone with potential for infarction. Children treated with steroids should be monitored for both glaucoma and sublenticular cataracts (55). These manifestations often attenuate once the exogenous steroids are eliminated. Hydroxychloroquine should be avoided if there is a family history of red-green color blindness. Orbital myositis may be an isolated finding or associated with widespread inflammatory myopathy. The isolated form is often seen with normal serum levels of muscle enzymes but can be documented by magnetic resonance imaging. Corticosteroid administration can be effective therapy (7).

### Other Disease Manifestations

Vasculopathy involving the central nervous system may be associated with depression and wide mood swings even in the absence of steroid therapy. Polyneuropathy is a rare finding and is considered to be a consequence of the vasculitic process (56). It is not usual for the child with definite juvenile dermatomyositis to present with Raynaud's phenomenon. Raynaud's symptoms are more frequently found as an isolated phenomenon, in overlap syndromes, or in those children who go on to develop scleroderma.

## EPIDEMIOLOGY

In childhood, there is a bimodal age distribution for polymyositis and dermatomyositis (at 5 to 9 years of age, 3.7 cases per million per year, and at 10 to 14 years, 4.3 cases per million per year) (57). Children with disease onset under the age of 7 years may have a milder course (15). In the United States, juvenile dermatomyositis is more frequently reported in whites (2), although children of African or Asian origin may be at increased risk for chronic myositis (58). In the United States, boys are affected twice the rate of girls. In the United Kingdom and Ireland, five times as many girls are diagnosed as boys, with an incidence of 1.9 per million children under age 16 years (59). A similar increase is reported for China (60). However, in Japan, the gender ratio was 1.3 males to 1 female, with no associated malignancy or interstitial lung disease (61). This is in contrast to data from a Chicago clinic population of 127 children with juvenile dermatomyositis, in which the female-to-male ratio was 1.7, or from a preliminary analysis of the National New Onset Juvenile Dermatomyositis Registry in which overall the female-to-male ratio was 2.17; for ages 5 years and below the ratio was 2.08.

The only long-term study of onset (39 patients observed between 1962 and 1982) showed that the use of corticosteroids reduced mortality but that calcinosis occurred in 56% of children treated after 1972. Three of the 56 developed moderate activity restriction. The other childhood-onset reports were based on 18 patients or less (62,63). In a 10-year follow-up examination of 12 children with childhood juvenile myositis, one of the entry criteria was the presence of normal muscle enzymes, eliminating those with persistent inflammatory disease. On physical examination, 58% had at least one residual finding and 78% of those with juvenile dermatomyositis had residual dermatologic sequelae. Ultrasound examination documented that 60% had possible residual fibrotic change in at least one muscle group, despite good muscle strength (63). In the other outcome study (average 18.5 years), 14 had been treated with corticosteroids. Although these adults had good educational achievements and employment status, the following was documented by physical examination: 35% had proximal muscle weakness, 18% had rash and no weakness, 41% had calcinosis, 18% had significant disability, and 33% had Raynaud's (62). Long-term data based on children who have been given a more contemporary type of aggressive medical therapy are not yet available. In none of the outcome studies have the children with myositis-associated antibodies been identified and excluded from the data analysis.

Some controversy exists concerning the season of year of disease onset of juveniles with dermatomyositis. The data appear to vary by geographic region and by year. In the north central region of the United States, children with definite juvenile dermatomyositis (diagnosed within 4 months of onset) were more likely to have their first symptoms in the months of January to June than at other periods of time in each of 7 years evaluated (1974 to 1980) (64). An investigation of 79 newly diagnosed patients with juvenile dermatomyositis from all regions of the United States (1989 to 1992) identified an increased frequency of disease onset in the spring and summer of some years (2), although another preliminary survey did not confirm this observation (14). In Canada, clustering of new cases of juvenile dermatomyositis was observed as well, suggesting an environmental influence (65). In the United Kingdom, several clusters of disease onset were identified, the largest of which was in April and May in 1992. The timing of clusters appeared to vary from year to year (59). A case-control study of children in the United States validated the impression of a significant increase in antecedent symptoms in the 3 months before diagnosis (66). It is not yet established if predilection for season of onset is the same for both adults and children living in the same region or if the peak onset of polymyositis is in the same time frame as that of dermatomyositis in either age group. A registry has been established through the National Institutes of Health to describe factors that surround the disease onset in children with juvenile dermatomyositis (67).

In addition to temporal seasonal differences, there may be regional differences in infectious agents associated with disease onset. Agents associated with the onset, and on occasion a flare of juvenile dermatomyositis, are group A β-hemolytic streptococci (14,68), hepatitis B (69), and RNA picornaviruses (66,70,71). Sera collected between 1974 and 1980 from newly diagnosed children from the Chicago area contained an increased frequency of both neutralizing and complement fixing antibodies to coxsackievirus B (72). These findings, however, were not reproduced by the same group of investigators in a study of 20 children with dermatomyositis from the same region with onset of disease in the years from 1987 to 1992 (71). Enteroviral RNA was identified in the muscle of patients from the United Kingdom with polymyositis and dermatomyositis (70,73), but other investigators have not found viral RNA in cases from the United States (71). Other infectious agents considered as triggers for juvenile dermatomyositis include *Toxoplasmosis gondii* (74,75) and hepatitis B (76). However, titers of antibodies to these organisms were not increased either in a regional study (64) or in a case-control national study of new onset juvenile dermatomyositis from 1987 to 1992 (71,77). Although Theiler's murine encephalomyelitis virus has been identified in adult patients with polymyositis, this agent has not been found in children with juvenile dermatomyositis (78). Taken together, the above data suggest that the etiology of juvenile dermatomyositis is multifactorial and includes a possible role for molecular mimicry. Evidence supporting this hypothesis is found in the report that an amino acid sequence in skeletal muscle myosin, which has homology with the streptococcal type 5 M protein, stimulates lymphocytes from children with recurrent dermatomyositis after streptococcal infections (68). Noninfectious exposures currently posited as causative agents in juvenile dermatomyositis include vaccines for measles, mumps, and rubella; hepatitis B; and diphtheria, pertussis, and tetanus (79). The median latency period from vaccination to onset of myositis is 45 days (80). Also implicated are drugs, including D-penicillamine (81), and growth hormone (82). Inflammatory myopathy can also develop after bone marrow transplantation as a consequence of a graft-versus-host reaction (83).

## LABORATORY TESTS IN INFLAMMATORY MYOPATHY

The laboratory evaluations used to establish the diagnosis of juvenile dermatomyositis and polymyositis in children are identical to those used in adults. Classically, patients have elevated serum levels of enzymes derived from skeletal muscle (creatine kinase, lactic acid dehydrogenase, aspartate aminotransferase, and aldolase), myopathic changes of electromyograms, and inflammatory changes in muscle biopsy (1). Up to 15% of patients will have normal levels of all enzymes, and electromyography may appear to be normal in a child despite an intense inflammatory infiltrate on muscle biopsy. This variability in laboratory testing in inflammatory myopathy may cause delay in diagnosis and hamper the management of the disease (84,85). No single muscle enzyme is reliably elevated in all children with juvenile dermatomyositis. Of those children with the rash and proximal muscle weakness of juvenile dermatomyositis, muscle biopsy and electromyogram have been found to be normal in 19% and 20%, respectively (2). Magnetic resonance imaging only identifies muscle inflammation of some cases (Fig. 2).

Electromyography often reveals insertional irritability, followed by spontaneous electrical activity at rest, is often observed. This pattern is not specific and also can be seen in the muscular dystrophies and in early acute myositis. Abnormal early full recruitment of muscle fibers with moderate effort occurs in about 45% of patients with juvenile dermatomyositis, and bizarre high-frequency discharges occur in 15% to 20%. Reduced motor unit activity is seen in Duchenne's muscular dystrophy and in juvenile dermatomyositis. Myasthenia gravis can coexist with an inflammatory myopathy, resulting in a greater degree of instability of motor unit potential than is found in uncomplicated inflammatory myopathies.

In juvenile dermatomyositis, vascular damage may occur in the absence of a prominent inflammatory component (86,87). The muscle pathology reflects vascular compromise and capillary dropout, with perifascicular atrophy of both type I and type II fibers (Fig. 4). Multiple satellite cells are frequently seen in atrophic fibers. Focal repair takes place concomitantly with fiber atrophy (88). Low-grade ischemia may also be related to expression of class I and class II major histocompatibility complex gene products, which are found primarily in the perifascicular area (89). There appears to be less primary involvement of vessels in children with polymyositis.

In new-onset untreated juvenile dermatomyositis, there is a marked increase in the number of CD8+ T cells that localize in the muscle compared with the decreased number of CD8+ T cells found in the peripheral blood (90). There is some evidence of oligoclonality of these muscle-associated lymphocytes, suggesting an antigen-driven process (91). CD14+ macrophages found on biopsy are associated with serum levels of neopterin, both of which decrease in response to therapy (92). In dermatomyositis, there appears to be a close relationship between CD4+ T cells and B cells and macrophages, suggesting a cytotoxic mechanism, perhaps directed against immune complex-modified endothelial cells (93). The interpretation of the histopathology is helped by having a description of the patient with respect to myositis-specific autoantibodies, duration of disease, previous

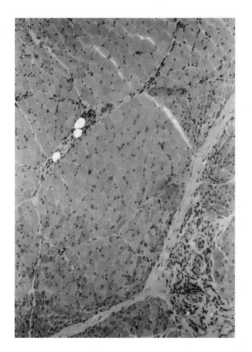

**FIG. 4.** Muscle biopsy of a child with juvenile dermatomyositis with symptoms for more than 4 months. The perifascicular atrophy is evident, with some increase in mature collagen. Capillary occlusion is evident with some muscle fiber size variation and a moderate mononuclear inflammatory infiltrate.

therapy, and evidence from electromyography, ultrasound, or magnetic resonance imaging indicating that the site biopsied was appropriate. A consistent scoring of the various tissue and vascular components at biopsy before initiating treatment will facilitate the evaluation of the response to therapy (94,95).

## Immunology

The humoral immune response may be altered in juvenile dermatomyositis. In early disease, IgM (46) or IgG (90) may be elevated or IgA deficiency may be present (46). Antinuclear antibodies are present in sera from 60% to 70% of newly diagnosed children. Rarely are other autoantibodies identified using an array of tissue and organ substrates (44) or standard tests (51). When present, the antinuclear antibodies is of speckled or cytoskeletal pattern in 60% to 70% of children and is often found in high titers (94,96).

An antibody specificity for heat shock protein 60 has been noted in the juvenile dermatomyositis (97). Antibodies to a 56-kDa nuclear protein (98) identified as annexin XI seen in a wide spectrum of connective tissue diseases have been found in juvenile dermatomyositis (99). Myositis-specific antibodies have been described but are rare in children compared with adults (100). The clinical picture of the few children recognized with anti-Jo-1 antibodies is similar to that of adults with the anti-synthetase syndrome (see Chapter 15). Manifestations include dyspnea on exertion and evidence of pulmonary fibrosis on both radiographic and histologic examination. Disease flares occur with the reduction of therapy (70). Most have severe arthritis. Some have "mechanic's hands" (101) (see Chapter 15).

Complement activation has been implicated in several studies of juvenile dermatomyositis. The C5b-9 membrane attack complex has been found localized to the intramuscular microvasculature (102) and correlates with the duration of the clinical disease (103). Immune complexes with complement activation appear to participate in the pathophysiology of this disease despite finding normal levels of total hemolytic complement, C3, and C4 in the blood. Increased levels of fibrinopeptide A and von Willebrand factor antigen have been reported (104).

Children with active untreated juvenile dermatomyositis tend to be lymphopenic (90). Despite this lymphopenia, there is a relative increase in the percent of CD19+ B cells. That increase correlates positively with clinical disease activity (105). In contrast, the percent of CD4+, CD8+, and CD25+ cells do not correlate with disease activity (106). The percentage of B cells falls in response to immunosuppression, often returning to normal ranges later than other serologic indicators. Some propose that the percentage of B cells can be used to guide doses and frequency of therapy (107). The CD4 to CD8 T-cell ratio is increased in peripheral blood.

Neopterin, a member of the pteridine family, is derived from GTP via guanosine triphosphate cyclohydrolase activity and is released from macrophages as a consequence of T-cell–dependent interactions involving interferon-$\gamma$ (108). Increased neopterin levels are associated with more active clinical disease activity scores in over 65% of cases (109–111). Increased neopterin levels were not associated with lymphocyte secretion of interferon-$\gamma$ in vitro (112) but reflect the CD14+ macrophage content on muscle biopsy (92). These data suggest an important role for macrophages in the pathogenesis of juvenile dermatomyositis. Support for this hypothesis comes from a study of serum and plasma from 64 children with a spectrum of active inflammatory myopathies (113). Elevation of interleukin-1 receptor agonist (IL1RA), soluble tumor necrosis factor receptor (sTNFR), soluble interleukin-2 receptor (sIL2R), and interleukin-10 suggested a role for monocyte–macrophage interaction.

## Genetic Associations

Records of patients with juvenile dermatomyositis in more than one family member are sporadic. The disease has been reported in monozygotic twins who developed muscle-related abnormalities two weeks after an upper respiratory infection (114). The association of the supratype A1, Cw7, B8, DR3 suggests a genetic link to disease susceptibility, and expression of HLA-DQA1*0501 has been implicated. The observed frequency of the C4a null allele suggests linkage disequilibrium in white patients with juvenile dermatomyositis compared with regional control subjects matched for HLA-DR3 (115). This observation was sustained when other racial groups in the United States were studied (116). Furthermore, analysis of family studies have confirmed the increased association of DAQ1*0501 with juvenile dermatomyositis (117). However, this association does not appear to hold for Czech children (118). The role of DQA1*0501 as an important susceptibility factor in the United States is strengthened by the observation that homozygosity for this allele is a risk factor for developing an inflammatory myopathy (119). Most recently, family studies involving 20 patients with juvenile dermatomyositis, 18 of their parents, and 49 unaffected siblings were performed. The HLA-DQA1*0501 gene was carried in 90% of the patients. Transmission of the DQA1*0501 was of maternal origin in 9 and paternal in 8 of 17 families (117). In addition, tumor necrosis factor α (TNF-α) polymorphism (5.5-kilobase [kb] fragment) was present in 85% of patients in that study. TNF-α synthesis by peripheral blood mononuclear cells is elevated in individuals positive for TNF2 (120,121). This may be a consequence of the linkage disequilibrium between the TNF2 allele and HLA extended haplotype, B8, DR3, that is common in juvenile dermatomyositis.

The TNF locus is placed in the class II region of the major histocompatibility complex on the short arm of chromosome 6, approximately 250 kb centromeric of the human HLA-B locus and 850 kb telomeric of the class II region containing DR3. Four polymorphisms have been described in the TNF locus. Two of these polymorphisms, located at −238 and −308, are in the region that regulates transcription of the cytokine TNF-α. TNF-α may contribute to the chronicity and vasculopathy of juvenile dermatomyositis and the complications of calcinosis and lipodystrophy (122). The TNF2 allele is identified by a G to A substitution at the *Ncor* I restriction site. There is recent evidence that different haplotypes are associated with a range of secretion of TNF-α by activated peripheral blood mononuclear cells (AA secrete more than GA > GG) (123,124).

There appears to be an association among the TNF alleles at -308 (GG, GA, AA), the disease course of juvenile dermatomyositis, the synthesis of TNF-α in vitro by patients' peripheral blood mononuclear cells and serum levels of TNF-α. Thirty-three children with definite juvenile dermatomyositis were studied. The disease course was defined as acute (single disease course less than 3 years) and chronic (mean disease duration, 5.0 years with either disease that required reinstitution of therapy or disease that had continued more than 3 years). TNF-α was not detectable in patients' sera. However, there was a significant difference in genotype frequency between the acute and chronic groups with a higher frequency of the TNF2 allele (AA, GA) in the chronic group. The endogenous TNF-α production in vitro for the acute and chronic groups was significantly different (121). Thus, the presence of the TNF2 allele and TNF-α production in vivo may be a significant predisposing factor for disease chronicity in juvenile dermatomyositis.

Calcinosis is significantly more prevalent on physical examination in children with dermatomyositis who carry the TNF2 allele. The prevalence was highest in AA group versus the GA versus the GG group (125). Whether the increased rate of calcinosis is related to the genotypes or the consequence of chronic inflammation is uncertain.

Partial lipodystrophy occurs in some children with dermatomyositis. This complication was observed in 9 of 46 children studied at various stages of treatment and disease activity. Seventeen had random insulin levels over 45 µU/mL, and 3 children had triglyceride levels two times the upper limit of normal. Of the ten children who have had oral glucose tolerance tests, four patients demonstrated insulin resistance consistent with partial lipodystrophy, with peak insulin levels ranging from 732 to 440 µU/mL (126). The DQA1*0501 and TNF allelic status was determined prospectively for 53 children with dermatomyositis. There was an increased prevalence of the DQA1*0501 allele with 90% AA, 78.5% GA, and 48.3% GG. Children positive for TNF2 allele and who had active disease of longer duration were more likely to have increased nonfasting insulin levels. This association further increased in those children with illness of more than 3 years' duration. Thus, altered insulin metabolism may be a consequence of the vasculopathy of chronic juvenile dermatomyositis, and increased production of TNF-α may play a role in the pathophysiology of both processes (127).

### Hematologic Findings

Acute phase reactants are often within normal limits except in children with acute and severe dermatomyositis. If they are elevated, one should check for other reasons, such as infected sites of calcinosis. The erythrocyte sedimentation rate and white blood cell count are also often within normal range. Lymphopenia is present often but is not commonly accompanied by an abnormal platelet count. A mild microcytic anemia may be present. Elevated levels of von Willebrand factor antigen provide a sensitive indicator of endothelial cell damage (128,129). Levels of the antigen may increase before a disease flare even when muscle enzyme levels are normal or remain elevated once the enzymes have normalized (104). Levels of von Willibrand factor antigen correlate with disease activity in over 60% of cases (130,131).

## DISEASE COURSE

The outcome of juvenile dermatomyositis has greatly improved since the 1960s when one third of the children died, one third were crippled, and one third recovered (132). For example, the reported mortality rate dropped to less than 3% in the United States and Japan by the 1980s (11). Since then, the disease course has been attenuated by early diagnosis and aggressive therapy (67,133). Several types of disease courses have been described: monocyclic, recurrent, and continuous (134). The frequency of calcinosis (which was associated with loss of mobility) has decreased from over 60% of cases (135) to about 23% at diagnosis (Table 1). The frequency of bone fracture in juvenile dermatomyositis has been markedly diminished by the use of high-dose intermittent intravenous methylprednisolone in conjunction with exogenous vitamin D (136). It is difficult to predict the child's outcome at the onset of their illness, although the magnitude of the initial serum levels of creatine kinase appears to be a correlate of disease severity (137). Several groups have found that prognosis is directly related to the degree of vascular involvement (135,138). Late disease recurrence after years of apparent inactivity has been reported (139), suggesting that need for periodic monitoring with more sensitive indicators of disease activity.

## DIFFERENTIAL DIAGNOSIS OF JUVENILE DERMATOMYOSITIS

The differential diagnosis of this inflammatory myopathy includes many of the major neuromuscular disorders of infancy and childhood and metabolic and infectious diseases that can be symptomatic at any age.

Gottron's sign can be mimicked by psoriatic lesions, accompanied by healing foci of hypopigmentation found in areas usually unaffected in juvenile dermatomyositis, such as the pretibial region. These rashes may clear with sun exposure. In contrast, sun exposure can precipitate symptoms and worsen rashes in juvenile dermatomyositis (140).

Other conditions associated with muscle cramps and contractures include hypothyroidism, uremia, and electrolyte imbalance such as hypokalemia, either iatrogenic or in conjunction with familial periodic paralysis. Pretibial tenderness is seen with erythema nodosum but is not a feature of juvenile dermatomyositis. Pain that awakens the child at night should be investigated for another cause, such as viral myositis, malignancy, osteoid osteoma, or osteomyelitis. Muscle weakness can be seen in adrenal dysfunction or after long-term high-dose steroid administration. In addition, thyroid, pituitary, and parathyroid dysfunction may be accompanied by skeletal complaints. Metabolic muscle diseases include defects of glycolysis (e.g., phosphofructokinase deficiency) and are associated with contractures, exercise intolerance, myoglobinuria, and an abnormal lactate response with a forearm ischemic exercise test. The child may have a defect in lipid metabolism such as a carnitine deficiency state (141), which may be exacerbated by nonsteroidal anti-inflammatory drugs. Exercise alone can induce changes that mimic inflammation on magnetic resonance imaging of muscle. Therefore, patients who are to be investigated with this technology should rest at least 30 minutes before testing (142). Children with spinal muscular atrophy do not usually have muscle pain on compression. Fatigue is common and is also exhibited by children with Duchenne or Becker dystrophies.

Acute infectious viral myositis in children, most frequently attributed to influenza A or B or coxsackievirus, is clinically differentiated from chronic myositis by its localization to the muscles of the calf, severe pain, and rapid resolution in 1 to 4 weeks (143). The myopathy may be characterized by myoglobinuria, electromyographic changes, and elevated creatine kinase. Children with human immunodeficiency virus or human T-cell leukemia virus type I illnesses may also have muscle complaints (5).

The calcinosis in juvenile dermatomyositis may be similar to that found in scleroderma or overlap syndrome (144). In addition, calcinosis must be differentiated from heterotopic calcinosis that may occur in children with progressive osseous heteroplasia, a distinct developmental disorder of heterotopic ossification characterized by patches of scattered dermal ossification followed by progressive ossification of deep connective tissue. The disease most often arises as a spontaneous mutation and is transmitted in an autosomal dominant Mendelian pattern (145). In these individuals, there may be evidence of both intramembranous and endochondral ossification, and a bony pattern may be seen on radiographic examination.

## THERAPY

There is continuing debate over the optimal medication, route of administration, and duration of treatment for childhood inflammatory myopathy (8,146). Recommendations are limited because of lack of long-term outcome data and the lack of comparisons of appropriate groups of children. For uncomplicated juvenile dermatomyositis, oral prednisone at 1 to 2 mg/kg is commonly used (8). Administration of vitamin D aids in proper absorption of calcium, which may be impaired by oral prednisone. Adequate hydration lessens the possibility of renal damage.

The child's linear growth may be temporarily arrested if the oral dosage of steroids used exceeds 4 mg/M$^2$. This, combined with increased weight secondary to both the prednisone and lack of exercise, proves a challenge for the teenager conscious of body image. Return to high-impact sports activities can be considered once the improvement in bone density takes place with disease control for the child, and the increased weight gain with oral prednisone may pose problems with compliance that is circumvented by the controlled intravenous administration of methylprednisolone.

High-dose intravenous intermittent (pulse) methylprednisolone has been used effectively for the treatment of juvenile dermatomyositis (39,147,148). Children treated with an intravenous course (30 mg/kg, 1 g maximal dose) plus low-dose daily prednisone (0.5 mg/kg/day) compared with standard treatment with oral prednisolone had a shorter disease course with respect to persistence of rash (1.5 versus 3.9 years) and weakness (1.5 versus 2.7 years) and did not have calcinosis, spine compression fracture, or growth retardation, although the frequency of cataracts was the same in both groups (136). Limited treatment with intravenous methylprednisolone alone was not effective in one study (149). When a subset of children with dermatomyositis who sustained a monocyclic disease course was subjected to a cost analysis, the group treated by the intravenous route had two fewer disease-free years, but their bill was about $10,000 higher than those given therapy orally (150). This cost of intravenous treatment has been brought down by shifting care away from the in-patient setting (M.S. Klein-Gitelman, personal communication, 1998).

If there is dysphagia or difficulty in handling secretions, the immediate use of both intravenous methotrexate and methylprednisolone is suggested. Methotrexate is given once a week at a starting dose of 15 mg/M$^2$ and intravenous methylprednisolone is given at 30 mg/kg/day. The frequency of the steroid administration is determined by the muscle biopsy findings and the rate of response. Low-dose oral steroids, 0.5 mg/kg/day, are given in the morning on the days that the methylprednisolone is not infused. The protocol for each child must be individualized. In general, an intensive course of intravenous methylprednisolone is used until there is normalization of the laboratory data, which is followed by a gradual reduction in therapy. High-dose intravenous methylprednisolone is not without adverse reactions. Analysis of a prospective log kept over a 5-year period by 213 children with various types of serious rheumatic disease who received a total of over 2,622 doses revealed that 22% experienced an adverse reaction, about half of which were behavioral changes ranging from euphoria to emotional lability. There was one case of anaphylaxis (151). Curiously, adverse reactions to intravenous methylprednisolone were closely associated with a record of previous accounts of cutaneous allergic eruptions to antibiotics (152).

In the adolescent, steroid therapy may exacerbate the age-related predisposition to acne. Administration of tetracycline, which is commonly used to treat acne, may lower the available levels of methotrexate, contributing to disease flare. With severe skin involvement, hydroxychloroquine (7 mg/kg/day) is given if there is no family history of red-green color blindness. With milder involvement, the cutaneous symptoms often resolve within several weeks, making the use of this drug less necessary. Topical agents to lessen dryness help the occasional puritis, as do topical steroids, which should be used sparingly (153). For breaks in the integument, a "skin substitute" (e.g., "second skin," DuoDerm) should be considered. Sepsis secondary to bacterial infection of calcinotic lesions must be treated aggressively.

Children who have severe onset or who do not respond to steroids have generally been treated with methotrexate (154). It appears that earlier initiation of this agent at doses of 15 mg once a week has reduced the morbidity of the disease (155) and permitted lower steroid dosages. Complaints of nausea can be circumvented by dividing the dose over a 24-hour period and supplementing with oral folic acid 1 to 2 mg/day. The function of the liver and bone marrow must be monitored. It is particularly important to inform the adolescent with juvenile dermatomyositis who is treated with methotrexate to avoid sun exposure and ingestion of alcohol.

If the child remains severely ill (sometimes despite normalization of muscle enzymes), evaluation of the immune system is useful in guiding the amount and duration of therapy (105). Intravenous cyclophosphamide therapy starting at 500 mg/M$^2$ every 3 weeks after adequate hydration plus MESNA for bladder protection can be considered. Serum levels of IgG must be checked on a periodic basis to ensure that they are adequate. If not, replacement therapy (0.4 gm/kg every 3 to 4 weeks) is needed to prevent recurrent infections.

When considering therapies other than steroids, high-dose intravenous gammaglobulin may initially help the rash (156,157), especially if given early in the disease course (158). A summary of case reports of the response of 27 children with dermatomyositis suggests that although intravenous gammaglobulin may be a good adjunct to other medical therapy, prolonged control of disease activity may not be achieved with this therapy alone. No data are available on plasmapheresis for children. The results of children with dermatomyositis treated with cyclosporin A appear to be encouraging (8). Evaluation of the efficacy of cyclosporin A has been proposed (159) but has been hampered by coexisting therapies (160).

At the moment there are no successful therapies for long-standing calcinosis in children with inactive disease. Magnetic resonance imaging may reveal inflammation associated with calcinosis, permitting more aggressive medical therapy that may result in regression of the calcinosis. Once the myositis is controlled, some of the calcific sites could be carefully appraised and, if not too extensive, excised while the child is still given adequate dosages of methotrexate. There are now less frequent recurrences of the calcicosis in the wound site.

Previous studies have documented decreased bone density and levels of osteocalcin (an indicator of bone mineral metabolism) in untreated active juvenile dermatomyositis (43). The young child with early onset of juvenile dermatomyositis appears to be the most at risk (161). In the adolescent, who often decreases intake of calcium-containing foods, administration of vitamin D and increasing the calcium intake may aid in calcium absorption from the gastrointestinal tract in the face of steroid therapy. This approach may decrease the occurrence of one of the most serious consequences of steroid therapy, osteopenia (55).

Combined medical and physical therapy is required in the early phase of the disease. Initially, patients benefit from gentle passive range of motion exercises. More intensive physical therapy is effective in later stages of the disease, once the inflammation has abated. Prevention of sunburn, both by avoidance and barriers (clothing, ultraviolet A/B paraminobenzoic acid (PABA)-free sunblocks over SPF 30), keeps inflammation in both muscle and skin in remission.

Recognition of the psychological factors that dominate the child's response to chronic illness is very important in achieving a good outcome. The mood swings that occur both as a result of the level of maturation and the administration of corticosteroids can be devastating if not recognized and appropriately treated. It is particularly important to allow the child to participate in decisions affecting therapy and to encourage age-appropriate independence, to establish their specific identity, and to master the tools needed for financial independence (162).

The outcome of juvenile dermatomyositis has improved with a reduction in morbidity and mortality, but little data are available concerning long-term follow-up. The limited available evidence suggests that those with onset of juvenile dermatomyositis in childhood do well in adulthood on socioeconomic and functional assessment.

## REFERENCES

1. Bohan A, Peter JB. Polymyositis and dermatomyositis. Parts 1 and 2. *N Engl J Med* 1975;292:344–347, 403–407.
2. Pachman LM, Hayford JR, Chung A, et al. Juvenile dermatomyositis at diagnosis: clinical characteristics of 79 children. *J Rheumatol* 1998;25:1198–1204.
3. Citera G, Espada G, Maldonado Cocco JA. Sequential development of two connective tissue diseases in juvenile patients. *J Rheumatol* 1993;20:2149–2152.
4. Miller ML, Levinson L, Pachman LM, Poznanski AK. Abnormal muscle MRI in a patient with systemic juvenile rheumatoid arthritis. *Pediatr Radiol* 1995;25:S107–S108.
5. Smadja D, Bellance R, Cabre P, et al. Clinical characteristics of HTLV-1 associated dermatopolymyositis. Seven cases from Martinique. *Acta Neurol Scand* 1995;92:206–212.
6. Serratrice G, Schiano A, Pellissier JF, et al. Les expressions anatomocliniques des pollymyosites chez l'enfant. *Ann Pediatr (Paris)* 1989;36:237–243.
7. Pollard ZF. Acute rectus muscle palsy in children as a result of orbital myositis. *J Pediatr* 1996;128:230–233.
8. Rider LG, Miller FW. Classification and treatment of the juvenile idiopathic inflammatory myopathies. *Rheum Dis Clin North Am* 1997;23:619–655.
9. Huang KW, Chen XH. Pathology of eosinophilic fascitis and relation to polymyositis. *Can J Neurol Sci* 1987; 4:632–637.
10. Masi AT, Hochberg MC. Temporal association of polymyositis-dermatomyositis with malignancy: methodologic and clinical considerations. *Mt Sinai J Med* 1988;55:471–478.
11. Hidano A, Keneka K, Arai Y. Survey of the prognosis for dermatomyositis with special reference to its associated malignancy and pulmonary fibrosis. *J Dermatol* 1986;13:233–241.
12. Sherry DD, Haas JE, Milstein JM: Childhood polymyositis as a paraneoplastic phenomenon. *Pediatr Neurol* 1993;9:155–156.
13. Sigurgeirsson B, Lindelöf B, Edhag O, Allander E. Risk of cancer in patients with dermatomyositis or polymyositis. A population-based study. *N Engl J Med* 1992;326:363–367.
14. Rider LG, Okada S, Sherry DD, et al. Epidemiologic features and environmental exposure associated with illness onset in juvenile idiopathic inflammatory myopathy (JIIM). *Arthritis Rheum* 1995;38:S362.
15. Rider LG, Okada S, Sherry DD, et al. Presentations and disease courses of juvenile idiopathic inflammatory myopathy (JIIM). *Arthritis Rheum* 1995;38:S362.
16. Kasteler JS, Callen JP. Scalp involvement in dermatomyositis. Often overlooked or misdiagnosed. *JAMA* 1994; 272:1939–1941.
17. Eisenstein D, Paller A, Pachman LM. Juvenile dermatomyositis presenting with rash alone. *Pediatrics* 1997; 100:391–392.
18. Cosnes A, Amaudric F, Gherardi R, et al. Dermatomyositis without muscle weakness. Long-term follow-up of 12 patients without systemic corticosteroids. *Arch Dermatol* 1995;131:1381–1385.
19. Silver RM, Maricq HR. Childhood dermatomyositis: serial microvascular studies. *Pediatrics* 1989;83: 278–283.
20. Pachman LM, Sundberg J, Kinder J, et al. Nailfold capillary studies in children with pediatric connective tissue diseases: systemic lupus erythematosus (SLE), juvenile dermatomyositis (JDMS), Raynaud's phenomenon (RP)—comparison with data from normal children. *Arthritis Rheum* 1996;39:R14.
21. Pachman LM, Sundberg J, Maduzia L, et al. Sequential studies of nailfold capillary vessels (NFC) in 10 children with juvenile dermatomyositis (JDMS): correlation with disease activity score (DAS) but not von Willebrand factor antigen (vWF:Ag). *Arthritis Rheum* 1995;38:S361.
22. Pachman LM, Mendez E, Kanuru J, et al. Nailfold capillary studies (NFC) in 50 untreated children with juvenile dermatomyositis (JDM). *Arthritis Rheum* 1998;40:S265.
23. Tucker LB, Sadegi-Neged A, Schaller JG. The association of acquired lipodystrophy with juvenile dermatomyositis. *Arthritis Rheum* 1990;33:S1496.
24. Kitson H, Malleson PN, Sanderson S, Cabral DA, Petty RE. Lipodystrophy in juvenile dermatomyositis patients: evaluation of clinical and metabolic abnormalities. *Arthritis Rheum* 1997;40:S140.
25. Commens C, O'Neill P, Walker G. Dermatomyositis associated with multifocal atrophy. *J Am Acad Dermatol* 1990;22:966–969.
26. Huang JL. Juvenile dermatomyositis associated with partial lipodystrophy. *Br J Clin Pract* 1996;50:112–113.

27. Quecedo E, Febrer I, Serrano G, et al. Partial lipodystrophy associated with juvenile dermatomyositis: report of two cases. *Pediatr Dermatol* 1996;13:477–482.
28. Kavanagh GM, Colaco CB, Kennedy CT. Juvenile dermatomyositis associated with partial lipoatrophy. *J Am Acad Dermatol* 1993;28:348–351.
29. Billings JK, Milgraum SS, Gupta AK, et al. Liopatrophic panniculitis: a possible autoimmune inflammatory disease of fat. Report of three cases. *Arch Dermatol* 1987;123:1662–1666.
30. Habib R, Levy M, Gubler MC, et al. Partial lipodystrophy associated with a type 3 form of membranoproliferative glomerulonephritis. *J Am Acad Dermatol* 1987;16:201–205.
31. Walport MJ, Davies KA, Botto M, Naughton MA, et al. C3 nephritic factor and SLE: report of four cases and review of the literature. *Q J Med* 1994;87:609–615.
32. Mahony D, Mahony S, Whelton MJ, McKiernan J. Partial lipodystrophy in coeliac disease. *Gut* 1990;31: 717–718.
33. Torrelo A, Espana A, Boixeda P, Ledo A. Partial lipodystrophy and dermatomyositis. *Arch Dermatol* 1991;127: 1846–1847.
34. Feldman BM, Ayling-Campos A, Luy L, Stevens D, et al. Measuring disability in juvenile dermatomyositis: validity of the childhood health assessment questionnaire. *J Rheumatol* 1995;22:326– 331.
35. Miller LC, Michael AF, Kim Y. Childhood dermatomyositis. clinical course and long term follow-up. *Clin Pediatr* 1987;26:561–568.
36. Pitt AM, Fleckenstein JL, Greenlee RG Jr, et al. MRI-guided biopsy in inflammatory myopathy: initial results. *Magn Reson Imag* 1993;11:1093–1099.
37. Keim DR, Hernandez RJ, Sullivan DB. Serial magnetic resonance imaging in juvenile dermatomyositis. *Arthritis Rheum* 1991;34:1580–1584.
38. Hernandez RJ, Sullivan DB, Chenevert TL. MR imaging in children with dermatomyositis: musculoskeletal findings and correlation with clinical and laboratory findings. *AJR Am J Roentgenol* 1993;161:359–366.
39. Yanagisawa T, Sueishi M, Nawata Y, Akimoto T, et al. Methylprednisolone pulse therapy in dermatomyositis. *Dermatologica* 1983;167:47–51.
40. Huppertz HI, Kaiser WA. Serial magnetic resonance imaging in juvenile dermatomyositis—delayed normalization. *Rheumatol Int* 1994;4:127–129.
41. Park JH, Vital TL, Ryder NM, et al. Magnetic resonance imaging and P-31 magnetic resonance spectroscopy provide unique quantitative data useful in the longitudinal management of patients with dermatomyositis. *Arthritis Rheum* 1994;37:736–746.
42. Perez MD, Abrams SA, Koenning G, et al. Mineral metabolism in children with dermatomyositis. *J Rheumatol* 1994;21:2364–2369.
43. Reed AM, Haugen M, Pachman LM, Langman CB. Abnormalities in serum osteocalcin values in children with chronic rheumatic diseases. *J Pediatr* 1990;116:574–580.
44. Pachman LM, Friedman JM, Maryjowski MC, et al. Immunogenetic studies in juvenile dermatomyositis. III. Study of antibody to organ-specific and nuclear antigens. *Arthritis Rheum* 1985;28:151–157.
45. Lian JB, Pachman LM, Gundberg CM, et al. Gamma-carboxyglutamate excretion and calcinosis in juvenile dermatomyositis. *Arthritis Rheum* 1982;25:1094–1100.
46. Pachman LM, Cooke N. Juvenile dermatomyositis: a clinical and immunologic study. *J Pediatr* 1980;96: 226–234.
47. Cuny C, Eicher JC, Collet E, et al. Cardiomyopathie dilatee revelant une dermatopolymyosite attitude therapeutique. *Ann Cardiol Angiol* 1993;42:155–158.
48. Isaeva LA, Deliagin VM, Bazhenova LK. Main manifestations of carditis in diffuse connective tissue diseases in children. *Cor Vasa* 1988;30:211–217.
49. Pachman LM. Juvenile dermatomyositis. *Pediatr Clin North Am* 1986;33:1097–1117.
50. Borrelli MP, Cordeiro MJ, Wroclawski P, et al. Ureteral necrosis in dermatomyositis. *J Urol* 1988;139:1275–1277.
51. Montecucco C, Ravelli A, Caporali R, et al. Autoantibodies in juvenile dermatomyositis. *Clin Exp Rheumatol* 1990;8:193–196.
52. Harris A, Webley M, Usherwood M, Burge S. Dermatomyositis presenting in pregnancy. *Br J Dermatol* 1995; 133:783–785.
53. Ohno T, Imai A, Tamaya T. Successful outcomes of pregnancy complicated with dermatomyositis. Case reports. *Gynecol Obstet Invest* 1992;33:187–189.
54. Fong LP, Yeung J. Spontaneous regression of retinal neovascularization in juvenile dermatomyositis. *Aust N Z J Ophthalmol* 1990;18:107–108.
55. Callen AM, Pachman LM, Hayford JR, et al. Intermittent high-dose intravenous methylprednisolone (IV pulse) therapy prevents calcinosis and shortens disease course in juvenile dermatomyositis (JDMS). *Arthritis Rheum* 1994;37:R10.
56. Vogelgesang SA, Gutierrez J, Klipple GL, Katona IM. Polyneuropathy in juvenile dermatomyositis. *J Rheumatol* 1995;22:1369–1372.
57. Medsger TA Jr, Dawson WN, Masi AT. The epidemiology of polymyositis. *Am J Med* 1970;48:715–723.
58. Benbassat J, Geffel D, Zlotnick A. Epidemiology of polymyositis-dermatomyositis in Israel. *Isr J Med Sci* 1980; 16:197–200.
59. Symmons DPM, Sills JA, Davis SM. The incidence of juvenile dermatomyositis: results from a nation-wide study. *Br J Rheumatol* 1995;43:732–736.

60. Wang Y-J, Lii Y-P, Lan J-l, Chi C-S, Mak S-C, Scian W-J. Juvenile and adult dermatomyositis among the Chinese: a comparative study. *Chin Med J (Taipei)* 1993;52:285–292.
61. Hiketa T, Matsumoto Y, Ohashi M, Sakaki R. Juvenile dermatomyositis: a statistical study of 114 patients with dermatomyositis. *J Dermatol* 1992;19:470–476.
62. Chalmers A, Sayson R, Walters K. Juvenile dermatomyositis: medical, social and economic status in adulthood. *Can Med Assoc J* 1982;126:31–33.
63. Collison CH, Sinal SH, Jorizzo JL, et al. Juvenile dermatomyositis and polymyositis: a follow-up study of long-term sequelae. *South Med J* 1998;91:17–22.
64. Christensen ML, Pachman LM, Schneiderman R, et al. Prevalence of coxsackie B virus antibodies in patients with juvenile dermatomyositis. *Arthritis Rheum* 1986;29:1365–1370.
65. Rosenberg AM. Geographical clustering of childhood dermatomyositis in Saskatchewan. *Arthritis Rheum* 1994;37:S402.
66. Pachman LM, Hayford JR, Hochberg MC, et al. New-onset juvenile dermatomyositis: comparisons with a healthy cohort and children with juvenile rheumatoid arthritis. *Arthritis Rheum* 1997;40:1526–1533.
67. Pachman LM, Mendez E, Chiu YI, et al. New onset juvenile dermatomyositis (JDM): increased time to diagnosis and therapy in minority children by physician report. *Arthritis Rheum* 1997;40:S333.
68. Martini A, Ravelli A, Albani S, et al. Recurrent juvenile dermatomyositis and cutaneous necrotizing arteritis with molecular mimicry between streptococcal type 5M protein and human skeletal myosin. *J Pediatr* 1992; 121:739–742.
69. Mihas AA, Kirby JD, Kent SP. Hepatitis B antigen and polymyositis. *J Am Med Wom Assoc* 1978;239:221–222.
70. Bowles NE, Dubowitz V, Sewry CA, Archand LC. Dermatomyositis, polymyositis, and coxsackie-B-virus infection. *Lancet* 1987;1004–1007.
71. Pachman LM, Litt DL, Rowley AH, et al. Lack of detection of enteroviral RNA or bacterial DNA in MRI directed muscle biopsies from twenty children with active untreated juvenile dermatomyositis. *Arthritis Rheum* 1995;38:1513–1518.
72. Christensen ML, Pachman LM, Schneiderman R, Patel DC, Friedman JM. Prevalence of coxsackie B virus antibodies in patients with juvenile dermatomyositis. *Arthritis Rheum* 1986;29:1365–1370.
73. Yousef GE, Isenberg DA, Mowbray JF. Detection of enterovirus specific RNA sequences in muscle biopsy specimens from patients with adult onset myositis. *Ann Rheum Dis* 1990;49:310–315.
74. Lapetina F. Toxoplasmosis and dermatomyositis: a causal or casual relationship. *Pediatr Med Chir* 1989;11: 197–203.
75. Schroter HM, Sarnet HB, Matheson DS, Seland TP. Juvenile dermatomyositis induced by toxoplasmosis. *J Child Neurol* 1987;2:101–104.
76. Peters AM, Heckmatt JZ, Hasson N, et al. Renal hemodynamics of cyclosporin A nephrotoxicity in children with juvenile dermatomyositis. *Clin Sci (Colch)* 1991;81:153–159.
77. Pachman LM, Hayford JR, Hochberg MC, et al. Seasonal onset in juvenile dermatomyositis (JDMS): an epidemiological study. *Arthritis Rheum* 1992;35:S88.
78. Rosenberg NL, Rotbart HA, Abzug MJ, et al. Evidence for a novel picornavirus in human dermatomyositis. *Ann Neurol* 1989;26:204–209.
79. Cotterill JA, Shapiro H. Dermatomyositis after immunization. *Lancet* 1978;2:1158–1159.
80. Shamim E, Rider LG, Perez M, et al. Demographic and clinical features of patients who develop myositis following immunization. *Arthritis Rheum* 1997;40:S204.
81. Swartz MO, Silver RM. D-Penicillamine induced polymyositis in juvenile chronic arthritis: report of a case. *J Rheumatol* 1984;11:251–252.
82. Yordam N, Kandemir N, Topaloglu H, et al. Myositis associated with growth hormone therapy. *J Pediatr* 1994; 125:671.
83. Adams C, August CS, Maguire H, et al. Neuromuscular complications of bone marrow transplantation. *Pediatr Neurol* 1995;12:58–61.
84. Rider LG, Miller FW. Laboratory evaluation of the inflammatory myopathies. *Clin Diagn Lab Immunol* 1995; 2:1–9.
85. Pachman LM. Imperfect indications of disease activity in Juvenile Dermatomyositis. *J Rheumatol* 1995; 2:193–197.
86. Banker BQ, Victor M. Dermatomyositis (systemic angiopathy) of childhood. *Medicine* 1966;45:261–289.
87. Emslie-Smith AM, Engel AG. Microvascular changes in early and advanced dermatomyositis: a quantitative study. *Ann Neurol* 1990;27:343–356.
88. Woo M, Chung SJ, Nonaka I. Perifascicular atrophic fibers in childhood dermatomyositis with particular reference to mitochondrial changes. *J Neurol Sci* 1988;88:133–143.
89. Karpati G, Pouliot Y, Carpenter S. Expression of immunoreactive major histocompatibility complex products in human skeletal muscles. *Ann Neurol* 1988;23:64–72.
90. O'Gorman MRG, Corrochano V, Roleck J, et al. Flow cytometric analysis of the lymphocyte subsets in peripheral blood of children with untreated active juvenile dermatomyositis. *Clin Diagn Lab Immunol* 1995;2: 205–208.
91. Pachman LM, O'Gorman MRG, Lawton TP, et al. Studies of muscle biopsies (MBx) from DAQ1*0501-untreated children with juvenile dermatomyositis (JDM) very early in their disease course: evidence of a TCR Vβ 8 motif and increased CD56+ NK cells. *J Rheumatol* 1997;40:S203.

92. Pachman LM, Maduzia L, Liotta M, et al. Serum neopterin (NEO) correlates with increased macrophages (CD14+) in MRI directed muscle biopsies in active juvenile dermatomyositis (JDMS). *Arthritis Rheum* 1996; 39:S191.
93. Engel AG, Arahata K. Mononuclear cells in myopathies: quantitation of functionally distinct subsets, recognition of antigen-specific cell-mediated cytotoxicity in some diseases, and implications for the pathogenesis of the different inflammatory myopathies. *Hum Pathol* 1986;17:704–721.
94. Pachman LM, Crawford S, Morello F, et al. MRI directed needle biopsy for the assessment of juvenile dermatomyositis (JDMS) response to therapy: comparison of initial and follow-up biopsies using a histological rating scale evaluating disease severity/chronicity. *Arthritis Rheum* 1996;39:R14.
95. Pachman LM, Crawford S, Morello F, et al. MRI directed muscle biopsy (Bx) for assessment of juvenile dermatomyositis (JDMS) response to therapy: comparison of initial and follow-up biopsies using a histological rating scale evaluating disease scverity/chronicity. *Arthritis Rheum* 1996;39:S191.
96. Pachman LM, Hardin JA, Cobb MA, Arroyave CM. The antinuclear antibody (ANA) in juvenile dermatomyositis (JDMS) is not Jo-1, suggesting that JDMS and polymyositis (PM) are different diseases. *Arthritis Rheum* 1984;27:S45.
97. Patterson BK, Lee C, Lane WC, et al. Antinuclear antibody (ANA) positive sera from juvenile dermatomyositis (JDMS) has specificity for heat shock protein 60 (HSP-60). *Pediatr Res* 1993;33:157A.
98. Cambridge G, Ovadia E, Isenberg DA, et al. Juvenile dermatomyositis: serial studies of circulating autoantibodies to a 56 kD nuclear protein. *Clin Exp Rheumatol* 1994;12:451–457.
99. Misaki Y, van Venrooij WJ, Pruijn GJ. Prevalence and characteristics of anti-56K/annexin XI autoantibodies in systemic autoimmune diseases. *J Rheumatol* 1995;22:97–102.
100. Rider LG, Miller FW, Targoff IN, et al. A broadened spectrum of juvenile myositis: myositis-specific autoantibodies in children. *Arthritis Rheum* 1994;37:1534–1538.
101. Rider LG, Targoff IN, Taylor-Albert ES, et al. Anti-Jo-1 autoantibodies define a clinically homogenous subset of childhood idiopathic inflammatory myopathy (IIM). *Arthritis Rheum* 1995;38:s362.
102. Kissel JT, Mendell JR, Rammohan KW. Microvascular deposition of complement membrane attack complex in dermatomyositis. *N Engl J Med* 1986;314:329–334.
103. Kissel JT, Halterman RK, Rammohan KW, Mendell JR. The relationship of complement-mediated microvasculopathy to the histologic features and clinical duration of disease in dermatomyositis. *Arch Neurol* 1991;48: 26–30.
104. Scott JP, Arroyave C. Activation of complement and coagulation in juvenile dermatomyositis. *Arthritis Rheum* 1987;30:572–576.
105. Eisenstein DM, O'Gorman MR, Pachman LM. Correlations between change in disease activity and changes in peripheral blood lymphocyte subsets in patients with juvenile dermatomyositis. *J Rheumatol* 1997;24: 1830–1832.
106. Eisenstein DM, O'Gorman MRG, Donovan M, Pachman LM. Percentage of B cells in peripheral blood of patients with JDMS. *Arthritis Rheum* 1995;38:R15.
107. Pachman LM. Juvenile dermatomyositis (JDMS): new clues to diagnosis and pathogenesis. *Clin Exp Rheumatol* 1994;12:S69–S73.
108. Barak M, Merzback D, Gruener N. The effect of immunomodulators on PHA or IFN-gamma induced release of neopterin from purified macrophages and peripheral blood mononuclear cells. *Immunol Lett* 1989;21: 317–322.
109. Pachman LM, Maduzia L, Chung A, et al. Juvenile dermatomyositis (JDMS): disease activity scores are correlated with levels of neopterin in serum. *Arthritis Rheum* 1995;38:R16.
110. Myones BL, Luckey JP, Hayford JR, Pachman LM. Increased neopterin levels in juvenile dermatomyositis correlate with disease activity and are indicative of macrophage activation. *Arthritis Rheum* 1989;52:S83.
111. DeBenedetti F, DeAmici M, Aramini L, et al. Correlations of serum neopterin concentrations with disease activity in juvenile dermatomyositis. *Arch Dis Child* 1993;69:232–235.
112. Chung D, Liotta M, Daugherty C, et al. In vitro synthesis of IFN-gamma by peripheral blood mononuclear cells (PBMCs) in active juvenile dermatomyositis (JDMS): lack of association with serum levels of neoptin (NEO). *Invest Med* 1996;44:368A.
113. Rider LG, Ahmed A, Beausang L, et al. Elevations of interleukin-1 receptor antagonist (IL1RA), sTNFR, sIL2R and IL-10 in juvenile idiopathic inflammatory myopathies (JIM) suggest a role for monocyte/macrophage and B lymphocyte activation. *Arthritis Rheum* 1998;41:S265.
114. Harati Y, Niakan E, Bergman EW. Childhood dermatomyositis in monozygotic twins. *Neurology* 1986;36: 721–723.
115. Reed AM, Pachman LM, Ober C. Molecular genetic studies of major histocompatibility complex genes in children with juvenile dermatomyositis: increased risk associated with HLA-DQA1*0501. *Hum Immunol* 1991;32: 235–240.
116. Reed AM, Stirling JD. Association of the HLA-DQA1*0501 allele in multiple racial groups with juvenile dermatomyositis. *Hum Immunol* 1995;44:131–135.
117. Reed AM, Pachman LM, Hayford JR, Ober C. Immunogenetic studies in families of children with juvenile dermatomyositis. *J Rheumatol* 1998;25:1000–1002.
118. Vavrincova P, Havelka S, Cerna M, Stastny P. HLA class II alleles in juvenile dermatomyositis. *J Rheumatol* 1993;20[Suppl 37]:17–18.

119. Rider LG, Gurley RC, Pandey JP, et al. Clinical, serologic, and immunogenetic features of familial idiopathic inflammatory myopathy. *Arthritis Rheum* 1998;41:710–719.
120. Abraham LJ, French MAH, Dawkins RL. Polymorphic MHC ancestral haplotypes affect the activity of tumor necrosis factor-alpha. *Clin Exp Immunol* 1993;92:14–18.
121. Pachman LM, Hong D, Liotta M, et al. Tumor necrosis factor alpha (TNF-α) allelic polymorphism at position-308: association of TNFA 2 with chronic disease course and increased endogenous in vitro production of TNF-α by unstimulated peripheral blood mononuclear cells (PBMCs) from children with juvenile dermatomyositis (JDM). *Pediatr Res* 1998;43:338A.
122. Pachman LM, Liotta M, Mendez E, et al. Peripheral blood mononuclear cells (PBMCs) from children with active juvenile dermatomyositis (JDM) produce endogenous TNF-α. *Arthritis Rheum* 1997;40:S78.
123. Bouma G, Crusius JBA, Pool MO, et al. Secretion of tumor necrosis factor alpha and lymphotoxin alpha in relation to polymorphisms in the TNF gene and HLA-DR alleles. Relevance of inflammatory bowel disease. *Scand J Immunol* 1996;43:456–463.
124. Wilson AG, Symons JA, McDowell TL, et al. Effects of a polymorphism in the human tumor necrosis factor α promotor on transcriptional activation. *Proc Natl Acad Sci USA* 1997;94:3195–3199.
125. Pachman LM, Hong D, Liotta M, et al. The TNFA 2 allele (AA, GA) is associated with calcinosis, a chronic disease course and increased in vitro production of TNF-α, but not TGF-β by peripheral blood mononuclear cells (PBMCs) from children with juvenile dermatomyositis (JDM). *Arthritis Rheum* 1998;41:S322.
126. Klein-Gitelman MS, Daaboul J, Oren PP, et al. Acquired lipodystrophy in juvenile dermatomyositis (JDM): who is at risk? *J Invest Med* 1997;45:342A.
127. Pachman LM, Klein-Gitelman MS, Daaboul J, et al. Increased non-fasting insulin levels in children with juvenile dermatomyositis (JDM) are associated with the TNFA2 allele (AA,GA) and increased disease duration. *Arthritis Rheum* 1998;41:S203.
128. Guzman J, Petty RE, Malleson PN. Monitoring disease activity in juvenile dermatomyositis: the role of von Willebrand factor and muscle enzymes. *J Rheumatol* 1994;21:739–743.
129. Bowyer SL, Ragsdale CG, Sullivan DB. Factor VIII related antigen and childhood rheumatic diseases. *J Rheumatol* 1989;16:1093–1097.
130. Bloom BI, Tucker LB, Miller LC, Schaller JG. Von Willebrand factor in juvenile dermatomyositis. *J Rheumatol* 1995;22:320–325.
131. Miller CH, Donovan JM, Maduzia L, et al. Relationship of von Willebrand factor antigen to disease activity in juvenile dermatomyositis. *Arthritis Rheum* 1995;39:R13.
132. Bitnum C, Daeschner CW, Travis LB, et.al. Dermatomyositis. *J Pediatr* 1964;64:101–131.
133. Ansell BA, Miller JJ III, Pachman LM, Sullivan DB. Controversies in Juvenile dermatomyositis. *J Rheumatol* 1990;17[Suppl 22]:1–6.
134. Spencer CH, Hanson V, Singsen BH, et al. Course of treated juvenile dermatomyositis. *J Pediatr* 1984;105:399–408.
135. Bowyer SL, Blane CE, Sullivan DB. Childhood dermatomyositis: factors predicting functional outcome and development of dystrophic calcification. *J Pediatr* 1983;103:882–888.
136. Pachman LM, Callen AM, Hayford JR, et al. Juvenile dermatomyositis (JDMS). Decreased calcinosis (Ca++) with intermittent high-dose intravenous methylprednisolone (IV pulse) therapy. *Arthritis Rheum* 1994;37:S429.
137. Van Rossum MAJ, Hiemstra I, Prieur AM, et al. juvenile dermato/polymyositis: a retrospective analysis of 33 cases with special focus on initial CPK levels. *Clin Exp Rheumatol* 1994;12:339–342.
138. Crowe WE, Love KE, Levinson JE, Hilton PK. Clinical and pathogenetic implications of histopathology in childhood polydermatomyositis. *Arthritis Rheum* 1982;25:126–139.
139. Lovell HB, Lindsley CB. Late recurrence of childhood dermatomyositis. *J Rheumatol* 1986;13:821–822.
140. Drake LA, Dinehart SM, Farmer ER, et al. Guidelines for care of dermatomyositis. *J Am Acad Dermatol* 1996;34:824.
141. Breningstall GN. Carnitine deficiency syndromes. *Pediatr Neurol* 1990;6:75–81.
142. Summers RM, Brune AM, Choyke PL, et al. Juvenile idiopathic inflammatory myopathy: exercise-induced changes in muscle at short time-inversion-recovery MR imagining. *Radiology* 1998;209:191–196.
143. Mejlszenkier JD, Safran AE, Healy JJ. The myositis of influenza. *Arch Neurol* 1973;29:441–443.
144. Lian JB, Skinner MS, Glimcher MJ, Gallop PM. Presence of gamma-carboxyglultamic acid in the proteins associated with ectopic calcification. *Biochem Biophys Res Commun* 1976;73:349–355.
145. Kaplan FS, Hahn GV, Zasloff MA. Heterotopic ossification: two rare forms and what they can teach us. *J Am Acad Orthopediatr Surg* 1994;2–5:288–296.
146. Malleson PN. Controversies in juvenile dermatomyositis. *J Rheumatol* 1990;17[Suppl 22]:1.
147. Laxer RM, Stein LD, Petty RE. Intravenous pulse methylprednisolone treatment of juvenile dermatomyositis. *Arthritis Rheum* 1987;30:328–334.
148. Miller JJ, III. Prolonged use of large intravenous steroid pulses in the rheumatic diseases of children. *Pediatrics* 1980;65:989–994.
149. Lang BA, Dooley J. Failure of pulse intravenous methylprednisolone treatment in juvenile dermatomyositis. *J Pediatr* 1996;128:429–432.
150. Klein-Gitelman M, Waters T, Pachman LM. A Comparison of the cost effectiveness of IV and PO corticosteroids in the treatment of juvenile dermatomyositis (JDMS). *Arthritis Rheum* 1996;39:R13.

151. Klein-Gitelman MS, Pachman LM. Improving costs for diagnosis and treatment of juvenile dermatomyositis (JDM). *J Rheumatol* (in press).
152. Klein-Gitelman MS, Pachman LM. Intravenus pulse corticosteroids (CS): adverse reactions are more variable than expected in children. *Arthritis Rheum* 1998;209:191–196.
153. Stonecipher MR, Callen JP, Jorizzo JL. The red face: dermatomyositis. *Clin Dermatol* 1993;11:261–273.
154. Jacobs JC. Methotrexate and azathioprine treatment of childhood dermatomyositis. *Pediatrics* 1977;59: 212–218.
155. Miller LC, Sisson BA, Tucker LB, et al. Methotrexate treatment of recalcitrant childhood dermatomyositis. *Arthritis Rheum* 1992;35:1143–1149.
156. Roifman CM, Schaffer FM, Wachsmuth SE, et al. Reversal of chronic polymyositis following intravenous immune serum globulin therapy. *JAMA* 1987;258:513–515.
157. Lang BA, Laxer RM, Murphy G, et al. Treatment of dermatomyositis with intravenous gammaglobulin. *Am J Med* 1991;91:169–172.
158. Basta M, Dalakas MC. High-dose intravenous immunoglobulin exerts its beneficial effect in patients with dermatomyositis by blocking endomysial deposition of activated complement fragments. *J Clin Invest* 1994;95: 1729–1735.
159. Heckmatt JZ, Hasson N, Saunders CE, et al. Effectiveness of cyclosporin for dermatomyositis. *Lancet* 1989;1: 1063–1066.
160. Pistoia V, Buoncompagni A, Scribanis R, et al. Cyclosporin A in the treatment of juvenile chronic arthritis and childhood polymyositis-dermatomyositis. Results of a preliminary study. *Clin Exp Rheumatol* 1993;11: 203–208.
161. Eisenstein DM, Shore R, Mendez E, et al. Bone mineral density and metabolism in 30 children with new onset, untreated juvenile dermatomyositis (JDM). *Arthritis Rheum* (in press).(abst)
162. White PH. Success on the road to adulthood: issues and hurdles for adolescents with disabilities. In: Athreya BH, ed. Pediatric rheumatology. Philadelphia: W.B. Saunders, 1997:697–707.

*Diseases of Skeletal Muscle,*
edited by Robert L. Wortmann.
Lippincott Williams & Wilkins, Philadelphia © 2000

# 6

# Pathogenesis of Idiopathic Inflammatory Myopathies

Ronald P. Messner

*Department of Medicine, Fairview—University of Minnesota Hospital and Clinics and
University of Minnesota Medical School, Minneapolis, Minnesota 55455*

The term idiopathic inflammatory myopathy applies to a group of diseases of unknown cause that cause proximal muscle weakness and have in common inflammatory changes in skeletal muscle. Despite not knowing the cause (or causes), considerable progress has been made in defining the pathologic processes involved. This information has led to a clearer understanding of the differences among the various diseases and has reinforced the belief that the driving pathologic processes are autoimmune in nature. The current hypothesis is that idiopathic inflammatory myopathies result from immune-mediated damage occurring in genetically susceptible individuals in response to an environmental stimulus. The strongest evidence for the importance of immune mechanisms comes from studies of the pathology of the inflamed muscle and the association with autoantibodies. Evidence for association with genes of the major histocompatibility locus is also strong. The link with environmental factors is as yet mostly theoretical.

## POLYMYOSITIS AND INCLUSION BODY MYOSITIS

The nature of the cellular infiltrates found in muscle in an idiopathic inflammatory myopathy provides strong evidence for immunologic mechanisms of muscle damage (Table 1). In polymyositis and sporadic inclusion body myositis, the inflammatory infiltrate is characterized by the presence of T cells that appear focused on the muscle fibers (1–3) (Table 1). The cellular infiltrate is most prominent in the endomysial area and is progressively less in the perimysial and perivascular areas. Cytotoxic CD8+ T lymphocytes are the dominant cell in the endomysial area where they are about twice as common as macrophages and B lymphocytes (Fig. 1). The ratio of CD8+ lymphocytes to other cells increases as you move from the perivascular area to the endomysium. Macrophages are equally distributed in the three areas, whereas the distribution of B lymphocytes is the reverse of that of the CD8+ cells. T cells and macrophages surround and can be identified invading nonnecrotic muscle fibers, suggesting cell-mediated cytotoxicity is an important factor in muscle damage. The population of cells invading muscle fibers is made up of mostly CD8+ T lymphocytes. In this area, the CD8+ cells are accompanied by macrophages, which are roughly half as common as the CD8+ cells, and a few CD4+ lymphocytes (4). The number of CD4+ T cells that can be identified invading muscle fibers is strikingly less than that in the endomysial area where they make up about one quarter of the cells in the inflammatory infiltrate. Thus, CD8+ T lymphocytes, the pri-

**TABLE 1.** *Characteristics of the pathologic processes*
*in idiopathic inflammatory myopathy*

|  | Polymyositis | Inclusion body myositis | Dermatomyositis |
|---|---|---|---|
| Cellular infiltrates |  |  |  |
|   T lymphocytes |  |  |  |
|     Endomysial | +++ | +++ | ++ |
|     Perimysial | ++ | + | + |
|     Perivascular | + | + | + |
|   T-cell antigen receptor |  |  |  |
|     $\alpha/\beta$ | Oligoclonal | Oligoclonal | Polyclonal |
|     CDR3 | Nonrandom | Random | Random |
|     CD45R | ++ (endomysial) | ++ (endomysial) | ++ (perivascular) |
|     LFA-1 | +++ | +++ | +++ |
|     Perforin and granzyme | ++ | ++ | − |
|   B lymphocytes |  |  |  |
|     Endomysial | +/− | +/− | + |
|     Perimysial | + | + | ++ |
|     Perivascular | + | + | +++ |
|   Macrophages | +/++ | +/++ | + |
|   NK cells | + | + | + |
| Muscle fibers |  |  |  |
|   Upregulated class I MHC | ++ | ++ | ++ |
|   Expressed class II MHC | − | − | − |
|   ICAM-1 | +++ | +++ | + |
|   Red rimmed vacuoles | − | ++ | − |
|   Amyloid | − | ++ | − |
| Muscle vasculature |  |  |  |
|   Capillary loss | − | + | ++ |
|   Increase ICAM-1 |  |  |  |
|     Inflamed areas | + | + | ++ |
|     Noninflamed areas | − | − | + |
|   Expression of VCAM-1 on arterioles | +/− | +/− | + |
|   Deposition of complement products | − | − | ++ |

CDR3, complementary determining region; CD45R, clusters of differentiation; NK, natural killers; MHC, major histocompatibility complex; ICAM-1, intercellular adhesion molecule; VCAM-1, vascular cell adhesion molecule.
From Ref. 3, with permission.

mary cells capable of carrying out antigen-directed cytotoxicity, are the dominant cells at the site of muscle fiber damage in polymyositis and sporadic inclusion body myositis.

Changes observed in muscle cells in polymyositis and sporadic inclusion body myositis are compatible with the hypothesis that damage to muscle is immune mediated (5). Muscle cells normally express low levels of major histocompatibility complex (MHC) class I but do not express MHC class II molecules. The expression of these molecules and that of intercellular adhesion molecule-1 (ICAM-1) can be induced on cultured myoblasts and myotubules by exposure to interferon-$\gamma$ (IFN-$\gamma$) alone or in combination with tumor necrosis factor-$\alpha$ (TNF-$\alpha$). MHC class I molecules are upregulated in polymyositis, sporadic inclusion body myositis, and dermatomyositis, probably as a result of release of cytokines from the infiltrating lymphocytes and macrophages. CD8+ T cells require recognition of class I molecules on the target cell to carry out their cytotoxic function. Although the expression of MHC class I is not in itself sufficient to initiate cytotoxic attack, upregulation of class I on myocytes in these patients provides the setting in which T-cell–mediated muscle damage can occur. The adhesion molecule ICAM-1 is also expressed on muscle in polymyositis and sporadic inclusion body myositis (6). ICAM-1 may also play a role in enabling cytotoxic lymphocytes to focus their attack on muscle fibers. MHC

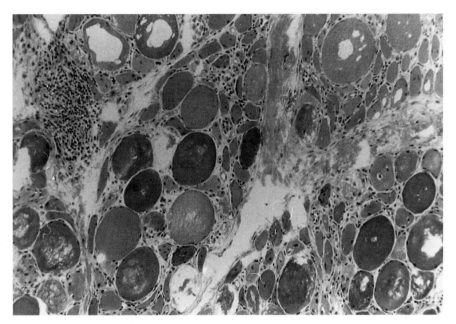

**FIG. 1.** Endomysial infiltrate in polymyositis.

class II molecules can be induced on muscle cultured in vitro, but expression of these molecules has not been found in biopsies of patients with idiopathic inflammatory myopathy. Experimental data indicate that myoblasts can be induced to express class II, can act as antigen-presenting cells, and can sensitize CD4+ T lymphocytes. These T cells can proliferate and under certain conditions carry out a cytotoxic attack on the myoblasts. Whether this occurs in idiopathic inflammatory myopathy is an open question.

A more detailed look at the infiltrating lymphocytes in idiopathic inflammatory myopathy further supports their role in mediating muscle damage. In polymyositis and sporadic inclusion body myositis, the activation marker HLA-DR is present on about one third of all lymphocytes found in the muscle and on about half of those cells that are invading muscle cells (5). Lymphocytes in the muscle almost all express the CD45RO surface marker, indicating antigen-primed memory T cells. The ratio of CD45RO cells to those with the CD45RA, a marker that denotes virgin uncommitted T cells, is increased in the muscle compared with the ratio in blood, providing further evidence that most lymphocytes are committed cells actively involved in an inflammatory process directed at muscle (3). Immunohistology has also identified a small subpopulation of the infiltrating lymphocytes, 4% to 8%, that bear the Ki-67 nuclear antigen that is associated with cellular proliferation. This observation suggests that a portion of the T cells in muscle have proliferated in situ in response to an antigen found in muscle (7).

Perhaps the most convincing pieces of evidence, that the T cells found in the muscle are directly involved in muscle damage, is the observation that CD8+ lymphocytes spread over the surface of muscle fibers and send narrow processes through the fiber membrane into the cytoplasm of the muscle cell. As the process develops, CD8+ cells and macrophages move through the fiber membrane and send these projections further into the fiber. Cytotoxic CD8+ T cells and adjacent muscle fibers also express the complementary adhesion molecules lymphocyte function-associated antigen-1 (LFA-1) and

ICAM-1 (6,8). The upregulation of these molecules on the infiltrating cytotoxic lympho-cyte and the opposing surfaces of the muscle fiber makes a strong case that the lympho-cytes are not found accidentally in this position but are actively attached to the muscle and directly involved in cytotoxic activity.

Cytokines are highly potent low-molecular-weight proteins that regulate the intensity and duration of the immune response. They are secreted by white cells and a few other cell types and exert short-range autocrine or paracrine action through specific receptors on the surface of the target cell. The ability of INF-γ to induce MHC molecules on mus-cle fibers and adhesion molecules on muscle endothelial cells is but one of many roles they may play in the immune attack on muscle. Unfortunately, their low concentration, and often transient secretion, makes them difficult to identify in tissue. This difficulty is reflected in the conflicting reports on their presence at sites of inflammation in idiopathic inflammatory myopathy. There is agreement that TGF-β is present in almost all biopsies of idiopathic inflammatory myopathy (9–12). The presence of TGF-β does not, however, appear to be specific because it is also found in Duchenne dystrophy and in some non-weak uninflamed controls (10,13). It is also difficult to determine the role played by TGF-β in idiopathic inflammatory myopathy without further information because it may en-hance or depress inflammation or promote fibrosis depending on other factors present in the local environment and the type of TGF-β receptors expressed on the tissue involved.

Interleukin (IL)-1 has been reported as absent (10), present in all idiopathic inflam-matory myopathy (12–14), and present only in dermatomyositis (15). Contradictory re-ports also exist for IL-2, IL-4, TNF-γ, and INF-α (5). One group of investigators who did not find strong evidence for the presence of proinflammatory cytokines did find evidence for the presence of chemokines (10). Chemokines are a group of small polypeptides that act as chemoattractants and regulate the expression of integrins in leukocyte membranes. Macrophage inhibiting protein-1α (MIP-1α), a member of the CC chemokine family that acts as a T- and B-lymphocyte chemoattractant and enhances the adhesion of CD8+ T cells to the extracellular matrix, was found in 13 of 14 biopsies from idiopathic inflam-matory myopathy and none from control subjects. Two other members of this chemokine family, MIP-1β and regulated on activation, normally T cell expressed and secreted (RANTES), were present but at lower frequency. RANTES, which is primarily secreted by T cells and attracts CD4+ T cells, macrophages, and eosinophils, was found only in treated patients. Overall the data on cytokines and chemokines in idiopathic inflamma-tory myopathy suggest that they may play a role but at present are not sufficient to define the exact nature or extent of that role.

It is unclear whether the immunologic mechanisms involved in idiopathic inflammatory myopathy are antigen driven and if so what antigens are involved. To date the identity of the key antigen or antigens is unknown, but study of the T-cell receptors displayed by the lymphocytes infiltrating the muscle in polymyositis and sporadic inclusion body myositis has provided evidence of a restricted immune response. This in turn implies the immune response seen in these patients is driven by an antigen or antigens present in the muscle.

The T-cell antigen receptor displayed by 95% of circulating lymphocytes is made up of one α and one β chain encoded by separate genes. These genes are divided into segments that encode different functional regions of the respective T-cell antigen receptor chain. These include the variable (V), joining (J), diversity (D), and constant (C) segments. Dur-ing T-cell maturation, these segments of each gene are independently and randomly com-bined (rearranged) to form the distinct functional receptor for that cell (Fig. 2). This process generates a very large number of different receptors capable of recognizing a di-verse array of antigens. Alpha chain diversity is generated by recombinations between V

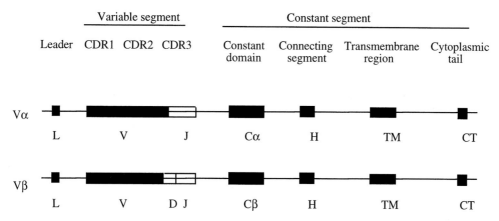

**FIG. 2.** Schematic representation of rearranged and α and β T-cell receptor genes.

and J regions, whereas that of the β chain in produced by VDJ rearrangements (16). The resulting T-cell antigen receptor recognizes antigen that is presented by MHC class I or II molecules. Three separate regions of the T-cell antigen receptor molecule, called complementary determining regions (CDR), are created in this process. The CDR1 and CDR2 regions recognize and bind to the MHC molecule, whereas the CDR3 contains the antigen recognition site (Fig. 3). CDR1 and CDR2 are formed by V regions of the α and β chains, whereas the much higher degree of diversity present in CDR3 is a product of different recombinations at the junctions between VJ or VDJ.

T-cell receptors can be grouped into families based on the V segments of their α and β chains. Because a given antigen–MHC complex will interact with a limited set of the rearranged V segments of the α and β chains, recognition of an antigen is shared by a subset of T cells with similar recombinations. Thus, response to a specific antigen is restricted (oligoclonal) with respect to the T-cell antigen receptor Vα and Vβ gene families and even more restricted with respect to the CDR3 sequence expressed in the responding T cells. Analysis of T-cell genes in a specific response should demonstrate this oligo-

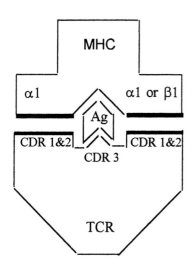

**FIG. 3.** Schematic representation of the interaction of the T-cell receptor (TCR) complementary regions with the major histocompatibility complex (MHC) molecule and the antigenic peptide during antigen recognition.

clonal pattern rather than the polyclonal pattern seen in a nonspecific response. Stimulation by superantigens involves binding of the superantigen to the less variable CDR1 and CDR2 regions of the T-cell antigen receptor and gives an intermediate response involving a larger number of cells, still restricted to a subset of T-cell antigen receptor gene families but less restricted in the CDR3 sequence.

Using monoclonal antibodies directed against specific T-cell antigen receptor families and/or polymerase chain reaction technology, it has been determined that T-cell antigen receptor genes in the T cells infiltrating muscle in polymyositis patients are oligoclonal, suggesting that the process is driven by a defined antigen(s) present in the muscle (5,17). It has also been suggested that two populations of T cells are found in the muscle, one that is clonally restricted that invades the muscle fibers in an antigen-directed cytotoxic response and a second that lies in the interstitium that is made up of heterogeneous nonspecific bystanders or regulatory cells (5). Similar analysis of biopsies from patients with sporadic inclusion body myositis has also shown restricted use of T-cell antigen receptor Vβ families. In this case, sequencing of the Vβ regions in most patients suggested antigen-driven clonal expansion but in one suggested a superantigen effect (17–19). Approximately 5% of circulating T cells display a T-cell antigen receptor made up of one γ and one δ chain. A single case in which the invading T cells carried the δ γ T-cell antigen receptor has been reported (20). In this instance the invading cells were essentially monoclonal and the muscle fibers expressed the 65-kDa heat shock protein. This type of response does not, however, appear to play a major role in idiopathic inflammatory myopathy because in most cases γ δ T-cell antigen receptor T cells make up a very small portion of the cells in the inflammatory infiltrate in the muscle (7).

Generation of cytotoxic T cells classically requires three signals: an antigen-recognition signal provided by presentation of an antigenic peptide on an MHC class I complex to the T-cell antigen receptor complex on a CD8+ T cell, a costimulatory signal provided by the interaction of B7 on the stimulating cell and CD28 on the lymphocyte, and the stimulatory action of IL-2 interacting with the IL-2 receptor, which is upregulated on the responding T cell by the first two steps (21). These three events combine to induce proliferation and differentiation into an antigen-activated cytotoxic T cell. This process is thought to take place primarily in lymph nodes where antigen-presenting cells and CD4+ Th1 type helper T cells provide the complex milieu necessary for this process. Effector cytotoxic T cells differ from native T cells in several ways. They are less dependent on a costimulatory signal for activation that is related to their expression of the CD45RO isoform of CD45. This allows them to respond to antigen–MHC complexes on cells that do not express B7. They double their expression of cell surface adhesion molecules CD2 and the integrin LFA-1. These molecules bind to LFA-3 and ICAMs on the stimulating or target cell and allow a strong bond to form between the two cells. Changes in these and other surface molecules also alter cytotoxic T-cell traffic patterns and allow them to home in on skin, mucosa, and sites of inflammation. They also begin to produce membrane-bound and soluble effector molecules. Once developed, cytotoxic T cells are thus free to roam about the body where they can seek out and attack their appropriate targets.

The effector function of a cytotoxic T cell is initiated by recognition of the antigen presented on a class I MHC complex on the target cell followed by binding of LFA-1 on the cytotoxic T cell to ICAMs on the target cell. Intracellular granules then move toward the surface of the cytotoxic T cells in contact with the target and are released into the space between the two cells. These granules contain TNF-β, perforin, and granzymes. Perforin creates pores in the target cell membrane that can disrupt its integrity, resulting in osmotic lysis and death by necrosis. These pores can also allow access of granzymes into the cytoplasm where they can trigger the apoptotic pathway in the target cell, leading to DNA fragmentation and death. Cytotoxic T cells also express the Fas ligand on their surface that can interact with Fas on the target cell membrane. This interaction also leads to apoptotic death of the target. Cell-mediated damage can also occur as a result of the activation of macrophages by CD4+ Th1 type T cells. In this pathway, antigen-sensitized Th1 cells respond to a specific antigen and release cytokines (such as IFN and TNF-β) and chemokines (such as IL-8 and MIF). These mediators in turn attract other lymphocytes and most importantly macrophages that then proceed to damage surrounding tissue through secretion of oxygen radicals, nitric oxide and TNF-α. In this type of response, less than 5% of the cells identified in the developed inflammatory infiltrate are specific for the initiating antigen.

In polymyositis and inclusion body myositis, the CD8+ T cells invading nonnecrotic muscle cells fit the profile of a committed cytotoxic T cell. The T-cell antigen receptor is oligoclonal, suggesting an antigen-driven response, and they display CD45RO and upregulation of LFA-1, indicating antigen-activated mature cells. With respect to the mechanism of cytotoxic T-cell activity, perforin and granzymes have been identified in the cells infiltrating the muscle, most often in CD8+ cells in the endomysial area (22), and the CD8+ T cells invading muscle fibers show reorientation of their granules to the contact surface with the muscle fiber (23), typical of an actively functioning cytotoxic T cell.

Fas ligand is present on the T cells and Fas is expressed on the muscles (24,25). Thus, all elements for necrotic and apoptotic cell death are in place at the muscle fiber surface in polymyositis and inclusion body myositis. Thus, it is somewhat surprising that no evidence has been found to indicate that muscle fiber damage in idiopathic inflammatory myopathy is related to apoptosis (26). It is equally surprising that pore-like structures suggestive of the effect of perforin have not been identified in muscle fibers that are under attack by cytotoxic T cells in polymyositis (27). Without these confirming data, it is not possible to state with certainty the exact mechanism of cell damage in idiopathic inflammatory myopathy. The lack of confirming data for these mechanisms may be due to methodologic problems that stem from differences between the very large multinucleated cells that make up muscle fibers and the mononucleated cells commonly used to assess target cell killing in laboratory or examined in most other diseases. The presence of multiple nuclei and huge volumes of cytoplasm in these large cells could make nuclear damage more difficult to find or confer a resistance to damage that alters the usual pattern of injury. It is also possible that muscle damage is not due to one mechanism but is the sum of several processes initiated by both cytotoxic T cells and macrophages, each of which plays a subtle but important role in the eventual death of the muscle fiber.

Although the pathologic process in sporadic inclusion body myositis has many similarities to polymyositis, sporadic inclusion body myositis has distinct pathologic characteristics that set it apart (28). Initially, polymyositis and sporadic inclusion body myositis are difficult to distinguish on routine light microscopy and histochemistry, but as the disease progresses the intensity of the inflammatory infiltrate in sporadic inclusion body myositis diminishes so that in the later stages little or no inflammation may be found. A second difference is the appearance of red rimmed vacuoles in the muscle fibers in inclusion body myositis that become progressively more common in mid- and late-stage disease (Fig. 4). A third difference seen on light microscopy is the presence of atrophic angular fibers that suggest a component of denervation. The most intriguing difference from the standpoint of pathogenesis is the presence of amyloid deposits in myofibers that are not found in other myopathies, with the exception of hereditary inclusion body myositis and oculopharyngeal muscular dystrophy.

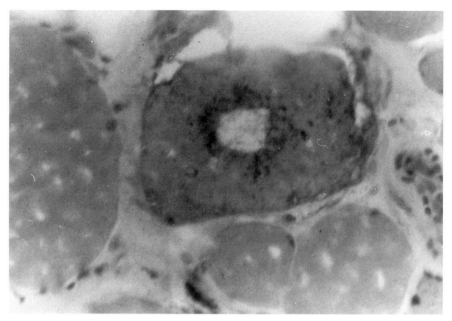

**FIG. 4.** Photomicrograph of lined or rimmed vacuole, a characteristic feature of inclusion body myositis.

Amyloid is a general term for protein deposits that are aggregated in β-pleated sheets and characteristically stain with Congo red. Using a sensitive fluorescence-enhanced Congo red staining technique, amyloid deposits can be found in all sporadic inclusion body myositis biopsies and in approximately 70% of the vacuolated muscle fibers (29,30). In sporadic inclusion body myositis, the amyloid deposits are made up of a group of proteins very similar to those found in the abnormal deposits seen in Alzheimer's disease (Table 2). The same protein deposits are found in patients with hereditary inclusion body myositis, but there is less formation of β-pleated sheets and less accumulation of hyperphosphorylated tau in hereditary inclusion body myositis compared with sporadic inclusion body myositis.

Accumulation of β-amyloid precursor protein appears to precede vacuolization and the formation of amyloid. The mRNA for β-amyloid precursor protein and prion protein are

**TABLE 2.** *Proteins characteristically of Alzheimer's disease that are found in the abnormal deposits in the vacuolated muscle fibers of patients with inclusion body myositis*

| Proteins | Localization in the abnormal deposits | | | |
| --- | --- | --- | --- | --- |
| | 6 to 10 nm amyloid-like fibrils | Amorphous structures | Floculomem-branous deposits | Paired helical filaments |
| β-Amyloid protein | + | + | + | − |
| β-Amyloid precurser protein | − | + | + | − |
| Ubiquitin | + | + | + | − |
| Hyperphosphorylated tau | − | − | − | + |
| Apoliprotein E | +/− | − | − | + |
| Prion protein | + | + | + | + |
| Nitonic acetylcholine receptor | − | + | + | + |

increased in vacuolated muscle fibers, indicating at least some of the accumulation is due to increased production (31). In an attempt to elucidate the mechanism underlying accumulation of these proteins, the gene for β-amyloid precursor protein was transferred into cultured human muscle fibers. The subsequent overproduction of this protein was accompanied by formation of 6- to 10-nm filaments, tubulofilamentous, amorphous deposits, and small Congophillic deposits similar to those seen in inclusion body myositis (32). A deficiency of cytochrome *c* oxidase was also seen in the effected fibers. These experiments suggest that overproduction of β-amyloid precursor protein may be an important step in initiating the cascade of events that leads to vacuolation and deposition of the other Alzheimer-related proteins in inclusion body myositis.

A buildup of these proteins in inclusion body myositis muscle may result from "junctionalization" of the fiber (28). The normal postsynaptic neuromuscular junction is characterized by a local buildup of the same proteins that accumulate in inclusion body myositis throughout the fiber. Perhaps under normal conditions these junctional proteins are synthesized under the control of adjacent specialized nuclei, but in inclusion body myositis this process spreads to involve nonjunctional nuclei as well. This change in regional control of specialized protein levels could be due to enhancement of a master gene that controls the whole sequence of proteins or to activation of a common promoter sequence common to the genes of proteins in this group. These changes in gene function could in turn be initiated by an inherited defect in control of the gene(s) in heredity inclusion body myositis or by an environmental agent such as a virus in sporadic inclusion body myositis. Alternatively, overproduction of only one protein may lead to the accumulation of the other proteins through disturbance of a feedback loop resulting in an increase of their production or a decrease in their catabolism.

## DERMATOMYOSITIS

In contrast to polymyositis and inclusion body myositis, dermatomyositis is characterized by a cellular infiltrate composed primarily of B lymphocytes and CD4+ T cells that appear focused on the vasculature. This pattern is more suggestive of damage mediated through humoral immune mechanisms. The cellular infiltrate is most prominent in the perivascular area and diminishes progressively in the perimysial and endomysial areas. B lymphocytes are much more prominent at all levels compared with polymyositis and inclusion body myositis. Macrophages are about equally distributed in the three areas, and the ratio of CD4+ to CD8+ lymphocytes is highest in the perivascular and lowest in the endomysial areas. CD8+ lymphocytes are present at the surface of the muscle fibers but are much less prominent than in polymyositis or sporadic inclusion body myositis, and invasion of muscle fibers by these cells is rarely seen in dermatomyositis. Perforin and granzymes are much less frequent in cells in the cellular infiltrate. This pattern is compatible with a process in which antigen-driven CD4+ helper lymphocytes provide help to B lymphocytes to generate antibodies that participate with complement in damage to the muscle vasculature.

The hypothesis that vascular damage is the key process leading to muscle damage in dermatomyositis is supported by the findings of numbers of capillaries per muscle fiber reduced in dermatomyositis compared with normal, polymyositis, or sporadic inclusion body myositis. This change occurs very early in the disease process (33) and is related to the perifascicular atrophy that is commonly seen in dermatomyositis muscle biopsies (Fig. 5). Capillary damage may be the initial lesion in dermatomyositis (33). Evidence of deposition of immunoglobulin and complement, including the terminal membrane attack

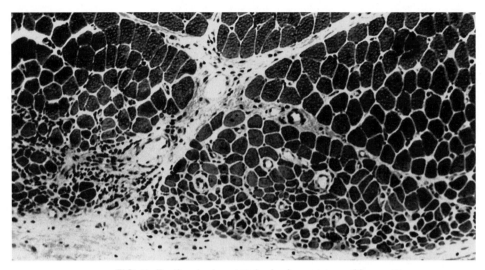

**FIG. 5.** Perifascicular atrophy in dermatomyositis.

complex of complement, in muscle arterioles and capillaries suggests that these vascular changes are due to immunologic mechanisms. These vessels also show upregulation of the adhesion molecule ICAM-1 and induction of expression of VCAM-1 (6,8). It is possible that the increase in expression of these adhesion molecules on muscle endothelial cells in dermatomyositis is related to the deposition of terminal complement components.

## WEAKNESS

Loss of muscle strength is the cardinal sign of idiopathic inflammatory myopathy. This weakness can certainly arise from loss of muscle fibers as the result of the attack of cytotoxic T cells or loss of their vascular supply. In many patients, however, the degree of weakness exceeds that expected from the extent of inflammation and damage seen on biopsy. These observations suggest that other factors also play a role in producing muscle weakness. One possibility is that mediators released by inflammatory cells interfere with membrane dynamics that are crucial to muscle function. Binding of calcium to sarcoplasmic reticulum is an important step in muscle contraction. Peripheral blood mononuclear cells from patients with active idiopathic inflammatory myopathy have been shown to release mediators that inhibit calcium binding by sarcoplasmic reticulum after coculture with autologous muscle (34). Direct study of muscle has also shown abnormalities in the sarcoplasmic reticulum. Sarcoplasmic reticulum membrane vesicles from muscle of patients with polymyositis and dermatomyositis accumulate less calcium than normal control subjects. Together these observations support the idea that changes in membrane dynamics may be important in the pathogenesis of weakness.

Maintenance of the membrane integrity essential for muscle contraction, and contraction itself, requires energy derived from an ATP-dependent process (see Chapter 2). Measurement of high-energy phosphate compounds in the muscles of patients with polymyositis and dermatomyositis by noninvasive magnetic resonance spectroscopy has shown that ATP pools are depleted more rapidly in patients than control subjects and also take longer to return to baseline ATP levels (35). These differences diminish with treatment along with improvement in strength (36), suggesting that altered energy metabolism is also an important component to their weakness. This theory is supported by studies in the murine model of myositis induced by coxsackievirus B1 (see below). Muscles from mice with this disease show utilization of the pentose phosphate shunt not seen in normal muscle and produce greater amounts of carbon dioxide and lactate than normal mouse muscle. These metabolic differences are accompanied by a 50% increase in activity of glucose-6-phosphate dehydrogenase and 6-phosphogluconate dehydrogenase and a 50% decrease in activity of myophosphorylase and myoadenylate deaminase (37).

Cytochrome *c* oxidase can be used as a marker for mitochondrial abnormalities. Cytochrome *c*-deficient fibers are rarely found in muscles of individuals under age 40 but are a common finding in individuals over age 65. They are more frequent in idiopathic inflammatory myopathy, especially in young patients with dermatomyositis and in inclusion body myositis (38). In dermatomyositis, the increase correlates with capillary loss, suggesting ischemia may be a cause, but they do not correlate with the degree of inflammation in dermatomyositis, polymyositis, or inclusion body myositis. Mitochondrial proliferation has been identified in nonregenerating muscle in idiopathic inflammatory myopathy in association with respiratory chain enzyme defects (39). Mitochondrial abnormalities are also suggested by the presence of multiple deletions in mitochondrial DNA. These deletions are not increased in age-matched control subjects in polymyositis or dermatomyositis but are increased in inclusion body myositis (40). The deletions are multiple and differ in different samples but tend to occur in regions similar to the areas where deletions are seen with aging and certain neurologic diseases characterized by multiple mitochondrial DNA deletions (41). At present, it is not clear whether these mitochondrial abnormalities represent primary or secondary phenomena or whether they play a role in the weakness experienced by patients with idiopathic inflammatory myopathy.

## AUTOANTIBODIES

Autoantibodies occur in most patients with polymyositis and dermatomyositis. Some of these, designated myositis-specific antibodies, are seen only in idiopathic inflammatory myopathy (see Chapter 15). Other antibodies are associated with idiopathic inflammatory myopathy and other autoimmune diseases. Their presence is prima facie evidence for humoral autoimmunity in these patients but has so far raised more questions than answers with regard to the etiology of the inflammatory process. As a group, myositis-specific antibodies are directed against intracellular proteins and ribonuclear proteins that are not usually expressed on the cell surface and are part of the basic machinery for protein synthesis in all cells. The anti-synthetase antibodies are the most common myositis-specific antibodies. Because the molecules targeted by myositis-specific antibodies are not exclusively found in muscle but are found in all cells, it is unlikely that myositis-specific antibodies are primary components of the mechanism of muscle injury. It is more likely that they are a secondary phenomena that reflect in some way the nature of the primary process. The association of myositis-specific antibodies with defined clinical subsets of idiopathic inflammatory myopathy reinforces the idea that they are important clues to the underlying mechanism. It has been suggested that they arise as a result of interaction of a virus with the synthetase during viral replication that breaks tolerance to the native protein by presenting it to the immune system in complex with the foreign viral protein (42). It is possible that a group of viruses is involved, each interacting with a different synthetase, thus explaining the fact that only one anti-synthetase antibody is found in an individual patient.

A search for viruses in muscle has so far been unrewarding, but it is possible that the initiating virus is eliminated while the immune response against the synthetase continues once self-tolerance is broken. It has also been suggested that these and other autoantibodies arise through molecular mimicry (43). In this hypotheses the synthetase is thought to share an antigenic epitope with an infectious or noninfectious environmental antigen. The immune response appropriately generated against the as yet unidentified foreign antigen then cross-reacts with the synthetase. This idea suffers form the variety of antigenically distinct proteins targeted by autoantibodies in polymyositis and dermatomyositis. Studies of the fine specificity of anti-synthetase antibodies have not resolved the issue. The antibodies usually react with conserved domains on the target molecule and frequently block its function. In some cases the antibody response recognizes multiple epitopes on the molecule (44). This situation is often found in an antigen-driven response directed against the molecule itself but could also be seen as a result of loss of tolerance and subsequent epitope spreading if the synthetase is the molecule sustaining a response initiated by a foreign antigen.

One recent attempt to clarify the relationship of anti-synthetase antibodies to idiopathic inflammatory myopathy was successful in inducing myositis by using DNA coding for the synthetase. Intraperitoneal immunization of mice with recombinant human histidyl-tRNA synthetase protein in adjuvant resulted in high titer antibodies to the protein but did not cause myositis. In contrast, intramuscular inoculation with naked cDNA of the human gene for histidyl-tRNA synthetase caused an inflammatory process in the muscle and low titer antibody to the synthetase (45). The inflammatory response included mononuclear cell infiltrates within necrotic fibers and surrounding endomysial tissue adjacent to normal and regenerating fibers that lasted up to 6 weeks after the last inoculation. No inflammation was found in muscle groups distant from the inoculation site or in the lung, indicating that peripheral tolerance to murine histidyl-tRNA was intact. Myositis was not seen in control subjects inoculated with the *HA* gene of influenza virus cloned into the same expression vector or in mice inoculated with the vector alone, indicating the myositis was specific for the synthetase DNA. The investigators speculate that local processing and presentation of the antigen to the immune system is crucial to development of the focal myositis produced in this model and that sustained production of the foreign protein provided an ongoing stimulus for the immune reaction against the muscle. Whether this model can be extended to the autologous synthetase remains to be seen.

## GENETICS

Many autoimmune diseases studied in experimental animals have a strong genetic component and association with genetic markers, particularly in the MHC antigens, and are found in a number of autoimmune diseases of humans. The theory that idiopathic inflammatory myopathy is primarily an autoimmune disease is supported by similar data (46). A clear association exists between polymyositis, dermatomyositis, and juvenile dermatomyositis and the MHC antigens HLA-B8 and DR3 in whites. Inclusion body myositis is also associated with DR3 in whites. This association may reflect the presence of an ancestral haplotype that has been associated with other autoimmune diseases, including systemic lupus and myasthenia gravis (46). There are insufficient data in other races to draw firm conclusions about MHC associations, but there is a suggestion that DR6 and DR3 may be associated with polymyositis in blacks. The myositis that occurs in mixed connective tissue disease in whites is associated with DR4 rather than DR3, but in this case the primary association appears to be the link between DR4 and the production of high titer antinuclear ribonucleoprotein antibodies that are present by definition in these patients (47). Production of myositis-specific antibodies also occurs on a restricted genetic background. The supertype specificity DR52, which is found on haplotypes DR3, DR5, DR6, and possibly DR8, is linked to the production of anti-tRNA synthetase antibodies (48,49). Antibodies to individual tRNA synthetases differ in their associations; anti-histidyl-tRNA synthetase antibody is linked to DR3 in whites and DR6 in blacks, whereas other antisynthetase antibodies are linked to DR2, DR8, or DQ1. Antibodies to Mi-2 and the nuclear antigen PM-Scl have different MHC associations (49,50). Overall, these data suggest that idiopathic inflammatory myopathy occurs in individuals with a restricted background of MHC genes and is modified in its clinical presentation by the presence of other MHC genes that influence the production of myositis-specific antibodies.

## ENVIRONMENTAL FACTORS

Reports of geographic clusters of myositis cases and the observation that subsets of patients defined by different myositis-specific antibodies tend to develop disease at different times of the year (51) have lent support to the idea that idiopathic inflammatory myopathy may be initiated by an infectious or noninfectious environmental agent. Many infectious agents have been suggested, including coxsackievirus, echovirus, adenovirus, *Toxoplasma*, and *Borrelia*. One clinical example of an association with a virus is the development of dermatomyositis with echovirus infection in children with X-linked hypogammaglobulinemia (52). Drugs such as D-penicillamine, cimetidine, and gemfibrozil have also been implicated as possible causes of idiopathic inflammatory myopathy. The development of a syndrome in patients on D-penicillamine that has all the features of polymyositis and resolves when the drug is withdrawn is the clearest example that a drug may induce idiopathic inflammatory myopathy (53). The human leukocyte antigen types of individuals with D-penicillamine–induced disease differ from those seen in the idiopathic polymyositis, suggesting that different host factors are involved in susceptibility to the two forms of the disease (54). The existence of these patients suggests a variety of environmental triggers of the disease that have yet to be discovered.

Because of their tropism for muscle, coxsackievirus have long been regarded as potential casual agents in the induction of chronic muscle diseases such as polymyositis, dermatomyositis, and chronic fatigue syndrome. The presence of antiviral antibodies in serum and the isolation of virus from patient stools provide evidence to support this link (55–57). Enterovirus has been identified in the muscles of patients with the disease in some studies, whereas others have found no evidence of its presence (58–61). Enterovirus infections are fairly common among the general population, so it is not surprising that some control subjects in these studies also test positive (62). Elevated titers of antibodies to *Toxoplasma* and *Borrelia* have been reported in idiopathic inflammatory myopathy, but no convincing evidence for the presence of either of these agents in idiopathic inflammatory myopathy has been provided. Associations have been claimed between idiopathic inflammatory myopathy and adulterated rapeseed oil, L-tryptophan, ciguatera toxin, silica, and silicone, but differences in clinical course, pathology, or questions about the cause and effect relationship make these cases less compelling.

Animal models have been used in an attempt to clarify the possible role of viruses in myositis. One well-studied model uses the Tucson strain of coxsackievirus B1. In this model, infection of neonatal mice leads to the development of acute viral myositis. Viral replication proceeds for about 2 weeks, after which time viral titers fall below detectable levels. Forty percent of the mice recover by 4 weeks with complete resolution of the acute inflammatory process in the muscle, restoration of normal muscle architecture, and strength. In 60% of the mice, the inflammatory process changes from acute to chronic and resembles that found in human polymyositis. The histopathologic picture includes ongoing muscle necrosis and regeneration accompanied by focal accumulation of mononuclear cell infiltrates. A characteristic waddling gait or hindlimb weakness is also observed and correlates positively with muscle inflammation (63). Development of the chronic inflammation is dependent on T cells. It does not develop in athymic nude nor neonatally thymectomized mice, and reconstitution of these resistant mice with spleen cells restores their susceptibility (64,65). Disease severity is associated with the MHC haplotype in susceptible inbred strains, which points to antigen-specific recognition as an important component of disease development (66). Electromyography supports a myopathic rather than a neurogenic origin for the disease (67). Chronic effects appear to be localized to the muscle, because the histology of other tissues, including brain and spinal cord, appears normal.

In the chronic phase of this model, virus cannot be cultured from the animal, but viral RNA persists in the muscle well beyond the time it can be cultured. By using the sensitive technique of reverse transcriptase-polymerase chain reaction, it has been shown that the time course of muscle inflammation parallels that of viral RNA persistence. Both are greatest at 4 weeks and decrease between 1 and 6 months. A low percentage (12%) of mice remain positive for viral RNA after 1 year (63,68). Persistence of viral RNA is also more prevalent in susceptible strains of mice compared with resistant strains (66). In situ hybridization reveals that persistent viral RNA is associated with three different patterns of histopathology (63): viral RNA lies in a subsarcolemmal location as an apparently silent infection of myofibers without associated inflammation or necrosis, viral RNA lies in necrotic myofibers that are surrounded by mononuclear cells, and viral RNA lies in an area with a severe loss of muscle fibers in cells that appear to be either proliferating satellite cells or cells that were infiltrating the damaged area. Molecular analysis of coxsackievirus B1 persistence indicates that the viral RNA is full length and does not contain any genomic mutations. However, it does exist in a double-stranded conformation that apparently confers stability but renders it noninfectious. Although the persistent RNA has the inherent capability to code for intact virus, it remains inactive under experimental conditions that are usually capable of reactivating infectious virus. These observations are compatible with the hypothesis that virus persistence may perpetuate an inflammatory response against muscle but that host factors are also required for full induction of the disease (68).

Encephalomyocarditis virus can also induce an inflammation in skeletal muscle that is characterized by a mononuclear cell infiltrate, perifascicular atrophy, myofiber degeneration, and regeneration (69). In this model, different inbred mouse strains also show different degrees of susceptibility to the disease. Viral RNA and muscle inflammation coincide and last for about 3 weeks after viral inoculation, suggesting that the inflammation is driven at least in part by the virus. Other models of enterovirus-induced inflammatory disease have described a variety of autoimmune phenomenon associated with prior coxsackievirus infection and viral RNA persistence. Among them, CVB3-induced myocarditis has been studied most extensively. Autoimmune manifestations vary depending on the host strain with immunopathic responses attributed to CD8+ cytotoxic T lymphocytes (cytotoxic T cells) in BALB/c mice, CD4+ T cells in DBA/2 mice, and both subsets in A mice (70). Other studies point to production of heart-reactive and myosin-reactive autoantibodies as mediators of immunopathology (71–73). It is of interest that these mouse strains ultimately develop immunopathic myocarditis and yet they arrive at this end point by different mechanisms. Because many of these studies used the same strain of virus, differences in the genetic composition of the host clearly plays a major role in the heterogeneity of the immunopathic response. In contrast, characteristics of the virus appear to be constant because myocardotic or amyocardiac viruses do not appear to change their pathogenicity in different hosts. This implies certain intrinsic characteristics of individual strains of the virus that are essential for expression of disease.

These animal models provide clear evidence that viral infection can cause chronic muscle inflammation and that a variety of autoimmune phenomena may be involved in the pathology. Despite the current negative clinical data from searches for virus in idiopathic inflammatory myopathy, the possibility remains that an agent such as a virus could initiate an immune reaction directed against virus in the muscle or cross-react with muscle and continue after the virus is eliminated. The myositis-specific anti-synthetase antibodies could be "footprints" of a previous viral infection. It is also possible that the different subsets of disease—polymyositis, dermatomyositis, sporadic inclusion body myositis, and the clinical subsets defined by myositis-specific antibodies—are the result of different environmental agents. Armed with better definition of the immunopathologic processes involved and the genetic factors that place individuals at risk, future searches for environmental triggers of idiopathic inflammatory myopathy may be more fruitful.

## REFERENCES

1. Arahata K, Engel AG. Monoclonal antibody analysis of mononuclear cells in myopathies. I. Quantitation of subsets according to diagnosis and sites of accumulation and demonstration and counts of muscle fibers invaded by T cells. *Ann Neurol* 1984;16:193–208.
2. Engel AG, Arahata K. Monoclonal antibody analysis of mononuclear cells in myopathies. II. Phenotypes of autoinvasive cells in polymyositis and inclusion body myositis. *Ann Neurol* 1984;16:209–215.
3. Mantegazza R, Bernasconi P, Confalonieri P, Cornelio F. Inflammatory myopathies and systemic disorders: a review of immunopathogenetic mechanisms and clinical features. *J Neurol* 1997;244:277–287.
4. Arahata K, Engel AG. Monoclonal analysis of mononuclear cells in myopathies. IV. Cell-mediated cytotoxicity and muscle fiber necrosis. *Ann Neurol* 1988;23:168–173.
5. Hohlfeld R, Engel AG, Goebels N, Behrens L. Cellular immune mechanisms in inflammatory myopathies. *Curr Opin Rheum* 1997;9:520–526.
6. De Bleeker JL, Engel AG. Expression of cell adhesion molecules in inflammatory myopathies and Duchenne dystrophy. *J Neuropathol Exp Neurol* 1994;53:369–376.
7. O'Hanlon TP, Miller FW. T cell-mediated immune mechanisms in myositis. *Curr Opin Rheum* 1995;7:503–509.
8. Cid M-C, Grau J-M, Casademont J, et al. Leukocyte/endothelial cell adhesion receptors in muscle biopsies from patients with idiopathic inflammatory myopathies (idiopathic inflammatory myopathy). *Clin Exp Immunol* 1996;104:467–473.
9. Lundberg I, Ulfgren A-K, Nyberg P, Andersson U, Klareskog L. Cytokine production in muscle tissue of patients with idiopathic inflammatory myopathies. *Arthritis Rheum* 1997;40:865–874.
10. Adams EM, Kirkley J, Eidelman G, Dohlman J, Plotz PH. The predominance of (CC) chemokine transcripts in idiopathic inflammatory muscle diseases. *Proc Assoc Am Physicians* 1997;109:275–285.
11. Confalonieri P, Bernasconi P, Cornelio F, Mangegazza R. Transforming growth factor-1 in polymyositis and dermatomyositis correlates with fibrosis but not with mononuclear cell infiltrate. *J Neuropathol Exp Neurol* 1997;56:479–484.
12. Tews DS, Goebel HH. Cytokine expression profile in idiopathic inflammatory myopathies. *J Neuropathol Exp Neurol* 1996;55:342–347.
13. Lundberg IE, Nyberg P.New developments in the role of cytokines and chemokines in inflammatory myopathies. *Curr Opin Rheum* 1998;10:521–529.
14. Belec L, Authier F-J, Chazaud B, Piedouillet C, Barlovatz-Meimon G, Gherardi RK. Interleukin (IL)-1b and IL-1b expression in normal and diseased skeletal muscles assessed by immunocytochemistry, immunoblotting and reverse-transcriptase-nested polymerase chain reaction. *J Neuropathol Exp Neurol* 1997;56:651–663.
15. Authier FJ, Mhir C, Chazaud B, et al. Interleukin-1 expression in inflammatory myopathies: evidence of marked immunoreactivity in sarcoid granulomas and muscle fibers showing Ischaemic an regenerative changes. *Neuropathol Appl Neurobiol* 1997;23:132–140.
16. Kuby J. *T-cell receptor*. New York: Freeman and Co., 1997.

17. Fyhr I-M, Moslemi A-R, Mosavi AA, Lindberg C, Tarkowski A, Olfors A. Oligoclonal expansion of muscle in-filtrating T cells in inclusion body myositis. *J Neuroimmunol* 1997;79:185–189.
18. O'Hanlon TP, Dalakas MC, Plotz PH, Miller FW. The alpha beta T-cell receptor repoitre in inclusion body myosi-tis: diverse patterns of gene expression by muscle infiltrating lymphocytes. *J Autoimmun* 1994;7:321–333.
19. Fyhr I-M, Moslemi A-R, Tarkowski A, Lindberg C, Oldfors A. Limited T-cell receptor V gene usage in inclusion body myositis. *Scand J Immunol* 1996;43:109–114.
20. Pluschke G, Ruegg D, Hohlfeld R, Engel AG. Autoaggressive myocytotoxic T lymphocytes expressing an un-usual gamma/delta T cell receptor. *J Exp Med* 1992;176:1785–1789.
21. Kuby J. *Cell-mediated and humoral effector responses*. New York: Freeman and Co., 1997.
22. Cherin P, Herson S, Crevon MC, et al. Mechanisms of lysis by activated cytotoxic cells expressing perforin and granzyme-B genes and the protein TIA-1 in muscle biopsies of myositis. *J Rheumatol* 1996;23:1135–1142.
23. Goebels N, Michaelis D, Engelhardt M, et al. Differential expression of perforin in muscle-infiltrating T cells in polymyositis and dermatomyositis. *J Clin Invest* 1996;97:2905–2910.
24. Behrens L, Bender A, Johnson MA, Hohlfeld R. Cytotoxic mechanisms in inflammatory myopathies: co-ex-pression of Fas and protective Bcl-2 in muscle fibers and inflammatory cells. *Brain* 1997;120:929–938.
25. Fyhr I-M, Oldfors A. Upregulation of fas/fas ligand in inclusion body myositis. *Ann Neurol* 1998;43:127–130.
26. Schneider C, Gold R, Dalakas MC, et al. MHC class I-mediated cytotoxicity does not induce apoptosis in mus-cle fibers nor in inflammatory T cells: studies in patients with polymyositis, dermatomyositis, and inclusion body myositis. *J Neuropathol Exp Neurol* 1996;55:1205–1209.
27. Arahata K, Engel AG. Monoclonal antibody analysis of mononuclear cells in myopathies. III. Immunoelectron microscopic aspects of cell-mediated muscle fiber injury. *Ann Neurol* 1986;19:112–125.
28. Askanas V, Engel WK. New advances in the understanding of sporadic inclusion-body myositis and hereditary inclusion-body myopathies. *Curr Opin Rheum* 1995;7:486–496.
29. Mendell JR, Sahenk Z, Gales T, Paul L. Amyloid filaments in inclusion body myositis. *Arch Neurol* 1991;48: 1229–1234.
30. Askanas V, Engel WK. Sporatic inclusion-body myositis and hereditary inclusion-body myositis: current con-cepts of diagnosis and pathogenesis. *Curr Opin Rheum* 1998;10:530–541.
31. Sarkozi E, Askanas V, Engel WK. Abnormal accumulation of prion protein mRNA in muscle fibers of patients with sporadic inclusion-body myositis and hereditary inclusion-body myositis. *Am J Pathol* 1994;145:1280–1284.
32. Askanas V, McFerrin J, Alvarez RB, Baque S, Engel WK. APP gene transfer into cultured human muscle induces inclusion-body myositis aspects. *Neuroreport* 1997;8:9–10.
33. Emslie-Smith AM, Engel AG. Microvascular changes in early and advanced dermatomyositis: a quantitative study. *Ann Neurol* 1990;27:343–356.
34. Kalvodouris AE. Mononuclear cells from patients with polymyositis inhibit calcium binding by sarcoplasmic reticulum. *J Lab Clin Med* 1986;107:23.
35. Newman ED, Kurland RJ. Magnetic response spectroscopy in polymyositis and dermatomyositis. Altered energy utilization during exercise. *Arthritis Rheum* 1992;35:199.
36. Park JH, Vital TZ, Ryder NM, et al. Magnetic resonance imaging and P-31 magnetic resonance spectroscopy provide unique quantitative data useful in the longitudinal management of patients with dermatomyositis. *Arthri-tis Rheum* 1994;37:736–746.
37. Chowdhury SA, Ytterberg SR, Wortmann RL. Abnormal energy metabolism in murine polymyositis. *Arthritis Rheum* 1989;32:S125.
38. Chariot P, Ruet E, Authier F-J, Labes D, Poron F, Gherardi R. Cytochrome *c* oxidase deficiencies in the muscle of patients with inflammatory myopathies. *Acta Neuropathol* 1996;91:530–536.
39. Campos Y, Arenas J, Cabello A, Gomez-Reino JJ. Respiratory chain enzyme defects in patients with idiopathic inflammatory myopathy. *Ann Rheum Dis* 1995;54:491–493.
40. Schroder JM, Molnar M. Mitochondrial abnormalities and peripheral neuropathy in inflammatory myopathy, es-pecially inclusion body myositis. *Mol Cell Biochem* 1997;174:277–281.
41. Moslemi A-R, Lindberg C, Oldfors A. Analysis of multiple mitochondrial DNA deletions in inclusion body myositis. *Hum Mutat* 1997;10:381–386.
42. Plotz PH, Rider LG, Targoff IN, et al. Myositis: immunologic contributions to understanding cause, pathogene-sis, and therapy. *Ann Intern Med* 1995;122:715–724.
43. Walker EJ, Jeffrey PD. Polymyositis and molecular mimicry, a mechanism of autoimmunity. *Lancet* 1986;2: 605–607.
44. Martin A, Shulman MJ, Tsui FWL. Epitope studies indicate that histidyl-tRNA synthetase is a stimulating anti-gen in idiopathic myositis. *FASEB J* 1995;9:1226–1233.
45. Blechynden LM, Lawson MA, Tabarias H, et al. Myositis induced by naked DNA immunization with the gene for histidyl-tRNA synthetase. *Hum Gene Ther* 1997;8:1469–1480.
46. Garlepp MJ. Genetics of the idiopathic inflammatory myopathies. *Curr Opin Rheum* 1996;8:514–520.
47. Kaneoka H, Hsu K-C, Takeda Y, Sharp GC, Hoffman RW. Molecular genetic analysis of HLA-DR and HLA-DQ genes among anti-U1-70-kd autoantibody positive connective tissue disease patients. *Arthritis Rheum* 1992;35: 83–94.
48. Arnett FC, Targoff IN, Mimori T, Goldstein R, Warner NB, Reveille JD. Interrelationship of major histocompat-ibility complex class II alleles and autoantibodies in four ethnic groups with various forms of myositis. *Arthri-tis Rheum* 1996;39:1507–1518.

49. Love LA, Leff RL, Fraser DD, et al. A new approach to the classification of idiopathic inflammatory myopathy: myositis-specific autoantibodies define useful homogeneous patient groups. *Medicine* 1991;70:360–374.
50. Oddis CV, Okano Y, Rudert WA, Trucco M, Duquesnoy RJ, Medsger TA. Serum autoantibody to the nucleolar antigen Pm-Scl. *Arthritis Rheum* 1992;35:1211–1217.
51. Leff RL, Burgess SH, Miller FW, et al. Distinct seasonal patterns in the onset of adult idiopathic inflammatory myopathy in patients with anti-Jo-1 and anti-signal recognition particle autoantibodies. *Arthritis Rheum* 1991;34: 1391–1396.
52. Crennan JM, Van Scoy RE, McKenna CH, et al. Echovirus polymyositis in patients with hypogammaglobuline-mia: failure of high dose intravenous gamma-globulin therapy and review of the literature. *Am J Med* 1986;81: 35–42.
53. Jenkins EA, Hull RG, Thomas AL. D-Penicillamine and polymyositis: the significance of the anti-Jo-1 antibody. *Br Soc Rheum* 1993;32:1109–1110.
54. Taneja V, Mehra N, Singh YN, Kumar A, Malaviya A, Singh RR. HLA-D region genes and susceptibility to D-pencillamine-induced myositis. *Arthritis Rheum* 1990;33:1445–1447.
55. Travers RL, Hughes GR, Sewall JR. Coxsackie B neutralization titers in polymyositis/dermatomyositis. *Lancet* 1977;1:1268.
56. Yousef GE, Bell EJ, Mann GF, et al. Chronic enterovirus infection in patients with postviral fatigue syndrome. *Lancet* 1988;1:146–150.
57. Schiraldi O, Iandolo E. Polymyositis accompanying coxsackie virus B2 infection. *Infection* 1978;6:32–34.
58. Leff RL, Love LA, Miller FW, et al. Viruses in idiopathic inflammatory myopathies: absence of candidate viral genomes in muscle. *Lancet* 1992;339:1192–1195.
59. Jongen PJH, Zoll GJ, Beaumont M, Melchers WJG, van de Putte LBA, Galama JMD. Polymyositis and dermatomyositis: no persistence of enterovirus or encephalomyocarditis virus RNA in muscle. *Ann Rheum Dis* 1993;52:575–578.
60. Fox SA, Finklestone E, Robbins PD, Mastaglia FL, Swanson NR. Search for persistent enterovirus infection of muscle in inflammatory myopathies. *J Neurol Sci* 1994;125:70–76.
61. Yousef GE, Isenberg DA, Mowbray JF. Detection of enterovirus specific RNA sequences in muscle biopsy specimens from patients with adult onset myositis. *Ann Rheum Dis* 1990;49:310–315.
62. Pallansch MA. Epidemiology of group B coxsackieviruses. In: Bendinelli M, Friedman H, eds. *Coxsackieviruses: a general update*. New York: Plenum, 1988:399–417.
63. Tam PE, Schmidt AM, Ytterberg SR, Messner RP. Viral persistence during the developmental phase of coxsackievirus B1-induced murine polymyositis. *J Virol* 1991;65:6654–6660.
64. Ytterberg SR, Mahowald ML, Messner RP. Coxsackievirus B1-induced polymyositis. Lack of disease expression in nu/nu mice. *J Clin Invest* 1987;80:499–506.
65. Ytterberg SR, Mahowald ML, Messner RP. T cells are required for coxsackievirus B1 induced murine polymyositis. *J Rheumatol* 1988;15:475–478.
66. Tam PE, Messner RM. Genetic determinants of susceptibility to coxsackievirus B1-induced chronic inflammatory myopathy: effect of host background and major histocompatibility complex genes. *J Lab Clin Med* 1996;128:279–289.
67. Strongwater SL, Dorovini-Zis K, Ball RD, Schnitzer TJ. A murine model of polymyositis induced by coxsackievirus B1 (Tucson strain). *Arthritis Rheum* 1984;27:433–442.
68. Tam PE, Schmidt AM, Ytterberg SR, Messner RP. Duration of virus persistence and its relationship to inflammation during the chronic phase of coxsackievirus B1-induced murine polymyositis. *J Lab Clin Med* 1994;123:346–356.
69. Cronin ME, Love LA, Miller FW, et.al. The natural history of encephalomyocarditis virus-induced myositis and myocarditis in mice. Viral persistence demonstrated by in situ hybridization. *J Exp Med* 1988;168:1639–1648.
70. Lodge PA, Herzum M, Olszewski J, Huber SA. Coxsackievirus B-3 myocarditis. Acute and chronic forms of the disease caused by different immunopathogenic mechanisms. *Am J Pathol* 1987;128:455–463.
71. Gauntt CJ, Higdon AL, Arizpe HM, et al. Epitopes shared between coxsackievirus B3 (CVB3) and normal heart tissue contribute to CVB3-induced murine myocarditis. *Clin Immunol Immunopathol* 1993;68:129–134.
72. Neu N, Craig SW, Rose NR, Alvarez F, Beisel KW. Coxsackievirus induced myocarditis in mice: cardiac myosin autoantibodies do not cross-react with the virus. *Clin Exp Immunol* 1987;69:566–574.
73. Wolfgram LJ, Beisel KW, Rose NR. Heart-specific autoantibodies following murine coxsackievirus B3 myocarditis. J Exp Med 1985;161:1112–1121.

*Diseases of Skeletal Muscle,*
edited by Robert L. Wortmann.
Lippincott Williams & Wilkins, Philadelphia © 2000

# 7

# Infections of Muscle

### Ronald P. Messner

*Department of Medicine, Fairview—University of Minnesota Hospital and Clinics and
University of Minnesota Medical School, Minneapolis, Minnesota 55455*

Infectious myositis represents the largest subset of inflammatory myopathies of known cause. Infection of muscle can occur with a variety of organisms and clinical presentations. Muscle pain, muscle tenderness, and fever are frequently present but are not universal. Appropriate diagnosis and treatment require a reasonable index of suspicion and knowledge of these different clinical patterns.

## BACTERIAL INFECTIONS

### Invasive Streptococcal Infections of Muscle

Invasive streptococcal infections (Table 1) have been on the rise in the past decade. Most involve group A streptococci, but group G streptococci have also been identified as a cause of this syndrome (1). The course of these infections may be rapid and very destructive. The dramatic course of some patients has led the lay press to describe them as "flesh-eating bacteria." Three major types of infection have been described: necrotizing fasciitis, myositis, and the streptococcal toxic shock syndrome, which may complicate either of the first two (2). In myositis, the infection spreads rapidly and diffusely through the muscle, causing edema and necrosis. These patients are clearly different form those with pyomyositis, who are characterized by local abscess formation in muscle. Toxins produced by group A streptococci are thought to be responsible for the invasive nature of this process. The surface M protein plays a role in decreasing phagocytosis of the bacteria, whereas streptococcal pyrogenic exotoxins are capable of producing the toxic shock syndrome. Acting as superantigens, they cross-link the T-cell receptor of the lymphocyte with the major histocompatibility molecule of antigen-presenting cells through attachment to the Vβ region of the T-cell receptor. This attachment bypasses the antigen-specific stimulation of a T cell and provides stimulation to as many as 40% of the T cells in the area, a

**TABLE 1.** *Typical clinical presentations of bacterial infections of muscle*

| Infection | Clinical findings |
|---|---|
| Invasive streptococci | Acute localized muscle pain, swelling, and tenderness with fever and bullous skin lesions |
| Pyomyositis | Tropical areas: young men with localized subacute muscle swelling and pain<br>Temperate areas: young and old immunocompromised men with localized subacute muscle swelling and pain |
| Tuberculosis | Slowly progressive single or multiple firm masses in muscle |

number both qualitatively and quantitatively different from the 0.01% of T cells activated through the conventional antigen-driven process. The outpouring of cytokines that results initiates toxic shock syndrome with fever, hypotension, and tissue injury (2).

Fortunately, myositis caused by these bacteria is rare but is deadly when it occurs, with a mortality rate of 80% to 100% compared with about 20% in necrotizing fasciitis. The infection may strike at any age. Males and females are equally affected, and there are no recognized specific predisposing factors. As in all invasive streptococcal infections, the source of the initial infection is found in only about half the patients. The primary symptom is pain in the affected muscle, which is rapidly followed by swelling, marked tenderness, fever, erythema over the area, and often a compartment syndrome. Bullae may also appear in the skin in the involved areas. The advent of associated toxic shock is heralded by hypotension and systemic signs of the adult respiratory distress syndrome, renal impairment, disseminated intravascular coagulation, or a macular rash that may desquamate. It is difficult to distinguish myositis from necrotizing fasciitis on clinical grounds. Involvement of muscle can be identified during surgical exploration and may also be seen on magnetic resonance imaging, the preferred modality for imaging soft tissue infections of the extremities (3). Treatment requires antibiotics and early surgery. Intravenous immunoglobulin is indicated if the streptococcal toxic shock syndrome is present. Experimental studies in animals has suggested that clindamycin is the antibiotic of choice, with erythromycin a good second choice (4). Although no solid data document its superiority, the acute and life-threatening nature of the situation has led to the use of a combination of antibiotics such as clindamycin and penicillin (2). Surgical drainage is key to survival and is best done early, before multisystem failure and spread of the infection to areas where debridement is more difficult.

## Pyomyositis

Pyomyositis is an entity characterized by the formation of abscesses in skeletal muscle. It was originally described in tropical areas of the world, including Africa, South America, the South Pacific, and the Caribbean, where it typically occurs in boys and young men (5). In this setting the lower limbs and pelvis are the most frequently effected sites, followed by the shoulder. *Staphylococcus aureus* is the infecting organism in over 90% of cases. The disease begins with cramping in the involved muscles and is followed by worsening pain, edema, and low-grade fever. Multiple sites occur in about 40% of cases and are usually asymmetric in location. Physical examination reveals a firm, hard, rubber-like induration in the affected muscle. Mild leukocytosis and eosinophilia may be present, but overt signs of inflammation are minimal. In this stage, termed the invasive stage, needle aspiration of the muscle does not yield pus. Two to 3 weeks after symptoms begin, the patient enters the suppurative stage with increasing signs of inflammation, including tenderness in the muscle, fever and leukocytosis, and pus on needle aspirate of the mass in the muscle. Positive blood cultures are rare. Most patients present to the physician at this stage. If the disease continues untreated, systemic signs of infection become prominent, with high fever, toxicity, and massive destruction of muscle. The abscesses seldom drain spontaneously due to their subfascial location. Septicemia with metastatic spread of the infection to the heart or pleura may occur in the late stage.

In temperate climates, including North America, pyomyositis has a somewhat different profile (6,7). The age range of patients is extended, with bimodal peaks at ages 20 to 40 and age 60. The male predominance is maintained, but the presence of underlying conditions is quite different. Although a significant number of patients in the tropics have coexistent parasitic infections, in temperate areas this association is rare. Instead, two thirds have an underlying human immunodeficiency virus (HIV) infection, diabetes, hemopoietic disorder, or other condition that results in immunosuppression (6). HIV infection is more common in younger patients, whereas diabetes and hematopoietic disorders occur more frequently in the older group. *S. aureus* still accounts for most cases, but other organisms may be involved. *Streptococcus* species are next most common, but a variety of gram-positive and gram-negative organisms has been reported. Accordingly, it is essential to obtain cultures from the abscesses to choose the appropriate antibiotic regimen.

Prompt diagnosis of pyomyositis requires a high index of suspicion because the disease can mimic other conditions and is frequently missed until treatment fails and further diagnostic tests are performed. Abscess in the calf can mimic deep vein thrombosis (8), in the paraspinal muscles presents with low back pain (9), and in the obturator muscle can cause sciatica (10). Routine laboratory tests are only moderately helpful. The erythrocyte sedimentation rate is usually elevated. Blood cultures are positive in about one third of the cases. Eosinophilia is rare, and muscle enzyme levels are usually normal. Magnetic resonance imaging provides the most sensitive technique to identify early pyomyositis, but computed tomography or ultrasonography can be useful, especially to guide needle aspiration to obtain material for culture. Patients diagnosed in the infiltrative stage may be successfully treated with intravenous antibiotics alone, but patients with abscess formation require percutaneous needle or, more commonly, surgical drainage (6,11).

## Tuberculosis

Infection of muscle with *Mycobacterium tuberculosis* is very rare and is estimated to occur in less than 0.02% of cases of tuberculosis. Muscle can become involved through extension from an adjacent focus such as bone or lymph node or less commonly through hematogenous spread. Tuberculous myopathy usually involves the extremities and evolves slowly over months to years. Typically, the muscle is swollen with a firm mildly tender mass that may on occasion be quite large. Multiple masses and involvement of multiple muscles may occur. Histologically, caseation is often present and cold abscesses may form. Less commonly, an inflammatory myositis with more diffuse interstitial granulation tissue or a reaction characterized by fibrosis and sclerosis may dominate the histologic picture (12). In one patient with dermatomyositis secondary to carcinoma, treatment with corticosteroids resulted in the hematogenous spread of coexistent pulmonary tuberculosis. The infection spread almost exclusively to muscle, with resulting muscle pain and recurrence of weakness. At autopsy, widespread muscle fiber degeneration and necrosis with a heavy macrophage infiltrate and many intracellular acid fast-bacilli were seen (13). Patients who are immunosuppressed, particularly those with acquired immunodeficiency syndrome (AIDS), may be more susceptible to tuberculous myopathy (14).

## PROTOZOAN INFECTIONS

### Toxoplasmosis

*Toxoplasma gondii* is a protozoan parasite that infects dogs, cats, cattle, sheep, and goats worldwide. It is transmitted to humans primarily through ingestion of cysts containing the organism in undercooked meat. Less commonly, it may be acquired through feces of the feline family or deer. In cats, *T. gondii* can form oocysts that mature after excretion from the animal to form sporozoites that contaminate soil, plants, and the hands of those touching contaminated material. When the sporozoite or the cyst containing bradyzoites from infected meat enters the intestine, it infects the gastrointestinal tract and multiplies. The resulting tachyzoites may infect leukocytes that disseminate throughout the body. Tachyzoites may infect any nucleated cell and many end up in skeletal muscle, causing cell lysis as they multiply. As the immune response matures, most tachyzoites are eliminated, but small numbers persist in muscle for years as bradyzoites in cysts. They may become reactivated if the host becomes immunosuppressed.

Most infections (Table 2) in immunocompetent humans are asymptomatic. Symptomatic infections usually present with lymphadenopathy and fatigue. Myalgia, fever, and headache may also be present. The disease is usually self-limited. More severe cases may involve the myocardium, liver, brain, lung, skin, and eye. In a small percentage of patients, myalgia and muscle stiffness are the primary symptom and may mimic idiopathic inflammatory myopathy. Muscle weakness may be profound, with creatine kinase levels 10 to 15 times normal and a myopathic pattern on electromyography. The use of steroids may cause transient improvement and further confuse the diagnosis (15). Diagnosis depends on demonstration of specific anti-toxoplasma antibodies using indirect hemagglutination or sandwich ELISA tests and demonstration of toxoplasma organisms in muscle biopsy tissue. Treatment is based on the severity of the symptoms and signs. Sulfadiazine and pyrimethamine act synergistically against reproducing tachyzoites. They do not, however, eliminate the parasites in cysts in the tissue. The addition of spiramycin is recommended when treating pregnant patients. In immunocompromised patients, especially those with AIDS, several other drugs have been used in combination with pyrimethamine, including clindamycin, azithromycin, clarithromycin, and atovaquone (16).

Histologic examination of muscle reveals inflammation in the perimysium and endomysium with aggregates of lymphocytes, histocytes, and an occasional giant cell (17). In patients with acute disease, tachyzoites may be seen in groups in intracellular vacuoles with Wright and Giemsa stain. Solitary tachyzoites are best seen with immunofluorescent or immunohistologic methods. Cysts containing thousands of bradyzoites that form later in the disease are between 10 and 200 μm in diameter. They are often found in areas of inflammation and are more easily recognized using the periodic acid–Schiff stain.

An association between toxoplasma and idiopathic inflammatory myopathy has been reported based on serologic evidence and case reports. In one study of 69 patients, those with polymyositis but not dermatomyositis were found to have higher frequency and titers with the Sabin-Feldman dye test than matched control subjects (18). Another study

**TABLE 2.** *Typical clinical presentations of parasitic and fungal infections of muscle*

| Infection | Clinical findings |
| --- | --- |
| Toxoplasmosis | Myalgia, muscle stiffness, and weakness; may mimic idiopathic inflammatory myopathy |
| Sarcocystis | Localized muscle pain, swelling, and weakness with eosinophilia |
| Microsporidia | Muscle pain, weakness, and fever in an immunocompromised patient |
| Trichinosis | Myalgia, periorbital edema, fever, and eosinophilia; may mimic idiopathic inflammatory myopathy |
| Toxocariasis | Myalgia and eosinophilia in a patient with pulmonary, CNS, and eye signs |
| Cysticerosis | Pseudohypertrophic myopathy with neurologic signs |
| Echinococcosis | Nontender tumor mass in muscle with liver and/or lung abnormalities |
| Fungal infections | Muscle pain and tenderness associated with fever and rash in an immunocompromised patient |

CNS, central nervous system.

found Sabin-Feldman dye tests were positive in half of 58 patients with polymyositis and dermatomyositis. Elevated IgM titers to toxoplasma occurred in one third of patients with polymyositis and one fifth of those with dermatomyositis compared with 0% to 3% in control subjects, suggesting active infection (19). A dozen patients with the diagnosis of both toxoplasmosis and idiopathic inflammatory myopathy have been reported in the English literature (20). Eight of these had skin rashes suggesting dermatomyositis. The diagnosis of toxoplasmosis was made on serologic tests in all, but only half had IgM antibodies and half had histologic confirmation of organisms in muscle. The response to therapy for toxoplasmosis was dramatic in only one case. Overall, it is difficult to determine whether toxoplasma infection was the cause of the inflammatory myositis, was reactivated by treatment or immunosuppressive effects of a coexistent idiopathic inflammatory myositis, or was an incidental finding in these patients.

## Sarcocystis

These organisms are parasitic protozoa related to *Toxoplasma* and are rare pathogens in humans. Infection, if and when it occurs, is usually asymptomatic. When it is symptomatic, it often presents with myositis (Table 2). These organisms infect birds, reptiles, and mammals and have an obligatory two-host life cycle. When infected muscle is ingested, sarcocysts increase by sexual reproduction in the intestine. Sporocysts are produced, excreted in the feces of the predator, and eaten by the prey species. In the prey species, the sporozoites penetrate the intestine and spread to multiply asexually in the endothelial cells of small blood vessels in many tissues where they again form sarcocysts. Striated muscle, kidney, and brain are most common tissues for sarcocyst formation. It is unclear whether humans play the role of the predator or prey species in this cycle. It is likely that they can fulfill both roles by eating either contaminated meat or vegetable matter.

Symptoms occur in humans when food contaminated by sporocysts is eaten and an infection typical of that seen in the prey species develops. Myalgia, localized pain, and swelling in muscle associated with weakness are common presentations. Low-grade fever, bronchospasm, eosinophilia, and elevation of muscle enzymes are also found (21,22). Diagnosis is made by muscle biopsy showing the cysts surrounded by an eosinophilic wall containing numerous spherical basophilic structures. The cysts are usually not accompanied by an inflammatory reaction. In chronic cases, however, they may have surrounding lymphocytes, histiocytes, and eosinophils (23). Sporocysts are sparse in the stool and require concentration for identification. There is no truly effective treatment for sarcocystis infection, but sulfonamide and pyrimethamine may be helpful.

## Microsporidia

This parasite is a very small unicellular protozoa that forms spores. It can infect most mammals, but human infection almost always occurs in immunocompromised individuals. Most human cases have been reported in HIV-positive patients. The organisms enter the host through the gastrointestinal tract or cut in the skin. The clinical picture varies according to the genus of microsporidia involved. *Encephalitazoon (E.bieneusi)* invades the small bowel, gallbladder, and nasal mucosa and is one of the most common enteric infections in AIDS patients. *E. intestinalis* and *E. hellum* are associated with disseminated infection, whereas *E. cuniculi* causes hepatitis, peritonitis, and nephritis (24).

Several patients have been described who presented with prominent muscle complaints. Fever, muscle weakness, and severe muscle pain were associated with elevated muscle enzymes in the blood. These patients were infected with *Pleistophora*, a genus found in cold-blooded vertebrates, or in one case with a new genus *Trachipleistophora* (*T. hominis*). In this case, discrete lesions were found in muscle with central degeneration of myofibers surrounded by fibers of normal size containing multiple polygonal vesicles each containing about 32 spores. Close to the center of the lesion, myofibers were packed with vesicles. In addition to muscle biopsy, microsporidia are hard to find in stool. Stained smears of the stool or concentrated urine may reveal the parasite, but assay by polymerase chain reaction (PCR) assay is much more sensitive (25). Intestinal biopsy with special stains may also reveal the organism. Treatment with albendazole, sulfadiazine, pyrimethamine, and folinic acid has been effective (24).

## NEMATODE INFECTIONS

### Trichinosis

*Trichinella* are capable of infecting over 100 different species of mammals and are found in all parts of the world except Australia and some Pacific islands. Human infection is usually acquired from eating uncooked domestic pork but may also be acquired from uncooked wild animals, including boar, and even marine mammals. Rarely, the meat of herbivores may be infected through contamination of their feed. Skeletal muscle plays a crucial role in the *Trichinella* life cycle. They are viviparous worms that complete a sexual cycle in a single host but require a second host to initiate another cycle. After ingestion of uncooked meat containing cysts, the cyst capsule is broken down by acid and pepsin and the larvae released. They lodge in the intestine where in a few hours they mature sexually and mate. A female worm may produce 1,000 to 50,000 larvae between the time when production begins 4 to 5 days after ingestion of the cyst until the adult worm is eliminated from the intestine weeks later. The new larvae penetrate through the intestine and travel through the mesenteric vessels and lymphatics to the heart, lungs, and other tissues. Most cause a transient infection and die; only those that reach the skeletal muscle find a compatible environment to form cysts in which they may persist in a viable state for years waiting for their current host to be eaten by another mammal so they can repeat the process (26).

Many infections are asymptomatic, but when symptoms occur they follow the progress of the larvae, beginning in the intestine with diarrhea, abdominal pain, and occasionally vomiting or constipation. This is followed by fever, myalgia, and periorbital and facial edema in almost all cases that develop symptoms. Muscle pain is most intense two to three weeks after infection. The migrating larvae prefer active muscle groups and frequently infect the tongue, diaphragm, and intercostal muscles. Muscles of the back and proximal limbs are also commonly involved. The clinical presentation can mimic polymyositis with myalgia, muscle tenderness, and weakness, which may be profound (27). An erythematous rash closely resembling that seen in dermatomyositis may appear. Myocarditis and heart failure may signal movement of the larvae through the heart, whereas cough and dyspnea may occur as larvae enter the lungs and diaphragm. The central nervous system is involved in 10% to 20% of cases, resulting in a wide variety of symptoms ranging from headache to seizures and cranial nerve palsies (28).

In the muscle, larvae penetrate muscle fibers and initiate a process in which the muscle cell is transformed into a nurse cell. The process in the muscle includes the loss of myofilaments and mitochondria, enlargement of nuclei, an increase in endoplasmic reticulum, production of a collagen capsule, and a network of surrounding blood vessels (29).

The capsule surrounding the nurse cell is made up of type IV and VI collagen synthesized by the nurse cell (30). The invaded cell survives, and the larva curled within it grows to a length of about 1 mm. The larva may remain viable inside the cell for many years. With time the host response to the nurse cell–parasite complex results in calcification of the capsule and, often, the worm itself.

Laboratory examination in the acute phase reveals leukocytosis, eosinophilia, increased IgE levels, elevation of muscle enzymes, and often hypergammaglobulinemia. Eosinophilia peaks in the third or fourth week and then slowly declines over months. Electromyography shows a myopathic picture similar to that seen in idiopathic inflammatory myopathies. The spinal fluid is usually normal but when central nervous system symptoms are present may reveal larva in up to one fourth of patients. Serum antibodies to *Trichinella* become positive at about 3 weeks after ingestion of the cysts and remain positive for several years. Biopsy of infected muscle showing encapsulated larvae will confirm the diagnosis. Treatment with mebendazole is the method of choice, with albendazole as a reasonable alternative drug. Corticosteroids may also be used to reduce acute symptoms (31).

## Cutaneous Larval Migrans

This parasite, *Ancylostoma cannium*, lives in the gut of dogs in the tropics and subtropics. Its eggs are passed in stool to the soil where they mature into larvae that are capable of penetrating the skin of humans. Children are most commonly infected. *A. cannium* cannot fully mature in humans and usually causes only a transient cutaneous infection with a red papule at the entry site and serpiginous erythematous pruritic tracks where they burrow through the epidermis. Eosinophilia is common, and occasionally Lofler's syndrome may occur. Invasion of muscle by the migrating worms is not common but may cause an inflammatory response rich in eosinophils that results in necrosis of muscle cells when it occurs.

## Toxocariasis (Visceral Larval Migrans)

*Toxocariasis cannis* and *Toxocariasis cati* are parasites of the intestines of dogs and cats. Their ova are released in the stool and remain viable in the soil for years. When ingested by humans, most frequently children, larvae penetrate the mucosa and move through the blood and lymph to the liver, lung, brain, eye, and muscle. Unable to complete their cycle in humans, they evoke an inflammatory response in the sites where they eventually come to rest.

Symptoms include fever, cough, pneumonitis, and occasionally headache, convulsions, and chorioretinitis. Eosinophilia is common. In the muscle, lymphocytes, eosinophils, histiocytes, and giant cells can be found along with muscle necrosis around the dead or dying larvae. The larvae are only 400 μm long and may be hard to find in pathologic sections of muscle biopsies. A capture ELISA test is recommended for serologic testing. Mebendazole and albendazole are both effective treatments (32).

## Dracunculiasis (Guinea Worm)

The life cycle of the Guinea worm includes humans and the *Cyclops* crustacean. It is common in Africa, the Middle East, and India. It is transmitted to humans in drinking water. Once ingested, the embryos migrate to the subcutaneous tissue, mature, and mate

(33). The males die and the female migrates into deeper tissue. When full of new embryos, the female migrates to the subcutaneous tissue of the extremities, forming a track through the connective tissue between muscles. An inflammatory reaction surrounds this track and resolves after she passes by. The worm may die on this journey, resulting in a local inflammatory reaction. Once the female reaches the subcutaneous tissue, she releases embryos, which causes a papule to form and often elicits a systemic febrile reaction. When the human host enters water, the blister breaks open and the embryos are released to infect crustaceans and restart the cycle. After release of the embryos, the adult worm may withdraw into the tissue or may protrude through the skin. Secondary infection of the exit site is relatively common. If left in the tissue, the adult worm eventually calcifies (34).

## CESTODE INFECTIONS

### Cysticercosis: *Taenia solium*

The pork tapeworm is rare in the United States but still common in many parts of the world, including Mexico and Central America, Eastern Europe, Africa, India, southeast Asia, and China. Eggs eaten by pigs release larvae that migrate to muscle and develop into cysticerci, which are thin-walled bladders containing a single infectious scolex. When a human eats uncooked contaminated pork, the scolex attaches to the wall of the gut, develops into an adult tapeworm, and releases eggs in the stool. Infected individuals contaminate their environment with the eggs. Under conditions of poor hygiene, eggs are ingested and can cause the dangerous tissue infection known as cysticercosis. Larvae emerge from the egg, penetrate the gut mucosa, enter the blood, and disseminate to various tissues. After about 2 months they complete development into a scolex. Cysticerci are primarily found in the central nervous system and skeletal muscle. In the brain they may cause a variety of symptoms, depending on their location, ranging from seizures and/or a meningoencephalitic syndrome to obstructive hydrocephalus.

Involvement of muscle is often asymptomatic but may cause myalgia, fever, and eosinophilia. These symptoms are often overshadowed by the neurologic symptoms. On rare occasions, muscle involvement may present as pseudohypertrophic myopathy with symmetric enlargement. Weakness may develop, causing confusion in light of the increased muscle bulk. This syndrome is also associated with nodules in the subcutaneous tissue and may effect the central nervous system and eye (35). When surgically incised, the bulging muscle is full of cysts. Inflammation is variable. In some cases none is found, whereas in others it occurs around the cysticerci. In some the muscle fibers themselves are inflamed. Swollen and atrophic fibers and fibrosis may be found (36). Radiologic demonstration of calcified cysts in muscle may suggest the diagnosis. The finding of eggs or proglottids in the stool confirms the presence of *T. solium* infection, and the presence of cysticerci on muscle biopsy is diagnostic. The adult worm may be eliminated from the gut with praziquantel treatment. For patients with multiple cysts, albendazole is the drug of choice (31).

### Echinococcosis

The definitive host for *Taenia echinococcus* is the dog or other carnivorous animals. In these animals the scolex attaches to the gut wall and forms the adult worm. Intermediate hosts such as humans and sheep become infected by ingestion of eggs shed by the definitive host. In the intermediate host, the hexacanth embryo is released and penetrates the intestinal mucosa after which it migrates to the liver and other organs where hydatid cysts are formed. The cycle is completed when the infected organ is ingested by a definitive host and an adult worm is again formed in the intestine and eggs are shed. The unilocular form due to *Echinococcus granulosus* is found primarily in sheep- and cattle-raising countries, including the Mediterranean, the Middle East, and Central and South America, whereas infection with *E. multilocularis* occurs in the cold areas of the northern hemisphere (37).

*E. granulosus* infection involves the liver in 50%, the lung in 10% to 40%, and other areas in 5% of patients. *E. multilocularis* is almost always found in the liver and involves the lung or brain in 5% to 10% of cases. Either type may involve muscle. The limb-girdle and paravertebral muscles are usually affected. Peripheral muscles are spared. Symptoms are due to expansion of the cysts. They present as a nontender tumor mass in the muscle, possibly associated with a dull ache in the area. The cysts may calcify and may be easily seen on radiographs. Serodiagnosis is available with purified echinococcus antigens, and PCR assays can distinguish the organism involved (37). The treatment of choice is surgical removal of the cysts. Albendazole can be used in inoperable cases and can reduce the risk of spread at surgery when started before the operation (31).

## FUNGAL INFECTIONS

Fungal infections presenting as muscle pain or weakness almost always occur in the setting of disseminated infection in an immunocompromised or granulocytopenic individual. Skin and muscle is frequently involved. A syndrome of fever, papular rash, and severe muscle pain with muscle tenderness occurs in disseminated candidiasis (38). A similar syndrome has been reported with disseminated *Scedosporium infaltum* infection (39). Pathology in these cases involves an infiltration of muscle with fungal hyphae. Muscle weakness and pain have been reported with subcutaneous lesions in disseminated *Candida bertholletiae* and with erythematous macules and palpable and nonpalpable purpura in disseminated *Fusarium proliferatum* infections (40). In both instances, hyphal infiltration of muscle is accompanied by a fungal vasculitis. Widespread infection of skeletal muscle with profound weakness can also occur in disseminated cryptococcal infection (41).

## VIRAL INFECTIONS

Typical clinical presentations of viral infections of muscle are presented in Table 3.

**TABLE 3.** *Typical clinical presentations of viral infections of muscle*

| Disorder | Clinical findings |
|---|---|
| Benign acute childhood | Transient calf pain and tiptoe walk after a URI, myositis |
| Acute viral myositis | Acute onset of muscle pain, weakness, and fever with adults myoglobinuria |
| Epidemic pleurodynia | Acute, severe, transient pleuritic lower chest or upper abdominal pain |
| Inflammatory myopathy in hypogammaglobulinemia | Slowly progressive proximal weakness in a patient with decreased gammaglobulins and signs of meningoencephalitis |
| Human immunodeficiency virus | Myalgia and proximal weakness typical of an inflammatory myopathy<br>Muscle wasting<br>Myalgia, weakness or pain with opportunistic infection, most commonly pyomyositis, tuberculosis, or microsporidia |

URI, Upper respiratory infection

## Acute Viral Myositis

### Benign Acute Childhood Myositis

This self-limited syndrome usually occurs in a small percentage of children infected during an epidemic of influenza. It is characterized by pain in the calves and occasionally the thighs. Symptoms increase with walking and often cause the child to crawl rather than walk. This syndrome follows about a week after the onset of an acute respiratory illness of fever, malaise, or rhinorrhea and lasts for about a week. The preceding respiratory illness may also include sore throat, headache, nausea, and abdominal pain. Examination of the muscles reveals tenderness to palpation and a tiptoe gait. The feet are held in plantar flexion, and dorsiflexion of the ankle causes pain. Strength is limited only by pain. The neurologic examination is normal. Muscle enzymes are mildly elevated in the serum, and rarely myoglobinuria may develop (42,43). Necrosis of scattered muscle fibers with little or no inflammatory infiltrate is seen on muscle biopsy. Viral cultures of the muscle have been negative in most cases. In the few cases that have been studied, viral particles have not been found in muscle (42). Although usually associated with influenza virus infection, this syndrome has also been reported in association with infection with other viruses, including adenovirus, coxsackievirus, parainfluenza virus, and respiratory syncytial virus. Treatment is supportive with rest, fluids, and nonaspirin analgesics.

### Acute Viral Myositis in Adults

This rare syndrome has been reported primarily in association with influenza infection. Unlike the childhood form it can be quite severe and lead to death. It is characterized by the acute onset of fever, myalgia, muscle weakness, and myoglobinuria. The muscle weakness may be proximal or diffuse. Examination reveals muscle tenderness in most patients and muscle swelling in about half. Renal failure may follow secondary to the myoglobinuria. Pulmonary congestion and cardiac dysfunction are seen in the most severe cases. Creatinine kinase reaches very high levels in the serum. Muscle biopsy reveals necrotic muscle fibers, which are found primarily in the periphery of the muscle fascicles, but few signs of inflammation (44). Death has been reported in 25% of the cases and is usually related to the cardiac, renal, or pulmonary complications. Most survivors recover completely in less than a month. A few follow a more prolonged course with recovery in several months. A similar syndrome has been reported in a few patients infected with coxsackievirus, Epstein-Barr virus, parainfluenza virus, cytomegalovirus, echovirus, herpes simplex virus, and HIV infection.

## Epidemic Pleurodynia (Bornholm Disease)

This illness is typically caused by coxsackievirus B, although some cases have been related to coxsackievirus A (45). These are single-strand RNA picornaviruses that spread through contact or waste water and cause epidemics in the spring and fall. Epidemic pleurodynia starts with an abrupt often severe pain in the lower chest and/or upper abdomen near the insertion of the diaphragm. The pain may refer to the back and shoulders. In some patients the neck and extremities are also involved. The pain increases with use of the muscles and is accentuated by breathing or coughing. The abdominal pain may mimic an acute abdomen. Some patients will have associated symptoms of aseptic meningitis, pericarditis, or orchitis. There are little data on the actual pathology, but muscle biopsies in a few patients have shown an acute inflammatory myopathy. The syndrome is self-limited with recovery in less than 10 days in most patients. Some patients may take longer to recover and complain of fatigue and myalgia for another month. There is no evidence for development of a chronic myopathy as a result of this syndrome.

## Chronic Viral Myositis

### *Enterovirus-induced Dermatomyositis-like Syndrome in Hypogammaglobulinemia*

A chronic inflammatory myopathy associated with skin changes is seen in about half of the patients with sex-linked hypogammaglobulinemia that develop echovirus infection with chronic meningoencephalitis (46). Myositis follows the onset of the meningoencephalitis by as much as several years. The weakness is slowly progressive and involves primarily proximal muscles. Myalgia is not a prominent symptom. The skin changes are quite varied. Edema, sometimes with a woody character, involving the trunk and extremities is the most common skin manifestation. Some patients have an erythematous rash that may be evanescent, whereas in others a violaceous telangiectatic rash has been noted on the extensor surfaces of the joints. The laboratory examination is typical of an inflammatory myopathy. Electromyography shows myopathic changes, and muscle enzymes are usually elevated. Muscle biopsy shows an inflammatory mononuclear infiltrate composed of lymphocytes and histiocytes that is primarily perivascular but is also described in the perimysial area. Degeneration, atrophy, and fibrosis complete the picture. Echovirus has been isolated from cerebrospinal fluid in all but one case in which coxsackievirus was found. Culture of muscle has been reported less frequently, but the same virus has been isolated from muscle and the cerebrospinal fluid in several patients.

Treatment is problematic. Corticosteroids are of no benefit. Treatment with intravenous gammaglobulin is superior to intramuscular administration, but neither can reliably reverse the process. The use of specific hyperimmune serum has met with some success as has the combined use of intravenous and intrathecal gammaglobulin. Unfortunately, about three fourths of the patients with this syndrome have died. The clear association of viral infection and chronic myositis in this syndrome sparked interest in the viral etiology of idiopathic inflammatory myopathy, but studies in patients with idiopathic myositis have as yet failed to convincingly document any association with a virus (see Chapter 6).

### *Hepatitis C Virus*

A number of reports have suggested an association between hepatitis C virus infection and polymyositis and dermatomyositis (64–66). A study of 53 patients with myositis revealed a prevalence of hepatitis C infection of 1.9% (67), a prevalence similar to the 1.4% reported for the general population in the United States (68). Further study is required to determine the relationship between this virus and myopathy.

## Human Immunodeficiency Virus

Skeletal muscle involvement in HIV infection can result from a variety of factors, which can be divided into four categories (47): HIV-associated myopathies, zidovudine (AZT) myopathy, HIV wasting syndrome, and opportunistic infections.

### HIV-associated Myopathies

HIV-associated myopathies can mimic the idiopathic inflammatory myopathy seen in HIV-negative patients. Clinical syndromes typical of polymyositis and inclusion body myositis have been described, as has a syndrome that matches acquired nemaline myopathy (47–49). An inflammatory myopathy also occurs in association with the diffuse infiltrative lymphocytosis syndrome (50). The pathology in HIV-associated inflammatory myopathy is essentially identical to that in HIV-negative inflammatory myopathy patients with the exception that CD4+ T lymphocytes are less frequent in the inflammatory infiltrate. As in the idiopathic inflammatory myopathies, activated CD8+ T cells are identified attacking muscle, CD45RO+ memory T cells are concentrated in the areas of inflammation, class I major histocompatibility complex molecules are upregulated on muscle cells, and adhesion molecules are upregulated in capillary and venular endothelial cells and on lymphocytes and monocytes at sites of inflammation (47,51). HIV does not directly infect muscle but is found occasionally in mononuclear cells in the inflammatory infiltrate (48,52). It is important to differentiate this type of inflammatory myopathy from that induced by drugs or opportunistic infections because it is responsive to treatment with corticosteroids (49).

Infection with human T-cell lymphotrophic virus type I is also associated with inflammatory myopathies that mimic idiopathic inflammatory myopathy. Clinical syndromes typical of polymyositis and inclusion body myositis have been described, as has a syndrome that combines myelopathy and polymyositis (52,53). These patients also display the virus in inflammatory cells surrounding muscle but not in myocytes.

### Zidovudine Myopathy

AZT is capable of inducing a mitochondrial myopathy that results in a syndrome clinically similar to an idiopathic inflammatory myopathy. Symptoms include proximal limb weakness and myalgia. Myopathic changes are found on electromyography, and elevated serum creatine kinase levels are increased. Symptoms generally resolve 4 to 6 weeks after discontinuation of the drug. The muscle pathology is distinctive and is characterized by ragged red fibers. Pale granular degeneration of fibers, increased neutral fat, and endomysial inflammation are typical findings (52). AZT inhibits reverse transcriptase and terminates DNA elongation when incorporated into a growing DNA strand (54). It also inhibits the mitochondrial DNA polymerase enzyme responsible for mitochondrial DNA replication. Muscles of patients with this syndrome demonstrate depletion of mitochondrial DNA, partial cytochrome $c$ oxidase deficiency, and reduced activity of respiratory chain complex II and III. Like AZT, analogues of AZT, didanosine and zalcitabine, cause cytotoxic effects in cultured muscle cells, but in patients they cause axonal myelopathy, not myopathy, suggesting that additional cofactors may play a role in producing the pathologic changes in nerve and muscle tissue (47,54).

### HIV Wasting Syndrome

A syndrome of wasting with loss of 10% or more of body weight occurs in about one fifth of all patients with AIDS and in one of four in the last 6 months of life. Weight loss is accompanied by loss of muscle mass, weakness and fatigue, and functional impairment. Early studies suggested that wasting was associated with a disproportionate loss of lean body mass compared with fat (55). In normal subjects during moderate energy restriction, loss of lean tissue varies inversely with baseline body fat. As energy balance becomes more negative, the proportion of weight lost from lean body mass increases (56). In AIDS, repeated bouts of infection episodes with rapid weight loss followed by weight gain are common. Frequently there is a downward trend in weight as recovery from each episode fails to regain the prior weight. There is also a trend to disproportionate loss of lean body mass because during refeeding, fat is replaced more rapidly than muscle (55). Wasting is associated with mortality, and death is common in AIDS when weight decreases to two thirds of normal (57).

Several factors contribute to wasting in AIDS, but the prime cause appears to be a decrease in energy intake with an increase in resting energy expenditure as an important cofactor. Reduced dietary intake may be due to depression, impaired taste, painful swallowing, nausea and vomiting, or malabsorption. Appetite suppression also occurs and may be due to the production of proinflammatory cytokines. Resting energy expenditure decreases when energy intake is reduced in normal individuals. In HIV infection, this relationship is altered. Resting energy expenditure is correlated with viral load. It is more variable than in normal subjects and is often elevated. Increases of 8% to 11% are seen, and the level may rise to 25% in AIDS and to 30% to 35% with superimposed infections. These changes are not sufficient themselves to cause wasting but are thought to contribute to the weight loss (57).

In the normal response to infection and inflammation a functional redistribution of body cell mass occurs. Protein is lost from the skeletal muscle, connective tissue, and the gut. The amino acids freed from this protein are then used for gluconeogenesis or synthesis of new protein in production of leukocytes, acute phase reactants, and tissue repair. The result is often a decrease in lean body mass and an increase in protein in other body compartments (57). The proinflammatory cytokines tumor necrosis factor-$\alpha$ and interleukin-1 appear to be involved in this redistribution of protein from muscle to other tissues. Inhibitors of these cytokines have been shown to reduce muscle protein catabolism in animal models. The mechanism through which these cytokines act is unclear as is their role in wasting in AIDS.

Hypogonadism can also contribute to wasting and loss of muscle strength in AIDS. The defect in sex hormone production may be primary or secondary to a hypothalamic defect. Replacement with anabolic preparations such as oxandrolone, oxymetholone, and nandrolone has resulted in weight gain and functional improvement in strength (57). Treatment with growth hormone has also resulted in an increase in lean body mass and body weight in patients with HIV-associated wasting (58), but the long-term effect on improvement in the quality of life of AIDS patients is not clear (59,60). Progressive resistance exercise training has been reported to be of some benefit in maintaining or improving lean body mass, muscle strength, and well-being in these patients (61).

### Opportunistic Infections

A wide variety of infections of muscle have been reported in HIV patients. Pyomyositis, usually due to *S. aureus* (62), tuberculosis, and microsporidial infections (63), are among the most common. As in any immunocompromised patient, a high index of suspicion and a timely workup, including muscle biopsy, culture, and imaging studies, are necessary to differentiate and appropriately treat these potentially reversible complications of the primary viral infection.

## MUSCLE INFECTION DUE TO SPIROCHETES

### Lyme Disease

Lyme disease typically begins with a flu-like illness and the characteristic rash of erythema migrans. In the following weeks to months, neurologic, cardiac, and musculoskeletal symptoms may occur, including both myalgia and arthritis. If left untreated, chronic arthritis, neurologic, and skin lesions may persist and progress over years. The causative organism, *Borrelia burgdorferi*, is a spirochete carried by ticks of the *Ixodes* group. These ticks feed on wild mice and deer that harbor the developing spirochetes. Acute infections are most common in temperate areas in the spring and summer.

Myalgia and generalized weakness occur in almost half of patients in the acute phase. These symptoms usually subside but in some patients may become severe and dominate the clinical picture even after conventional treatment. It is not clear that myalgia without evidence of myositis represents persistence of the spirochete. *Borrelia* are difficult to identify in tissue, but several studies have failed to identify the organisms in muscle of these patients, and only a few cases with positive tests for *B. burgdorferi* DNA have been found (69). This syndrome does not appear to respond to antibiotic therapy (70). In contrast, other patients develop clear myositis characterized by severe muscle pain. This complication is usually associated with arthritis or neurologic involvement. Gallium scan or computed tomography shows changes consistent with inflammation, and biopsy reveals infiltration of lymphocytes, plasma cells, and macrophages with atrophy of fibers in the involved area and organisms found in the site of inflammation (71). Myositis has also been noted with the diffuse fasciitis associated with peripheral eosinophilia that may occur in this disease. *B. burgdorferi* organisms have been identified by both silver stain and PCR in the superficial and deep dermis, fascia, fat, and skeletal muscle in these patients (72).

### Leptospirosis

This infection is most prevalent in the tropics. It is spread by urine from infected humans and animals. It gains entrance through cuts in the skin or mucous membranes, most often as the result of contact with contaminated water. Onset is abrupt, with headache, fever, myalgia, nausea, and vomiting. Jaundice and decreased renal function soon appear. Involvement of the eye and meninges may also occur. Invasion of muscle with moderate to severe pain occurs in about half the patients and may progress to rhabdomyolysis (73). The calf muscles are effected most often. Pectoral, back, and abdominal muscles may also be effected. Involvement of the abdominal muscles may mimic an acute abdomen. Elevation of the serum creatine kinase accompanies muscle damage. Biopsy reveals focal necrosis, regeneration, and often hemorrhage. Inflammation is scant in most cases but may be marked in patients with extensive necrosis. Identification of organisms with silver stain on muscle biopsy can suggest the diagnosis, which is confirmed by serologic testing. Muscle injury in this disease heals without scarring or fibrosis.

### Syphilis

Involvement of muscle is quite uncommon in syphilis. Rarely, patients develop gummata in muscle that presents as firm masses. A diffuse myositis associated with fibrosis of muscle tissue that presents as gradually progressive weakness can also occur (74).

# REFERENCES

1. Wagner JG, Assimacopoulos AP, Stoehr A, et al. Acute group G streptococcal myositis associated with strepto-coccal toxic shock syndrome: case report and review. *Clin Infect Dis* 1996;23:1159–1161.
2. Weiss KA, Laverdiere ML. Group A streptococcus invasive infections: a review. *Can J Surg* 1997;40:18–25.
3. Towers JD. The use of intravenous contrast in MRI of extremity infection. *Semin Ultrasound CT MR* 1997;18: 269–275.
4. Stevens DL. Invasive group A streptococcal disease. *Infect Agents Dis* 1996;5:157–166.
5. Chiedozi C. Pyomyositis: review of 205 cases in 112 patients. *Am J Surg* 1979;137:225–259.
6. Gomez-Reino JJ, Aznar JJ, Pablos JL, et al. Nontropical pyomyositis in adults. *Semin Arthritis Rheum* 1994;23: 396–405.
7. Patel SR, Olenginski TP, Perruquet JL, Harrington TM. Pyomyositis: clinical features and predisposing condi-tions. *J Rheumatol* 1997;24:1734–1738.
8. Wang KC, Fang CM, Chen WJ, et al. Pyomyositis of the calf muscles mimicking distal deep venous thrombosis: a case report. *Am J Orthop* 1997;26:358–359.
9. Cecil M, Dimar JRN. Paraspinal pyomyositis, a rare cause of severe back pain: case report and review of the lit-erature. *Am J Orthop* 1997;26:785–787.
10. Gurbani SG, Cho CT, Lee KR, Powell L. Gonococcal abscess of the obturator internal muscle: use of new diag-nostic tools may eliminate the need for surgical intervention. *Clin Infect Dis* 1995;20:1384–1386.
11. Christin L, Serosi G. Pyomyositis in North America: case reports and review. *Clin Infect Dis* 1992;15:668–677.
12. Kim JH, Wallerstein S, Thoe M, et al. Myopathy in tuberculosis: two presumptive cases and a review of the lit-erature. *Mil Med* 1997;162:221–224.
13. Davidson GS, Voorneveld CR, Krishnan N. Tuberculous infection of skeletal muscle in a case of dermato-myositis. *Muscle Nerve* 1994;17:730–732.
14. Lupatkin H, Brau N, Flomenberg P, Simberkoff MS. Tuberculous abscesses in patients with AIDS [see com-ments]. *Clin Infect Dis* 1992;14:1040–1044.
15. Montoya J, Jordan R, Lingamneni S, et al. Toxoplasmic myocarditis and polymyositis in patients with acquired toxoplasmosis diagnosed during life. *Clin Infect Dis* 1997;24:676–683.
16. Weiss LM. Toxoplasmosis. In: Rakel RE, ed. *Conn's current therapy*. Philadelphia: W.B. Saunders, 1998: 154–159.
17. Banker B. Parasitic myositis. In: Engle A, Franzini-Armstrong C, eds. *Myology*. New York: McGraw-Hill, 1994: 1438–1460.
18. Phillips P, Kassan S, Kagen L. Increased toxoplasma antibodies in idiopathic inflammatory muscle disease: a case-controlled study. *Arthritis Rheum* 1979;22:209–214.
19. Magid S, Kagen S. Serologic evidence for acute toxoplasmosis in polymyositis-dermatomyositis: increased fre-quency of specific anti-toxoplasma IgM antibodies. *Am J Med* 1983;73:313–320.
20. Ytterberg S. The relationship of infectious agents to inflammatory myositis. *Rheum Dis Clin North Am* 1994;20: 995–1015.
21. Van den Enden E, Praet M, Joos R, et al. Eosinophilic myositis resulting from sarcocystosis. *J Trop Med Hyg* 1995;98:273–276.
22. Mehrotra R, Bisht D, Singh PA, et al. Diagnosis of human sarcocystis infection from biopsies of the skeletal mus-cle. *Pathology* 1996;28:281–282.
23. Beaver P, Gadil R, Morea P. Sarcocystis in man: a review and report of five cases. *Am J Trop Med Hyg* 1979;28: 819–844.
24. Field AS, Marriott DJ, Milliken ST, et al. Myositis associated with a newly described microsporidian, *Tra-chipleistophora hominis*, in a patient with AIDS. *J Clin Microbiol* 1996;34:2803–2811.
25. Curry A. Microsporidians. In: Cox FEG, ed. *Parasitology*. London: Arnold, 1998:411–423.
26. Despommier D. Nematodes: trichurida and dioctophymatida, enoplean parasites. In: Schmidt GDAR, ed. *Foundations of parasitology*. Boston: W.C. Brown, 1995.
27. Santos Duran-Ortiz J, Garcia-de la Torre I, Orozco-Barocio G, et al. Trichinosis with severe myopathic involve-ment mimicking polymyositis. Report of a family outbreak. *J Rheumatol* 1992;19:310–312.
28. Taratuto AL, Venturiello SM. Trichinosis. *Brain Pathol* 1997;7:663–672.
29. Roberts L, Janovy J. Nematodes: trichurida and dioctophymatida, enoplean parasites. In: Schmidt GDAR, ed. *Foundations of parasitology*. Dubuque: W.C. Brown, 1996:385–403.
30. Polvere RI, Kabbash CA, Capo VA, et al. *Trichinella spiralis*: synthesis of type IV and type VI collagen during nurse cell formation. *Exp Parasitol* 1997;86:191–199.
31. Pearson RD. Intertinal parasites. In: Rakel RE, ed. *Conn's current therapy*. Philadelphia: W.B. Saunders, 1998: 535–543.
32. Despommier DD. Thichinella and toxocara. In: Cox FEG, Wakelin J, eds. *Parasitology*. London: Arnold, 1998: 597–607.
33. Muller R. Dracunculiasis. In: Cox FEG, ed. *Parasitology*. London: Arnold, 1998:661–665.
34. Markell EK, Voge M, John DT. *Medical parasitology*, 7th ed. Philadelphia: W.B. Saunders, 1992.
35. Jacob LC, Mathew NT. Pseudohypertrophic myopathy in cysticercosis. *Neurology* 1968;18:767–771.
36. Sawhney BB, Cnopra JS, Banerji AK, Wahi P. Pseudohyperthophic myopathy in cysticercosis. *Neurology* 1976; 26:270–272.

37. Taratuto AL, Venturiello SM. Echinococcosis. *Brain Pathol* 1997;7:673–679.
38. Jarowski CI, Fialk MA, Murray HW, et al. Fever, rash and muscle tenderness: a distinctive clinical presentation of disseminated candidiasis. *Arch Intern Med* 1978;138:544–546.
39. Farag SS, Firkin FC, Andrew JH, et al. Fatal disseminated *Scedosporium inflatum* infection in a neutropenic immunocompromised patient. *J Infect* 1992;25:201–204.
40. Helm TN, Longworth DL, Hall GS, et al. Case report and review of resolved fusariosis. *J Am Acad Dermatol* 1990;23:393–398.
41. Hurd DD, Staub DB, Roelofs RI, Dehner LP. Profound muscle weakness as the presenting feature of disseminated cryptococcal infection. *Rev Infect Dis* 1989;11:970–974.
42. Farrell MK, Partin JC, Bove KE, et al. Epidemic influenza myopathy in Cincinnati in 1997. *Pediatrics* 1980;96:545–551.
43. McIntyre PG, Doherty C. Acute benign myositis during childhood: report of five cases. *Clin Infect Dis* 1995;20:722.
44. Gamboa ET, Eastwood AB, Hays AP, et al. Isolation of influenza virus from muscle in myoglobinuric polymyositis. *Neurology* 1979;29:1323–1335.
45. Ikeda RM, Knodracki SF, Drabkin PD, et al. Pleurodynia among football players at a high school: an outbreak associated with coxsackievirus B1. *JAMA* 1993;270:2205–2206.
46. Crennan JM, Van Scoy RE, McKenna CH, Smith TF. Echovirus polymyositis in patients with hypogammaglobulinemia. Failure of high-dose intravenous gamma-globulin therapy and review of the literature. *Am J Med* 1986;81:35–42.
47. Chariot P, Gherardi R. Myopathy and HIV infection. *Curr Opin Rheum* 1995;7:497–502.
48. Cupler EJ, Leon-Monzon M, Miller J, et al. Inclusion body myositis in HIV-1 and HTLV-1 infected patients. *Brain* 1996;119:1887–1893.
49. Masanes F, Pedrol E, Grau JM, et al. Symptomatic myopathies in HIV-1 infected patients untreated with antiretroviral agents—a clinico-pathological study of 30 consecutive patients. *Clin Neuropathol* 1996;15:221–225.
50. Salahuddin K, Cohen PR, Williams F, et al. The diffuse infiltrative lymphocytosis syndrome: clinical and immunogenetic features in 35 patients. *AIDS* 1996;10:385–391.
51. Carota A, Pizzolato GP, Redard M, et al. Adhesion molecules in HIV-related and idiopathic polymyositis: immunohistochemical studies. *Clin Neuropathol* 1997;16:312–318.
52. Dalakas MC. Inflammatory and toxic myopathies. *Curr Opin Neurol Neurosurg* 1992;5:645–654.
53. Evans BK, Gore I, Harrell LE, et al. HTLV-I associated myelopathy and polymyositis in a US native. *Neurology* 1989;39:1572–1575.
54. Benbrik E, Chariot P, Bonavaud S, et al. Cellular and mitochondrial toxicity of zidovudine (AZT), didanosine (ddI) and zalcitabine (ddC) on cultured human muscle cells. *J Neurol Sci* 1997;149:19–25.
55. Mulligan K, Bloch AS. Energy expenditure and protein metabolism in human immunodeficiency virus infection and cancer cachexia. *Semin Oncol* 1998;25:82–91.
56. Forbes GB. Lean body mass-body fat interrelationships in humans. *Nutr Rev* 1987;45:225–231.
57. Moldawer LL, Sattler FR. Human immunodeficiency virus-associated wasting and mechanisms of cachexia associated with inflammation. *Semin Oncol* 1998;25:73–81.
58. Schambelan M, Mulligan K, Grunfeld C, et al. Recombinant human growth hormone in patients with HIV-associated wasting. *Ann Intern Med* 1996;125:873–882.
59. Windisch PA, Papatheofanis FJ, Matuszewski KA. Recombinant human growth hormone for AIDS-associated wasting. *Ann Pharmacother* 1998;32:437–445.
60. McNurlan MA, Garlic PJ, Steigbigel RT, et al. Responsiveness of muscle protein synthesis to growth hormone administration in HIV-infected individuals declines with severity of disease. *J Clin Invest* 1998;100:2125–2132.
61. Evans WJ, Roubenoff R, Shevitz A. Exercise and the treatment of wasting: aging and human immunodeficiency virus infection. *Semin Oncol* 1998;25:112–122.
62. Vassilopoulos D, Chalasani P, Jurado RL, et al. Musculoskeletal infections in patients with human immunodeficiency virus infection. *Medicine (Baltimore)* 1997;76:284–294.
63. Windsor JJ. Microsporidial infections in humans: current practice and developments in laboratory diagnosis. *Br J Biomed Sci* 1997;54:216–221.
64. Uneo Y, Kondo K, Kidokoro N, et al. Hepatitic C infection and polymyositis. *Lancet* 1995;346:319–320.
65. Weidensaul D, Iman T, Holyst M-M, et al. Polymyositis, pulmonary fibrosis, and hepatitis C. *Arthritis Rheum* 1995;38:437–439.
66. Gomez A, Solans R, Simeon CP, et al. Dermatomyositis, hepatocarcinoma, and hepatitis C: comment on article by Weidernsaul et al. [letter]. *Arthritis Rheum* 1997;40:394–395.
67. Monger RM, West SG. Inflammatory myopathy and hepatitis C virus infection. *Arthritis Rheum* 1998;41:1323–1325.
68. Shapiro CN. Epidemiology of viral hepatitis. In: *Proceedings of the American Association for the Study of Liver Diseases*. Chicago: American Association for the Study of Liver Diseases, 1994:41.
69. Frey M, Jaulhac B, Piemont Y, et al. Detection of *Borrelia burgdorferi* DNA in muscle of patients with chronic myalgia related to Lyme disease. *Am J Med* 1998;104:591–594.
70. Steere AC. Musculoskeletal manifestations of Lyme disease. *Am J Med* 1995;98:44S–48S.

71. Atlas E, Novak SN, Duray PH, Stere AC. Lyme myositis: muscle invasion by *Borrelia burgdorferi. Ann Intern Med* 1988;109:245–246.
72. Granter SR, Barnhill RL, Duray PH. Borrelial fasciitis: diffuse fasciitis and peripheral eosinophilia associated with *Borrelia* infection. *Am J Dermatopathol* 1996;18:465–473.
73. Solbrig ML, Sher LH, Kula RW. Rhabdomyolysis in leptospirosis (Weil's disease). *J Infect Dis* 1987;156:692–693.
74. Durstan JH, Jefferies FJ. Syphilitic myositis. *Br J Vener Dis* 1975;51:141.

*Diseases of Skeletal Muscle,*
edited by Robert L. Wortmann.
Lippincott Williams & Wilkins, Philadelphia © 2000

# 8

# Sarcoidosis

## David B. Hellmann

*Department of Medicine, Johns Hopkins University School of Medicine,
Baltimore, Maryland 21205*

Sarcoidosis is a multisystem granulomatous disease of unknown cause that most commonly affects young adults and can present with pulmonary symptoms, constitutional symptoms, extrathoracic inflammation, or with asymptomatic hilar adenopathy (1–6). Although relatively infrequent, skeletal muscle disease can be the initial manifestation of sarcoidosis. In patients with extrathoracic involvement, sarcoidosis can mimic other inflammatory myopathies, vasculitic syndromes, and collagen vascular diseases.

## CLINICAL PRESENTATIONS

Although the presentation of sarcoidosis can be extremely variable, most patients present in one of four ways (Table 1): with pulmonary symptoms (40% to 45%), with constitutional symptoms (20% to 30%), with inflammation at an extrathoracic site (25%), or with asymptomatic hilar adenopathy (5% to 12%) (1–3,5,6). The clinical features of sarcoid myopathy must be considered in the context of other disease manifestations.

**TABLE 1.** *Clinical features or sarcoidosis*

| Feature | Frequency (%) |
|---|---|
| Respiratory | |
|   Cough | 30 |
|   Sputum | 11 |
|   Hemoptysis | 4 |
|   Breathlessness | 28 |
|   Chest pain | 15 |
| Constitutional symptoms | |
|   Fatigue | 27 |
|   Malaise | 15 |
|   Weight loss | 28 |
|   Fever | 17 |
| Extra-thoracic inflammation | |
|   Lymphadenopathy | 73 |
|   Skin lesions | 32 |
|   Erythema nodosum | 8 |
|   Liver disease | 21 |
|   Eye disease | 21 |
|   Joint disease | 5–15 |
|   Neurologic disease | 5 |
|   Myositis (symptomatic) | 4 |

From Refs. 2 and 3, with permission.

Approximately two of three patients will eventually have pulmonary symptoms (3). Cough is the most common pulmonary symptom (Table 1) and can be mild or severe. Typically, the cough is dry as sputum production is exiguous. Hemoptysis is usually absent initially but may be recurrent, massive, and life-threatening in patients who develop mycetomas, cavitary lesions colonized with aspergillus, sometimes called fungus balls. Breathlessness varies in severity and correlates poorly with chest x-ray findings (3). More than 90% of patients have an abnormal chest radiograph.

Many patients with sarcoidosis experience constitutional symptoms (Table 1), and approximately one fourth of patients present with fever, weight loss, or malaise. The presence of fever is strongly associated with hepatic disease, manifested by hepatomegaly, elevation of the alkaline phosphatase, and hepatic granulomas (3). Peripheral lymphadenopathy is common (Table 1). Lymph nodes in sarcoidosis are usually 1 to 5 cm in size, nontender, and distributed symmetrically in the cervical, submandibular, axillary, epitrochlear, and inguinal regions (3).

Skin disease occurs in about one third of patients, and the different cutaneous manifestation help define distinct subsets of patients (2,3). Erythema nodosum, for example, affects whites more frequently than blacks and occurs early, often in association with hilar adenopathy and periarthritis (a triad known as Löfgren's syndrome). This syndrome carries an excellent prognosis with a high likelihood of complete sustained remission (2,3,6). In contrast, plaques, nodules, ulcers, and scaling lesions are associated with chronic sarcoidosis (Fig. 1) (2,3). One typical pattern of cutaneous sarcoidosis known as lupus pernio consists of violaceous plaques over the nose, cheeks, and ears. The cutaneous lesions of some patients with sarcoidosis may suggest dermatomyositis.

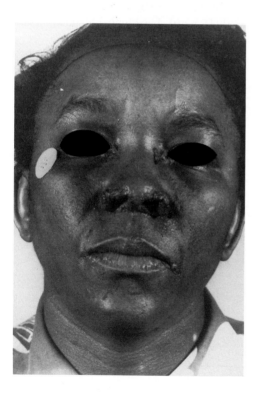

**FIG. 1.** A woman with nodular lesions in inner canthi of the eyes, on alae nasae, and around the mouth and on the lips. (From Ref. 18, with permission.)

The most common ocular manifestation of sarcoidosis is anterior uveitis, manifested by the triad of red eye, photophobia, and blurred vision (3,7). Posterior uveitis, asymptomatic conjunctional nodules, keratoconjunctivitis, and lachrymal gland enlargement may also occur (2,3). Sarcoidosis involving the nasal mucosa or nasal cartilage can produce a saddle nose deformity, thereby mimicking Wegener's granulomatosis (2,3,6). Sarcoidosis can also affect the larynx and trachea (2,6). Parotid gland enlargement from sarcoidosis mimics Sjögren's syndrome (2,3,6).

Sarcoidosis of visceral organs can have protean manifestations. Sarcoidosis of the liver results most frequently in hepatomegaly and fever (1–3). Cardiac disease most frequently presents as ventricular arrhythmia with or without cardiomyopathy (1–3). Severe pulmonary sarcoidosis can be complicated by cor pulmonale. Renal disease in sarcoidosis consists of nephrocalcinosis, renal calculus, membranous granulonephritis, and renal insufficiency (1–3,6).

Two forms of arthritis occur in sarcoidosis (4,6,8–14). The first is an acute arthritis that occurs typically within the first 6 months, often in association with erythema nodosum (Löfgren's syndrome) (4,6,9,14). This disease is more a periarthritis than a true synovitis. The acute arthritis affects a variable number of joints but typically is oligoarticular. Monarthritis is rare with the acute form. The chronic arthritis of sarcoidosis typically begins 6 months or more after the disease onset. It is usually oligoarticular but may be monarticular and may result in characteristic cystic changes of bones (4,6,9). Chronic digital sarcoid arthropathy can lead to dactylitis and is also frequently associated with overlying cutaneous lesions.

The most frequent manifestation of neurosarcoidosis is a peripheral VIIth nerve palsy, which can be bilateral (3). Other neurologic signs include basilar meningitis, seizures, central nervous system vasculitis, hydrocephalus, intracranial mass lesions, and neuroendocrine disorders such as hypopituitarism or diabetes insipidus (1–3,15,16). Peripheral nervous system manifestations include mononeuritis multiplex.

## LABORATORY FEATURES

Mild anemia is common, but hematocrits below 30% are unusual in the absence of some other cause (1–3,6). Leukopenia (WBC < 4,000/mm$^3$) occurs in approximately one fourth of patients, eosinophilia (>5% eosinophils) in a third, and hypercalcemia in a fifth (1–3,6). The erythrocyte sedimentation rate is not markedly elevated except in patients with Löfgren's syndrome. Most patients have polyclonal gammopathy and many are hyperuricemic. The serum creatinine is normal in the absence of renal disease or hypercalcemia. Pulmonary function tests are abnormal in most patients with type II or type III x-rays (Table 2) (1–3,6). A restrictive pattern is most common, but an obstructive pattern occurs in patients having extensive endobronchial disease.

**TABLE 2.** *Classification of chest x-ray findings in sarcoidosis*

| Type | Findings | Frequency (%) |
|------|----------|---------------|
| O | Normal | 10–15 |
| I | Hilar adenopathy | 50 |
| II | Hilar adenopathy plus pulmonary (alveolar, interstitial, or reticulonodular) infiltrates | 25 |
| III | Pulmonary infiltrates or fibrosis without adenopathy | 10–15 |

## DIAGNOSIS

No single finding or test result establishes the diagnosis of sarcoidosis. Rather, the diagnosis of sarcoidosis requires a compatible clinical picture, histologic evidence of non-caseating granulomas, and exclusion of other causes. The serum angiotensin-converting enzyme level, which is elevated in 60% of patients with sarcoidosis, cannot be used diagnostically because of its lack of specificity (3,6). Bronchial alveolar lavage in sarcoidosis shows a lymphocytosis with an elevated CD4/CD8 ratio, but the findings are not specific (3,6,17).

The Kveim-Siltzbach test has been performed at some centers to help support the diagnosis of sarcoidosis. The test is performed by injecting interdermally homogenized spleen or lymph node material from a patient with sarcoidosis. Biopsy of the skin site 4 to 6 weeks later demonstrated noncaseating granulomas in many patients with sarcoidosis, especially those who have lymphadenopathy. The test is not widely performed because the material has not been approved by the Food and Drug Administration and transmission of retroviral agents has been a concern (18).

## SKELETAL MUSCLE DISEASE

Sarcoid myopathy was first described in 1907 by Licharew, who presented to the Moscow Dermatological Society the case of a 17-year-old girl with focal nodular lesions in skeletal muscle (19). In 1914, Block first detailed the microscopic features of sarcoid granulomas in muscle (Fig. 2) (16). Involvement of skeletal muscles in sarcoidosis was initially thought to be rare (1,20,21). For example, Longcope and Freiman's (1) series of 160 patients from the Johns Hopkins Hospital and Massachusetts General Hospital reported in 1952 noted only a single patient with sarcoid nodules in the muscles of the forearm. However, subsequent series have noted that blind biopsy of asymptomatic muscles in patients with sarcoidosis revealed granulomas in 50% to 80% of patients (22–27). Symptomatic muscle disease has proven to be much less common, affecting only up to 2% to 3% of patients (2).

Symptomatic disease generally presents in one of three ways: chronic myositis, nodular focal myositis (as occurred in Longcope and Freiman's patient) and an acute myositis (Table 3).

Chronic myositis is by far the most common disease manifestation of sarcoidosis involving skeletal muscle. Although sarcoidosis typically is a disease of young people, chronic myositis from sarcoidosis chiefly affects postmenopausal women (28). In other clinical respects, the disease mimics polymyositis with weakness and pain most commonly affecting the proximal muscles (8,20,28,29). Involvement of pelvic girdle and thigh muscles is most common followed by the shoulder girdle and deltoid muscles (30). Involvement of the facial or bulbar muscles (30–32) or the respiratory muscles (33,34) is rare. The muscles usually appear normal upon inspection, but pseudohypertrophy has been described (21,35). Atrophy and contractures are uncommon at presentation but may develop months or years later. In the precorticosteroid era, some cases were initially diagnosed as "muscular dystrophy," but the late onset and the absence of family history help to distinguish muscle involvement with sarcoidosis (19,36,37). Distal muscle involvement has been described but perhaps erroneously, because some of these patients also have peripheral neuropathy. Approximately two thirds of the patients have active sarcoidosis in other organs, but skeletal muscle involvement may be the presenting manifestation in one third of cases (19,38).

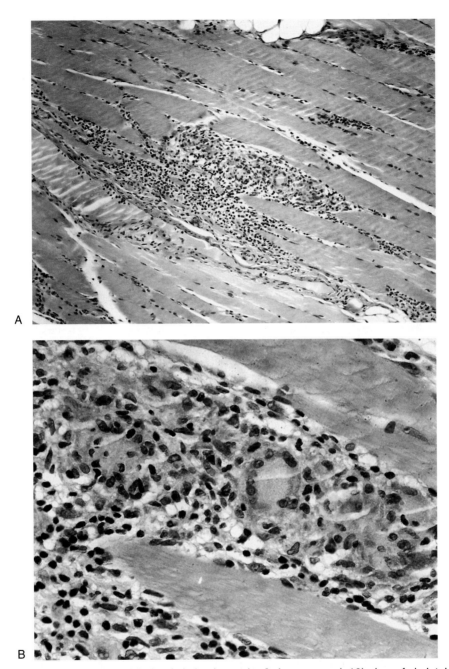

**FIG. 2.** Histology of sarcoidosis of skeletal muscle. **A:** Low-power (×10) view of skeletal muscle with scattered foci of granulomatous inflammation. **B:** High-power (×100) view of well-demarcated noncaseating granulomas with histiocytes and multinucleated giant cells. (Courtesy of Frederic Askin, M.D.)

**TABLE 3.** *Manifestations of sarcoidosis of skeletal muscles*

| Form | Prevalence |
|------|------------|
| Asymptomatic granulomas in skeletal muscle | Common prevalence (50% to 80% of cases) |
| Chronic myositis | Uncommon |
| Focal nodular myositis | Rare |
| Acute myositis | Rare |

Laboratory abnormalities in sarcoid myositis are similar to those of other inflammatory myopathies. Electromyography is usually abnormal, showing a myopathic pattern in over 90% (28). Serum creatine kinase levels are elevated in only a third (28). Muscle biopsy virtually always reveals granuloma but also shows concomitant myopathic changes. The granulomas most often occur in a perivascular distribution and are located between muscle fibers (21,28,39–41) (Fig. 2). Some biopsies show extensive destruction of fibers, presumably related to compression (28). Other specimens show widespread muscle degeneration and regeneration unassociated with nearby granuloma. Immunohistochemical studies have shown that the granuloma in muscle, as in other organs affected by sarcoidosis, consist chiefly of CD4+ T cells (23). In sarcoid myositis, granuloma and affected muscle fibers frequently express interleukin-1 (42).

Treatment with prednisone at doses of greater than 20 mg/day appears to be effective. Contractures have been reported but more frequently can be attributed to delayed rather than ineffective therapy. The optimal duration of therapy needed has not been determined. Whether the serum creatine kinase levels mirror the degree of tissue inflammation in those patients with elevated levels is not known.

Nodular myositis is the second most common form of skeletal muscle involvement in sarcoidosis (28). Typically, small tender nodules develop at musculotendinous junctions without a specific distribution pattern (40). Sometimes the nodule in the muscle results from extension of an overlying cutaneous sarcoid lesion. Affected patients usually do not have weakness, but patients may experience myalgias and cramps. Involvement of muscles of the extremities has been most common, but involvement of the diaphragm (1) or abdominal wall muscles (43) has been reported. A few patients develop contractures. Prednisone appears to be effective therapy if initiated early.

Acute myositis is the least common form of symptomatic muscle disease in sarcoidosis (26,30,37,40). The disease is characterized by the development over a few days to 2 weeks of diffuse myalgia, muscle tenderness, and proximal weakness. Acute arthritis and erythema nodosum often accompanies this presentation. In about half of the patients, myositis develops de novo. In the remainder, it appears as an exacerbation of chronic myositis. In contrast to the patients with chronic myositis, those with early acute myositis are usually less than 36 years old (28). Acute myositis can be recurrent, isolated to a single muscle or muscle group, and cause pseudohypertrophy (35).

In acute myositis, the electromyogram usually reveals changes consistent with an inflammatory myopathy (26,37). The histologic pattern of acute and chronic myositis appear identical. Although experience with treatment is limited, prednisone does appear effective. Spontaneous improvement can also occur (35).

## DIFFERENTIAL DIAGNOSIS OF MUSCLE DISEASE IN SARCOIDOSIS

Both the acute and chronic forms of sarcoid myositis can mimic polymyositis because each can cause myalgia, proximal muscle weakness, elevated serum creatine kinase levels, and myopathic patterns on electromyography. Rarely, co-occurrence of dermatomyositis or polymyositis and sarcoidosis has been reported (44–48). Predominance of CD4+ T cells infiltrating the muscle is seen not only in sarcoidosis but also in dermatomyositis. In contrast, CD8+ T cells predominate in polymyositis and inclusion body myositis (23,49). Sarcoid myositis has also been associated with other diseases, including primary biliary cirrhosis (50), scleroderma (51), inclusion body myositis (52,53), and myasthenia gravis (54).

Finding noncaseating granuloma in skeletal muscle is not specific for diagnosis of sarcoidosis (22,55). Other conditions that can cause tissue granuloma include tuberculosis, fungal infections, carcinoma, and thymoma (28). Thus, the diagnosis of sarcoidosis in skeletal muscle requires a compatible clinical presentation, characteristic histologic changes, and exclusion of other disorders (3).

## EPIDEMIOLOGY

The incidence and prevalence of sarcoidosis vary greatly among geographic regions and ethnic groups (3,56). The peak incidence occurs between the ages of 20 and 40 (3), but onset can occur as early as 7 years or as late as 74 years (2). The prevalence appears to be highest in African Americans living in the southern Atlantic states and in whites living in Scandinavian countries. The prevalence of sarcoidosis in African Americans (1 per 2,500 individuals) is eight times higher than in American whites (3,56,57). Women are affected slightly more commonly than men (3).

## PATHOGENESIS

Although the cause of sarcoidosis is unknown, several lines of evidence indicate that the host immune response plays a central role in the pathogenesis of the disease (57,58). The pathologic hallmark of sarcoidosis is noncaseating granulomatous inflammation (1–3). The granulomas consist of a central follicle of epithelial cells accompanied by multinucleated giant cells surrounded by macrophages, lymphocytes, and fibroblasts (3,39). Studies in the lung have shown that an alveolitis, comprised of activated CD4+ Th1 T cells and activated macrophages, precedes the development of granuloma (59–61). In sarcoidosis, the granulomas disseminate widely (Table 4) and can injure tissues by compressing tissues; by secreting and activating inflammatory cells that release destructive enzymes and oxygen radicals; by elaborating cytokines that produce fever, fatigue, and other constitutional symptoms; and by releasing cytokines that promote fibrosis (3,57,60). In addition, activated

**TABLE 4.** *Frequency of granulomas in different tissues*

| Tissue | Frequency (%) |
| --- | --- |
| Lungs | 86 |
| Lymph nodes | 86 |
| Liver | 86 |
| Spleen | 63 |
| Heart | 20 |
| Kidney | 19 |
| Bone marrow | 17 |
| Pancreas | 6 |
| Adrenals | <1 |

From Refs. 1–3 and 5, with permission.

macrophages within granulomas accelerate the conversion of 25-hydroxyvitamin D to 1,25-hydroxyvitamin D. The more potent 1,25-hydroxyvitamin D promotes intestinal absorption of calcium and can cause hypercalcemia (62,63).

Abnormalities of both the cellular and humeral immunity have been identified in sarcoidosis. The cellular immune response is hyperactive in tissues and hypoactive in the peripheral blood (13). Most patients with sarcoidosis have lymphopenia and a low helper to suppressor T cell ratio in peripheral blood (0.8 to 1 in patients compared with 1.8 to 1 in normal individuals) (6,61). In addition, most patients with sarcoidosis have cutaneous anergy (5,6,61). The humeral immune response, in contrast, is increased. Most patients show polyclonal hypergammaglobulinemia, and nearly a third develop autoantibodies such as a rheumatoid factor or an antinuclear antibody (5,6,61).

The clustering in certain regions and among specific ethnic groups with the occasional aggregation of cases in families implicates infection, a toxin, or genetically determined differences in the immune response as potentially important in the pathogenesis of sarcoidosis (64). That alveolar T cells are oligoclonal reinforces the argument that sarcoidosis represents an immune response to a specific, perhaps environmental trigger (64–66). Despite reports of disease in multiple family members, genetic studies have failed to identify any human leukocyte antigen hepatotypes that are consistently associated with sarcoidosis (67).

## MANAGEMENT

The treatment of sarcoidosis depends on the extent and intensity of tissue inflammation (3,6). Some patients, such as those with asymptomatic hilar adenopathy, require no treatment. Patients with Löfgren's syndrome frequently respond to nonsteroidal anti-inflammatory drugs or low-dose prednisone (less than 20 mg/day) (3). Acute arthritis may respond to colchicine or nonsteroidal agents. Skin disease other than erythema nodosum responds to chloroquine or intralesional injections of corticosteroids (3,6,68–71).

Prednisone is the mainstay of treatment for patients with severe involvement of internal organs, such as the lung, brain, heart, or skeletal muscle (3,6). Some have advocated initiating treatment with 40 mg/day and dividing doses, if necessary, to control fever (3). Subsequently, the prednisone dose is reduced by 5 mg every 2 weeks until 15 mg/day is reached (3). If objective improvement does occur, the dose is continued for 6 to 8 additional months before attempting a further slow taper (3). Methotrexate at doses of 10 mg/week has been effective in patients with pulmonary sarcoidosis who cannot tolerate prednisone (72–74). The value of methotrexate in treating sarcoidosis of skeletal muscle has not been systematically evaluated. Use of cyclosporine in patients with sarcoid myositis has not been studied, but this agent has produced contradictory results in patients with pulmonary sarcoidosis (75).

## REFERENCES

1. Longcope WT, Freiman DG. A study of sarcoidosis: based on a combined investigation of 160 cases including 30 autopsies from the Johns Hopkins Hospital and Massachusetts General Hospital. *Medicine* 1952;31:1–132.
2. Mayock RL, Bertrand P, Morrison CE, Scott JH. Manifestations of sarcoidosis: analysis of 145 patients, with a review of nine series selected from the literature. *Am J Med* 1963;35:67–89.
3. Bascom RA, Johns CJ. The natural history and management of sarcoidosis. In: Stollerman GH, ed. *Advances in internal medicine*. Vol. 31. Chicago: Yearbook Medical Publishers, 1986:213–241.
4. Kaplan H. Sarcoid arthritis: a review. *Arch Intern Med* 1963;112:924–935.

5. Stobo JD, Hellmann DB. Sarcoidosis. In: Cohen AS, Bennet JD, eds. *Rheumatology and immunology*, 2nd ed. Orlando, FL: Grune and Stratton, 1986:301–309.
6. Hellmann DB. Sarcoidosis. In: Klippel JH, Weyand CM, Wortmann RL, eds. *Primer on the rheumatic diseases*, 11th ed. Arthritis Foundation, Atlanta 1997:325–327.
7. Jabs DA, Johns CJ. Ocular involvement in chronic sarcoidosis. *Am J Ophthalmol* 1986;102:297–301.
8. Myers GB, Gottlieb AM, Mattman PE, et al. Joint and skeletal muscle manifestations in sarcoidosis. *Am J Med* 1952;12:161–169.
9. Gumpel JM, Johns CJ, Shulman LE. The joint disease of sarcoidosis. *Ann Rheum Dis* 1967;26:194–205.
10. Spilberg I, Siltzbach LE, McEwen C. The arthritis of sarcoidosis. *Arthritis Rheum* 1969;12:126–137.
11. Shaw RA, Holt PA, Stevens MB. Heel pain in sarcoidosis. *Ann Intern Med* 1988;15:675–677.
12. Palmer DG, Schumacher HR. Synovitis with non-specific histological changes in synovium in chronic sarcoidosis. *Ann Rheum Dis* 1984;43:778–782.
13. Glennas A, Kvien TK, Melby K, et al. Acute sarcoid arthritis: occurrence, seasonal onset, clinical features and outcome. *Br J Rheumatol* 1995;34:45–50.
14. Kellner H, Späthling S, Herzer P. Ultrasound findings in Löfgren's syndrome: is ankle swelling caused by arthritis, tenosynovitis or periarthritis? *J Rheumatol* 1992;19:38–41.
15. Stern BJ, Krumholz A, Johns C, et al. Sarcoidosis and its neurological manifestations. *Arch Neurol* 1985;42:909–917.
16. Chapelon C, Ziza JM, Piette JC, et al. Neurosarcoidosis: signs, course and treatment of 35 confirmed cases. *Medicine* 1990;69:261–276.
17. Nagai S, Izumi T. Bronchoalveolar lavage. Still useful in diagnosing sarcoidosis? *Clin Chest Med* 1987;18:787–797.
18. Johns CJ, Michele T. The clinical management of sarcoidosis: a 50-year experience at the Johns Hopkins Hospital. *Medicine* 1999;78:65–111.
19. Harvey JC. A myopathy of Boeck's sarcoid. *Am J Med* 1959;27:356–363.
20. Silverstein A, Siltzbach LE. Muscle involvement in sarcoidosis. *Arch Neurol* 1969;21:235–241.
21. Douglas AC, Macleod JG, Matthews JD. Symptomatics arcoidosis of skeletal muscle. *J Neurol Neurosurg Psychiatry* 1973;36:1034–1040.
22. Hunninghake GW, Gilbert S, Pueringer R, et al. Outcome of the treatment for sarcoidosis. *Am J Respir Crit Care Med* 1994;149:893–898.
23. Takanashi T, Suzuki Y, Yoshino Y, Nonaka I. Granulomatous myositis: pathologic re-evaluation by immunohistochemical analysis of infiltrating mononuclear cells. *J Neurol Sci* 1997;145:41–47.
24. Uddenfeldt P, Bjelle A, Olsson T, et al. Musculo-skeletal symptoms in early sarcoidosis. Twenty-four newly diagnosed patients and a two-year follow-up. *Acta Med Scand* 1983;214:279–284.
25. Wallace SL, Lattes R, Malia JP, Ragan C. Muscle involvement in Boeck's sarcoid. *Ann Intern Med* 1958;48:497–511.
26. Phillips RW, Phillips AM. The diagnosis of Boeck's sarcoid by skeletal muscle biopsy. Report of four cases. *Arch Intern Med* 1956;98:732–736.
27. Stjernberg N, Cajander S, Truedsson H, Uddenfeldt P. Muscle involved in sarcoidosis. *Acta Med Scand* 1981;209:213–216.
28. Wolfe SM, Pinals RS, Aelion JA, et al. Myopathy in sarcoidosis: clinical and pathologic study of four cases and review of the literature. *Semin Arthritis Rheum* 1987;16:300–306.
29. Schmirigk K, Uldall B. The disease of Besnier-Boeck-Schaumann and granulomatous polymyositis. *Eur Neurol* 1968;1:137–157.
30. Dyken PR. Sarcoidosis of skeletal muscle. A case report and review of the literature. *Neurology* 1962;12:643–651.
31. Crompton MR, MacDermot V. Sarcoidosis associated with progressive muscular wasting and weakness. *Brain* 1961;84:62–74.
32. McConkey B. Muscular dystrophy in sarcoidosis. *Arch Intern Med* 1958;102:443–446.
33. Pringle CE, Dewar CL. Respiratory muscle involvement in severe sarcoid myositis. *Muscle Nerve* 1997;20:379–381.
34. Ost D, Yeldandi A, Cugell D. Acute sarcoid myositis with respiratory muscle involvement. Case report and review of the literature. *Chest* 1995;107:879–882.
35. Matteson EL, Michet CJ. Sarcoid myositis with pseudohypertrophy. *Am J Med* 1989;87:240–241.
36. Coërs C. The histological features of muscle sarcoïdosis. *Acta Neuropathol* 1967;7:242–252.
37. Alpert JN, Groff AE, Bastian FO, Blum MA. Acute polymyositis caused by sarcoidosis: report of a case and review of the literature. *Mt Sinai J Med* 1979;46:486–488.
38. Hinterbuchner CN, Hinterbuchner LP. Myopathic syndrome in muscular sarcoidosis. *Brain* 1964;87:355–366.
39. Sheffield EA. Pathology of sarcoidosis. *Clin Chest Med* 1997;18:741–754.
40. Jamal MM, Cilursu AM, Hoffman EL. Sarcoidosis presenting as acute myositis. Report and review of the literature. *J Rheumatol* 1988;15:1868–1871.
41. Hewlett RH, Brownell B. Granulomatous myopathy: its relationship to sarcoidosis and polymyositis. *J Neurol Neurosurg Psychiatry* 1975;38:1090–1099.
42. Authier FJ, Mhiri C, Chazaud B, et al. Interleukin-1 expression in inflammatory myopathies: evidence of marked immunoreactivity in sarcoid granulomas and muscle fibres showing ischaemic and regenerative changes. *Neuropathol Appl Neurobiol* 1997;23:132–140.

43. Levine CD, Miller JJ, Stanislaus G, et al. Sarcoid myopathy: imaging findings. *J Clin Ultrasound* 1997;25: 515–517.
44. Hart Y, Schwartz MS, Bruckner F, McKeran RO. Relapsing dermatomyositis associated with sarcoidosis [letter]. *J Neurol Neurosurg Psychiatry* 1988;51:311–313.
45. Itoh J, Akiguchi I, Midorikawa R, Kameyama M. Sarcoid myopathy with typical rash of dermatomyositis. *Neurology* 1980;30:1118–1121.
46. Callen JP. Sarcoidosis appearing initially as polymyositis. *Arch Dermatol* 1979;115:1336–1337.
47. Lipton JH, McLeod BD, Brownell AKW. Dermatomyositis and granulomatous myopathy associated with sarcoidosis. *Can J Neurol Sci* 1988;15:426–429.
48. Kubis N, Woimant F, Polivka, et al. A case of dermatomyositis and muscle sarcoidosis in a Caucasian patient. *J Neurol* 1988;245:50–52.
49. Tajima Y, Shinpo K, Itoh Y, et al. Infiltrating cell profiles of sarcoid lesions in the muscles and peripheral nerves: an immunohistological study. *Intern Med* 1997;36:876–881.
50. Hughes P, McGavin CR. Sarcoidosis and primary biliary cirrhosis with co-existing myositis. *Thorax* 1997;52: 201–202.
51. Groen H, Postma DS, Kallenberg CGM. Interstitial lung disease and myositis in a patient with simultaneously occurring sarcoidosis and scleroderma. *Chest* 1993;104:1298–1300.
52. Danon MJ, Perurena OH, Ronan S, Manaligod JR. Inclusion body myositis associated with systemic sarcoidosis. *Can J Neurol Sci* 1986;13:334–336.
53. Schimrigk K. Demonstration of inclusion bodies in the musculature of patients with muscle sarcoidoses and polymyositis. *Eur Neurol* 1968;1:50–59.
54. De Bleecker J, van Aken L, van Landegem W, et al. Myasthenia gravis and sarcoidosis: report of 2 cases. *Eur Neurol* 1996;36:326–327.
55. Lynch PG, Bansal DV. Granulomatous polymyositis. *J Neurol Sci* 1973;18:1–9.
56. Hosoda Y, Yamaguchi M, Hiraga Y. Global epidemiology of sarcoidosis. What story do prevalence and incidence tell us? *Clin Chest Med* 1997;18:681–694.
57. Thomas PD, Hunninghake GW. Current concepts of the pathogenesis of sarcoidosis. *Am Rev Respir Dis* 1987; 135:747–760.
58. Newman LS, Rose CS, Maier LA. Sarcoidosis. *N Engl J Med* 1997;336:1224–1234.
59. Keogh BA, Hunninghake GW, Line BR, Crystal RG. The alveolitis of pulmonary sarcoidosis: evaluation of natural history and alveolitis-dependent changes in lung function. *Am Rev Respir Dis* 1983;128:256–265.
60. Crystal RG, Roberts WC, Hunninghake GW, et al. Pulmonary sarcoidosis: a disease characterized and perpetuated by activated lung T-lymphocytes. *Ann Intern Med* 1981;94:73–94.
61. Kataria YP, Holter JF. Immunology of sarcoidosis. *Clin Chest Med* 1997;18:719–739.
62. Mason RS, Frankel T, Chan Y, et al. Vitamin D conversion by sarcoid lymph node homogenate. *Ann Intern Med* 1984;100:59–61.
63. McFadden RG, Vickers KE, Fraher LJ. Lymphocyte chemokinetic factors derived from human tonsils: modulation by 1,25-dihydroxyvitamin D3 (calcitriol). *Am J Respir Cell Mol Biol* 1991;4:42–49.
64. Moller DR. Etiology of sarcoidosis. *Clin Chest Med* 1997;18:695–706.
65. Forman JD, Klein JT, Silver RF, et al. Selective activation and accumulation of oligoclonal Vβ-specific T cells in active pulmonary sarcoidosis. *J Clin Invest* 1994;94:1533–1542.
66. Tamura N, Moller DR, Balbi B, et al. Preferential usage of the T-cell antigen receptor ≠o-chain constant region Cβ1 element by lung T-lymphocytes of patients with pulmonary sarcoidosis. *Am Rev Respir Dis* 1991;143: 635–639.
67. Rybicki BA, Maliarik MJ, Major M, et al. Genetics of sarcoidosis. *Clin Chest Med* 1997;18:707–717.
68. Morse SI, Cohn ZA, Hirsch JG, Schaedler RW. The treatment of sarcoidosis with chloroquine. *Am J Med* 1961; 779–784.
69. O'Leary TJ, Jones G, Yip A, et al. The effects of chloroquine on serum 1,25-dihydroxyvitamin D and calcium metabolism in sarcoidosis. *N Engl J Med* 1986;315:727–730.
70. Johns CJ, Zachary JB, Ball WC Jr. A ten-year of corticosteroid treatment of pulmonary sarcoidosis. *Hopkins Med J* 1974;134:271–283.
71. Winterbauer RH, Kirtland SH, Corley DE. Treatment with corticosteroids. *Clin Chest Med* 1997;18:843–851.
72. Kaye O, Palazzo E, Grossin M, et al. Low-dose methotrexate: an effective corticosteroid-sparing agent in the musculoskeletal manifestations of sarcoidosis. *Br J Rheumatol* 1995;34:642–644.
73. Lower EE, Baughman RP. Prolonged use of methotrexate for sarcoidosis. *Arch Intern Med* 1995;155:846–851.
74. Baughman RP, Lower EE. Steroid-sparing alternative treatments for sarcoidosis. *Clin Chest Med* 1997;18: 853–864.
75. Newman LS, Rose CS, Maier LA. Sarcoidosis. *Lancet* 1997;336:1224–1234.

*Diseases of Skeletal Muscle,*
edited by Robert L. Wortmann.
Lippincott Williams & Wilkins, Philadelphia © 2000

# 9

# Metabolic Diseases of Muscle

## Robert L. Wortmann

*Department of Internal Medicine, University of Oklahoma College of Medicine,
Tulsa, Oklahoma 74129*

A wide variety of conditions can be classified as metabolic myopathies. These have in common an underlying abnormality in muscle that interferes with that tissue's ability to produce or maintain adequate levels of energy. The study of metabolic muscle disease is relatively new. Myophosphorylase deficiency, the first described myopathy, was predicted in 1951 (1) and the enzymatic defect identified in 1959 (2). Subsequently, additional defects of carbohydrate metabolism and disorders of lipid and purine metabolism have been recognized. The sequence of mitochondrial DNA was reported in 1981 (3). This sequencing and subsequent research have yielded opportunities to diagnose and understand the most recently categorized metabolic disorders, the mitochondrial myopathies. Surely, additional metabolic diseases of muscle await discovery.

Clinically, these conditions must be considered when evaluating patients with proximal muscle weakness, myoglobinuria, or exercise intolerance due to fatigue, myalgias, or cramps. The evaluation of such patients requires an awareness of potential diagnoses, an understanding of energy metabolism of normal muscle, and an acknowledgment that much remains to be learned about this area before more successful therapies will be available.

The metabolic diseases of muscle can be divided between those that are primary or inherited and those that are secondary or associated with an acquired condition (Table 1).

**TABLE 1.** *Classification of metabolic diseases of muscle*

Primary (inherited)
  Sarcoplasmic biochemical defects
    Disorders of glycogen metabolism
    Disorders of glycolysis
    Purine nucleotide cycle block
  Mitochondrial defects
  Disorders of fatty acid transport
  Substrate utilization defects
  Tricarboxylic acid cycle defects
  Disorders of respiratory chain[a]
  Abnormal oxidation-phosphorylation coupling[a]
  Disorders of ion channels and electrolyte flux
  Sodium, chloride, and calcium channelopathies
  Abnormalities of calcium distribution
Secondary (acquired)
  Endocrine diseases
  Metabolic disorders
  Nutritional abnormalities
  Electrolyte disturbances

[a]The terms "mitochondrial myopathy" or "mitochondrial encephalmyopathy" are often applied to these.

The primary forms are generally classified according to the altered biochemistry or intercellular component involved rather than by clinical presentation.

## DISORDERS OF GLYCOGEN METABOLISM

The discovery in 1959 of myophosphorylase deficiency was the first report of a biochemical abnormality in an inherited myopathy (2). This observation occurred 8 years after McArdle (1) had deduced that "a gross failure of the breakdown in muscle of glycogen to lactate acid" was responsible for life-long exercise intolerance in a 30-year-old man. Subsequently, additional inborn errors of glycogen metabolism associated with muscle dysfunction have been reported and grouped under the term glycogen storage diseases. These have in common the accumulation of excess glycogen in muscle tissue and can be subclassified between defects in glycogen metabolism (synthesis or degradation) and defects of glycolysis (Table 2).

Most individuals with glycogen storage disease are well at rest and perform mild exercise without difficulty, because free fatty acids are the major source of energy under those conditions. In most individuals, the enzymatic block causes problems under conditions when carbohydrate is relied on for generation of ATP. This inability to replenish depleted high-energy phosphate stores results in exercise intolerance, cramping, contracture, and muscle necrosis. This is the most common and easily understood presentation. For reasons that are not understood, some patients present with the gradual onset of proximal muscle weakness.

**TABLE 2.** *Glycogen storage disease that involves skeletal muscle*

| Type | Enzyme deficient | Age at onset | Clinical presentation |
|---|---|---|---|
| Abnormal glycogen metabolism | | | |
| II | Acid maltase ($\alpha$–1,4-1,6–glucosidase) | Infantile | Floppy baby |
| | | Childhood | Cardiomyopathy |
| | | Adult | Proximal weakness |
| | | | Respiratory problems |
| III | Debrancher enzyme (amylo-1-6-glycosidase) | Infantile | Hepatosplenomegaly |
| | | Adult | Failure to thrive |
| | | | Distal weakness |
| | | | Myoglobinuria |
| IV | Brancher enzyme ($\alpha$-1,6-glucosyl-transglycolase) | Childhood | Cirrhosis |
| | | Juvenile | Progressive weakness |
| | | Adult | Neuropathy |
| V | Myophosphorylase | Children | Exercise intolerance |
| | | Juvenile | Myoglobinuria |
| | | Adult | Proximal weakness |
| VI | Phosphorylase b kinase | Childhood | Hepatomegaly |
| | | Adult | Exercise intolerance |
| | | | Myoglobinuria |
| Abnormal glycolysis | | | |
| VII | Phosphofructokinase | Childhood | Exercise intolerance |
| | | Adult | Myoglobinuria |
| | | | Proximal weakness |
| | | | Hemolytic anemia |
| IX | Phosphoglycerate kinase | Childhood | Hemolytic anemia |
| | | Adult | Exercise intolerance |
| | | | Myoglobinuria |
| X | Phosphoglycerate mutase | Adult | Exercise intolerance |
| | | | Myoglobinuria |
| XI | Lactate dehydrogenase | Adult | Exercise intolerance |
| | | | Myoglobinuria |

## Acid Maltase Deficiency

Acid maltase ($\alpha$–1,4-1,6-glucosidase) is an enzyme found in lysosomes that catalyzes the release of glucose from maltose, oligosaccharides, and glycogen. Its precise role in cellular metabolism is not known. The gene for this enzyme is located in the q23-q25 region on chromosome 17 (4), and the deficiency is transmitted through autosomal recessive inheritance (5).

Three different clinical syndromes have been described. These differ in age of presentation, organ involvement, and prognosis (6). The infantile form (Pompe's disease) causes symptoms of muscle weakness, hypotonia, and congestive heart failure that begin shortly after birth and progress to death within the first 2 years of life. This form is characterized by massive glycogen deposits in cardiac, hepatic, neural, and muscular tissues. The second variety presents in early childhood, generally sparing the heart and liver. The major manifestation is muscle weakness that is more proximal than distal and that may affect the diaphragm. Death usually occurs before age 30 as a result of respiratory failure.

Adult forms cause few problems before age 20. The weakness tends to involve proximal muscles and the torso. Individual muscles or even parts of muscles can be affected, but craniobulbar muscles are spared. Weakness of respiratory muscles with respiratory failure may dominate the clinical picture. Atypical presentations have also been described (7–9). The myopathic form is slowly progressive and is easily confused with polymyositis or limb-girdle muscular dystrophy.

The serum creatine kinase level is usually elevated but can be normal or only minimally increased. Electromyography is always abnormal, although variably so. Characteristic changes are practically diagnostic and include an unusually intense electrical irritability in response to movement of the needle electrode and myotonic discharges in the absence of clinical myotonia. In some individuals, however, the changes are indistinguishable from those observed in some cases of polymyositis. Acid maltase deficiency causes a vacuolar myopathy (Table 3). The vacuoles have a high glycogen content and stain for acid phosphatase. Small foci of acid phosphatase activity may also be found in muscle fibers that do not contain vacuoles. Glycogen is readily seen in involved muscle by electron microscopy, but the excess glycogen is not confined to just vacuolar structures (see Chapter 18, Fig. 23). The vacuolar changes in muscle from patients with acid maltase deficiency tend to be less widespread and less striking in adults compared with children, and other causes of vacuolar myopathy must be excluded (Table 3). Assay of acid maltase in muscle, lymphocytes, cultured fibroblasts, or urine can be used to confirm the diagnosis.

**TABLE 3.** *Diseases associated with vacuoles in skeletal muscle*

| | |
|---|---|
| Metabolic | Acid maltase deficiency |
| | Phosphofructokinase deficiency |
| | Carnitine deficiency states |
| | Periodic paralysis |
| | Paramyotonia congenita |
| Toxic | Alcohol |
| | Colchicine |
| | Chloroquine |
| | Zidovudine |
| Inflammatory | Inclusion body myositis |
| | Dermatomyositis |
| Infections | Echovirus |
| Neurologic | Duchenne's muscular dystrophy |
| | Oculopharyngeal dystrophy |
| | Distal myopathy |
| | Lafara's disease |

Several important questions concerning acid maltase deficiency remain unanswered. Why does glycogen collect in nonlysosomal locations and why is it not degraded by cytosolic enzymes? What causes the muscular symptoms, because the pathways of glycogen and glucose metabolism for energy production are intact? Why are peripheral muscles involved in some individuals and respiratory muscles affected in others?

Treatment centers around nutrition. Nocturnal respiratory support is useful. High-protein diets (30% to 47% of total calories) have been effective in some patients, as have low-carbohydrate diets supplemented with epinephrine injections or a regular diet supplemented with branched-chain amino acids (6,10–12). Resistive respiratory muscle exercise may be helpful for those with respiratory muscle involvement.

## Myophosphorylase Deficiency

Myophosphorylase deficiency (McArdle's disease) is considered the prototypic myopathic glycogen storage disease (1,2). Most cases have an autosomal recessive pattern of inheritance, although autosomal dominant inheritance has been reported (13,14). A nonsense mutation at codon 49 of exon 1 for the muscle glycogen phosphorylase gene located on chromosome 11q13 has been found in half of white patients who are homozygous and about one-third of those who are heterozygous (15,16). Additional mutations have been reported.

The cardinal clinical feature of myophosphorylase deficiency is exercise intolerance associated with pain, fatigue, stiffness, or weakness. The degree of exercise intolerance varies. Symptoms typically follow activities of high intensity and short duration or those that require less intense effort for longer intervals and resolve with rest. In fact, most affected individuals function well, provided they adjust their activities to a level below their individual threshold for symptoms. When they exceed their exercise tolerance, they become symptomatic. In addition to stiffness and weakness, painful muscle cramps are sometimes associated with muscle necrosis, myoglobinuria, and potentially reversible acute renal failure. Most affected individuals readily learn to adjust their activity levels once they realize they can exercise longer if they allow a brief rest immediately after the first sensation of muscle pain. This is referred to as the "second wind" phenomenon and is attributed to the combination of increased blood flow stimulated by the increased muscular activity and the ability of alternative energy substrates (amino acids and fatty acids) to be mobilized and used to generate energy (17,18).

Myophosphorylase deficiency may become symptomatic at any age. Rarely, the deficiency affects infants, causing progressive muscle weakness, respiratory insufficiency, and death (19). Other children manifest psychomotor development delay and proximal weakness (20). However, most individuals become symptomatic between the ages of 10 and 30 years of age (21). In those individuals, some symptoms usually are noted in childhood, but many are often overlooked and recognized only in retrospect. For unknown reasons, severe cramps and myoglobulinuria are rare before adolescence. Some individuals complain only of being tired and having poor stamina, whereas others develop progressive muscle weakness that tends to be proximal and may be misdiagnosed as polymyositis (22). The development of fixed proximal muscle weakness later in life is attributed to recurrent exertional muscle injury (23). These symptoms may develop so insidiously that diagnosis is not made until after age 75.

Magnetic resonance spectroscopy confirms the muscle biochemistry predicted by the known enzymatic block (24). Concentrations of ATP and creatine phosphate are normal at rest. With exercise, however, the expected decrease in pH is not seen and the recovery of energy-rich metabolites to baseline levels is delayed. The lack of pH change is due to the ability to form lactic acid, and the decreased intolerance for aerobic exercise is attributed to limited generation of pyruvate that interferes with normal oxidative metabolism (25). Exercise studies demonstrate decreased maximum oxygen consumption and small arteriovenous oxygen differences, confirming a defect in oxidative metabolism due to impaired substrate availability (26).

Elevated levels of serum creatine kinase are found in over 90% of individuals with myophosphorylase deficiency (27). These levels escalate dramatically during symptomatic episodes. Electromyographic studies are usually normal unless myoglobinuria is present. However, nonspecific abnormalities, including increased insertional activity, an increased number of polyphasic potentials, and evidence of muscular irritability with fibrillations and positive waves, have been reported. The cramps that develop after vigorous activity or ischemic exercise are electrically silent (1).

A useful, but nonspecific, tool used to study individuals suspected of being deficient in myophosphorylase activity is the forearm ischemic exercise test (see Chapter 14 for protocol and discussion). This test exploits the abnormal biochemistry that results from the absence of myophosphorylase activity. Normal muscle generates lactate from the degradation of glycogen when anaerobic conditions are produced (see Chapter 2). Additionally, ammonia, inosine, and hypoxanthine concentrations increase significantly, providing evidence of excessive purine nucleotide breakdown (28,29). The glycolytic pathway is blocked when myophosphorylase activity is absent, and consequently lactate cannot be released into the circulation. In normal individuals, venous lactate levels increase three- to sixfold shortly after ischemic exercise, but in myophosphorylase-deficient individuals, levels do not change.

The diagnosis of myophosphorylase deficiency is made by analysis of muscle tissue. Classic changes observed with light microscopy include thick deposits of glycogen at the periphery and thinner linear deposits within cells. The amounts of deposits vary widely, and in milder cases deposits may not be obvious. Deposition is readily appreciated with electron microscopy (Fig. 1). The absence of histochemical staining for myophosphorylase activity secures the diagnosis. False-positive results can be seen in patients with low

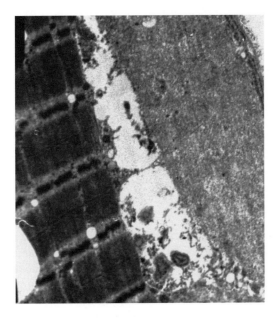

**FIG. 1.** Electron microscopy demonstrating abnormal glycogen deposition adjacent to the sarcolemia and among the myofilaments.

residual activity or when the fetal isoform or the muscle isoform of the enzyme is transiently expressed in regenerating fibers after rhabdomyolysis (30,31).

Although no specific treatment is available for myophosphorylase deficiency, aerobic exercise training and high-protein diets have had positive effects (32,33). Myophosphorylase is the major repository of vitamin $B_6$ in the body, accounting for 80% of the total body pool. Some myophosphorylase-deficient patients show signs of subclinical vitamin $B_6$ deficiency and have reported greater resistance to fatigue with oral vitamin $B_6$ supplementation (34). Simply making the diagnosis is useful for patients and their family members because it allows them to better understand the basis for their symptoms, how best to conduct their activities of daily living, and to understand their prognosis.

### Other Defects in Glycogen Metabolism

Deficiencies of brancher and debrancher enzymes have been reported but are rare. Brancher enzyme deficiency causes cirrhosis and fatal hepatic failure in childhood. The liver disease can be associated with hypotonia and contracture or exercise intolerance and cardiopathy (35). Histologically, this deficiency is characterized by deposition of an abnormal periodic acid–Schiff-positive polysaccharide. A mild juvenile variant characterized by slowly progressive myopathy has been described (36) as has an adult-onset polyglucosan body disease with upper motor neuron signs and peripheral neuropathy (37).

Debrancher enzyme splits the terminal glucose residues from the phosphorylase-limited dextran that remains after the action of myophosphorylase. The deficiency is inherited as an autosomal recessive trait, localized to chromosome 1p21 (38). Deficiency of debrancher enzyme results in phosphorylase-limited dextran accumulation and deposition in muscle, liver, and blood cells. In childhood, this defect presents with hepatosplenomegaly, fasting hypoglycemia, and failure to thrive. Less frequently, individuals may develop slowly progressive muscle weakness with exercise intolerance, distal muscle wasting, and rarely myoglobinuria beginning after age 20 years (39,40). There may also be associated neuropathy. These individuals have elevated serum creatine kinase levels and fail to generate lactate after forearm ischemic exercise.

Phosphorylase b kinase helps to regulate glycogen metabolism through the activation of myophosphorylase and inhibition of glycogen synthetase. The enzyme consists of four subunits and is under complex regulation, allowing for variable inheritance and heterogeneous clinical pictures. These include an X-linked deficiency that causes hepatomegaly, fasting hypoglycemia, and growth retardation (41); a myopathy presenting in childhood with hypotonia or exercise intolerance with extremity weakness and myoglobinuria (42); a fatal infantile cardiomyopathy (43); and an autosomal recessive form that presents with various combinations of myopathy and hepatomegaly in adults (44,45). In contrast to patients with other glycogen storage diseases, serum creatine kinase levels are not uniformly elevated, and the lactate response to forearm ischemic exercise is normal or only minimally blunted.

### Defects in Glycolysis

#### *Phosphofructokinase Deficiency*

The clinical manifestations of phosphofructokinase deficiency (Tarui's disease) can be identical to those of myophosphorylase deficiency with exercise intolerance, cramps, and episodes of myoglobinuria with or without proximal muscle weakness. However, phosphofructokinase deficiency also causes hemolytic anemia, which may be seen with or without myopathy, and in some cases seizures, cortical blindness, corneal opacifications, and mental retardation.

Isoenzymes of phosphofructokinase vary in subunit composition. The muscle enzyme consists of M subunits, and the erythrocyte enzyme contains M and L subunits. Phosphofructokinase deficiency is inherited as an autosomal recessive trait, with the M subunit mapped to chromosome 1. The L subunit has been localized to chromosome 21 (46). Defects in the L subunit cause only hemolysis, but defects involving M subunits can affect both muscle and erythrocytes with enzyme activity completely lacking in muscle and at 50% in red blood cells. Considerable heterogeneity exists at molecular and clinical levels (47–49).

Patients diagnosed as adults (as old as age 65 years) in retrospect recall having had problems with either exercise intolerance or cramps in their youth. Phosphofructokinase-deficient individuals differ from myophosphorylase-deficient individuals in that the second wind phenomenon is less common and exercise intolerance is more likely to be associated with nausea and vomiting. The lack of second wind is attributed to a block in oxidative metabolism that prevents lipolysis and prevents release of free fatty acid (50). Because of this mechanism, the consumption of glucose may actually lower oxidative capacities by depriving muscles of its major source of energy and induce an "out-of-wind" phenomenon (51).

Most have elevated serum creatine kinase levels at rest and about one third develop myoglobinuria. Electromyographic findings are either normal or provide nonspecific results consistent with myopathy or inflammation. Venous lactate levels fail to raise with forearm ischemic exercise. $^{31}$P-magnetic resonance spectroscopy demonstrates an absence of pH change and the appearance of a phosphomonoester peak, representing the hexose phosphates that accumulate as would be predicted because of the enzyme block (52). The appearance of a phosphomonoester peak is found in other inborn errors of glycolysis but is not seen in myophosphorylase deficiency.

Histochemical analysis of muscle tissue is needed to confirm the diagnosis. In addition to increased glycogen deposition and decreased phosphofructokinase activity, deficient muscle also contained an abnormal polysaccharide similar to that seen in brancher enzyme deficiency (40). Hemolysis associated with myopathic disease may be subclinical, causing only an increased reticulocyte count, or severe, causing jaundice and gallstones. Hyperuricemia and gout commonly develop, probably because of the high levels of purine nucleotides released with hemolysis and during exercise (53,54). Therapeutic recommendations are similar to those for myophosphorylase deficiency and with the additional recommendation that affected individuals avoid exercise after high-carbohydrate meals (51,55).

### Other Defects in Glycolysis

Deficiencies of phosphoglycerate kinase (56,57), phosphoglycerate mutase (58), and lactate dehydrogenase (59,60) have been described. The most common manifestation of phosphoglycerate kinase deficiency is hemolytic anemia, sometimes associated with seizures and mental retardation. However, adolescent-onset variety with exercise intolerance, myalgia, and myoglobinuria has been reported (56,57). Phosphoglycerate mutase deficiency presents in adulthood with intolerance to strenuous exercise, cramps, and myoglobinuria (58). The clinical manifestations reported for lactate dehydrogenase deficiency and similar to those reported for young men with phosphoglycerate mutase deficiency (59,60). These genetic defects all cause a failure of lactate release after ischemic exercise and require histochemical staining or enzyme analysis of muscle for diagnosis.

## DISORDERS OF LIPID METABOLISM

Plasma free fatty acids are the major source of energy while fasting, at rest, and exercising at lower intensity and for longer durations. Abnormalities involving the processing of fatty acids for energy may lead to abnormal accumulations of lipid between myofibrils. The disorders of lipid metabolism are due to biochemical defects that occur in mitochondria (Table 4). Those that result from defective fatty acid transport or defects in β-oxidation are often referred to as lipid storage diseases. The term mitochondrial myopathy is more often used to represent defects of the respiratory chain and oxidative phosphorylation.

### Lipid Storage Diseases

Defects in the pathways of fatty acid oxidation interfere with energy production in most organs. Therefore, individuals with a lipid storage myopathy may have other tissues involved as well. Most defects described to date can affect skeletal muscle, heart, liver, kidney, and mental status. The most common symptoms in patients with a lipid storage disease are myalgia and weakness. Infants typically present with failure to thrive or hypotonia, whereas adults present with progressive proximal muscle weakness or with episodic rhabdomyolysis. The predominance features, degree of disorder, and combinations of organs involved vary widely among individuals, suggesting environmental factors may also play a role in these diseases.

The reason for the variation in clinical presentations is not understood. However, the laboratory features of these diseases can be attributed to the accumulation of potentially toxic intermediates proximal to the enzymatic blocks and to the resultant decreased availability of energy-producing substrates. When the liver is involved, disorders of fatty acid oxidation will lead to fasting hypoglycemia, elevated serum levels of free fatty acids, and hypoketosis. Because of the altered metabolism, the liver cannot make ketone bodies. Hypoglycemia results from the increased use of glucose for energy that is required to compensate for the decreased availability of energy from lipids. A second factor that con-

**TABLE 4.** *Disorders of metabolism that occur in mitochondria*

| Defect | Deficiency |
|---|---|
| Fatty acid transport | Carnitine |
| | Primary |
| | Secondary |
| | Carnitine palmitoyltransferase |
| Substrate utilization | Pyruvate carboxylase |
| | Pyruvate dehydrogenase complex |
| | Long-chain, medium-chain, and short-chain fatty acid acyl-CoA dehydrogenases |
| Tricarboxylic acid cycle | Fumarase |
| | α-Ketoglutarate dehydrogenase |
| Respiratory chain | Complex I |
| | Complex II |
| | Complex III |
| | Complex IV |
| | Complex V |
| | Multiple or combined components |
| | Primary |
| | Secondary |
| Oxidative–phosphorylation coupling | Luft's syndrome |

tributes to hypoglycemia is impaired hepatic glyconeogenesis. These abnormalities may lead to rapid metabolic decompensation with multiorgan failure, encephalopathy, and coma. Other laboratory abnormalities may include lactic acidosis and elevated serum ammonia levels. The former is due to increased anaerobic glycolysis, and the latter to rapid ATP depletion and increased activation of the purine nucleotide cycle (see Chapter 2).

## Carnitine Deficiency States

Fatty acids produce energy by being processed through pathways located in mitochondria. Short- and medium-chain fatty acids enter mitochondria freely but long-chain fatty acids require a carrier for transfer into these organellae. Carnitine serves that carrier function and helps to regulate coenzyme A (CoA)/acyl-CoA ratios in mitochondria. Sources of carnitine include the diet, with red meat and dairy products containing large quantities, and de novo synthesis from lysine and methionine in liver, brain, and kidney. Carnitine is transported from the blood by an active process into muscle, where 98% of the body stores are maintained. The major route of carnitine elimination is in the urine.

The first recognized case of muscle carnitine deficiency was reported in 1973 by Engel and Angelini (61). Soon thereafter, Karpati et al. (62) reported another form of carnitine deficiency, a systemic variety. Today, carnitine deficiencies can be classified as either primary or secondary. Primary deficiencies have a genetic basis and can be further divided between myopathic and systemic forms. Secondary deficiencies are those that result from other disorders or that result from genetic defects in other pathways of intermediary metabolism (Table 5) (63).

### *Primary Carnitine Deficiencies*

Myopathic carnitine deficiency is characterized by progressive muscle weakness that generally begins in childhood (64,65). The weakness is proximal in distribution but can involve facial and pharyngeal muscles as well. Less common features include exertional myalgias, myoglobinuria, and cardiomyopathy. Over 50% of patients have elevated serum creatine kinase levels, and most have myopathic changes (polyphasic motor unit potentials of small amplitude and short duration) on electromyography. Serum carnitine concentrations are usually normal, a finding consistent with the evidence indicating that a

---

**TABLE 5.** *Carnitine deficiency states*

Primary deficiencies
  Muscle carnitine deficiency
  Systemic carnitine deficiency
Secondary deficiencies
  Organic acidurias
  Respiratory chain defects
  Methylenetetrahydrofolate reductase deficiency
  Renal Fanconi syndrome
  Hemodialysis
  Cirrhosis
  Myxedema
  Adrenal insufficiency
  Hypopituitarism
  Pregnancy
  Valproic acid or pivampicillin therapy

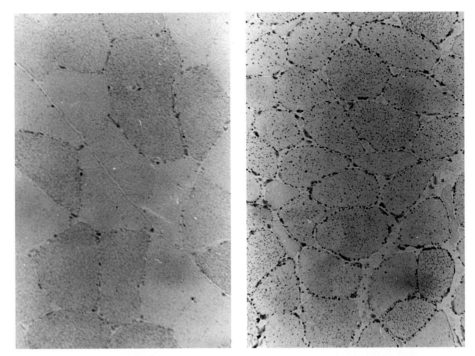

**FIG. 2.** Oil red O staining for fat. On the left, normal staining; on the right, increased staining. Increased fat in muscle is a nonspecific finding and can result from lipid storage disease, mitochondrial myopathy, ischemia, or obesity.

defect in carnitine transport into muscle cells underlies this form of the disease. The only histologic abnormality in muscle is increased lipid deposition (Fig. 2) (see Chapter 18, Fig. 7). This is a nonspecific finding because similar changes can result from ischemia and obesity. The diagnosis is made by biochemical analysis of muscle tissue.

The first reported patient with systemic carnitine deficiency was an 11-year-old boy with progressive muscle weakness and a history of recurrent attacks that resembled Reye's syndrome (62). The attacks began with vomiting and were followed by coma, hepatosplenomegaly, liver function abnormalities, and hypoglycemia. This defect results from inheritance of nonfunctional high-affinity carnitine receptors (66). Onset of this autosomal recessive disorder is almost always in early childhood. Typically, the systemic features are the major manifestations, but cardiac muscle involvement with congestive heart failure may predominate. Carnitine concentrations are reduced in skeletal muscle, heart, liver, and serum.

### Secondary Carnitine Deficiencies

Many individuals previously believed to have primary carnitine deficiencies have been found to have a secondary deficiency resulting from another metabolic defect (63,67). Carnitine deficiency can be secondary to genetic defects in other reactions in intermediary metabolism or other disorders. These include the organic acidurias (disorders of straight-chain fatty acids and branched-chain amino acids that cause infantile lactic acidosis) (68), selective defects of each respiratory chain complex (63), and methylenetetrahydrofolate reductase deficiency (69). Secondary carnitine deficiency has also been observed in patients with renal failure requiring chronic hemodialysis (but not chronic peritoneal dialysis), end-stage cirrhosis with cachexia, myxedema, adrenal insufficiency, hypopituitarism, and pregnancy and with valproic acid or pivampicillin therapy (70–73).

Attempts at treatment should include a diet rich in carbohydrates and medium-chain fatty acids and avoidance of fasting. During acute attacks, therapy should be designed to prevent hypoglycemia and correct any electrolyte and acid-base imbalances that develop. Despite the theoretic likelihood that all types of carnitine deficiency could be effectively treated with dietary supplementation, in reality the response is variable.

Dietary supplementation with L-carnitine is given at a dose of 100 mg/kg/day for children and 2 to 4 g in divided doses for adults. In general, individuals with a primary deficiency are more likely to have a good response. Some patients have benefited from corticosteroid therapy and propranolol. Intravenous infusion of L-carnitine (20 mg/kg) at the end of dialysis treatments has been shown to decrease post-dialysis symptoms, improve exercise capacity, increase one's sense of well-being, and possibly increase muscle mass in patients requiring chronic hemodialysis (73). Treatment with riboflavin alone or in combination with L-carnitine has proven beneficial to individuals with other defects of lipid metabolism. This addition is worth considering, although a benefit in carnitine deficiency has not been demonstrated (74–76).

### Carnitine Palmitoyltransferase Deficiency

In 1973, DiMauro and Melis-DiMauro (77) reported a deficiency of carnitine palmitoyltransferase in two brothers with recurrent myoglobinuria. Symptoms typically include attacks of myalgia, cramps, stiffness, or tenderness, with myoglobulinuria. Attacks usually develop after prolonged exercise or fasting at times when fatty acids are the major source of cellular energy. Cold exposure, infection, high fat intake, and emotional stress and the use of ibuprofen or diazepam, general anesthesia, surgery, and pregnancy may also be important contributing and precipitating factors (78–80). Approximately 80% of those with the autosomal recessive trait who are symptomatic are male.

Mild attacks may be experienced in childhood, but severe attacks usually do not occur until the teenage years or later. Intermittent episodes of severe muscle cramping and passage of rose or darkish urine may be ignored or puzzling. This enzyme deficiency may be the most common cause of exercise-induced rhabdomyolysis, myoglobinuria, and proximal muscle pain and weakness in young adult males (81). Middle-aged women may present with chronic history of diffuse aching and fatigue provoked by fasting, high fat intake, or prolonged exertion (82). About one forth of individuals develop renal failure with episodes of myoglobinuria. Respiratory failure may result during severe attacks.

The clinical picture of carnitine palmitoyltransferase differs from that of the glycogen storage disease that also causes episodic myoglobinuria. Individuals with carnitine palmitoyltransferase deficiency can perform brief intervals of intense exercise, do not experience warning signs of a second wind or out-of-wind phenomenon, and cannot abort attacks with rest. It is typically easier for them to run a 300-yard dash than walk 18 holes of golf.

Serum creatine kinase levels are usually normal except during episodes of symptomatic rhabdomyolysis or with prolonged fasting. Serum lactate concentrations increase in a normal fashion after forearm ischemic exercise. Electrophysiologic studies and muscle tissue are entirely normal between attacks. Lipid accumulation is rarely observed in muscle. The diagnosis is made by measuring carnitine palmitoyltransferase activity in muscle. Recently, proton magnetic resonance spectroscopy has been used to measure acetylation of the carnitine pool (82). This may prove to be a very useful noninvasive method for diagnosis.

Based on the known biochemistry, it would be predicted that carnitine palmitoyltransferase deficiency and carnitine deficiency would cause similar abnormalities. However, this is not the case. Fixed weakness is quite unusual in carnitine palmitoyltransferase deficiency, but the disease may present in adulthood with features characteristic of some mitochondrial myopathies. These include exercise intolerance associated with external ophthalmoplegia and ragged red fibers in skeletal muscle (83). Why the clinical and histologic features of these deficiencies differ is not understood.

Management consists primarily of education, although the combination of oral supplementation of L-carnitine and riboflavin may be of some benefit (75). Avoidance of both prolonged strenuous exercise and fasting will prevent most attacks. Infection may not be preventable, but the need for adequate rest during an infection must be emphasized. Treatment with frequent feedings of a high-carbohydrate diet low in long-chain fatty acids supplemented with medium-chain fatty acids and L-carnitine has been beneficial (82). Myoglobinuria constitutes a medical emergency because it may lead to renal failure. The renal failure is reversible if recognized and treated appropriately (see Chapter 13).

## Defects in β-Oxidation

Fatty acids are metabolized in mitochondria through β-oxidation. The first step of this process is catalyzed by the flavoprotein containing acyl-CoA dehydrogenases. These include long-chain acyl-CoA dehydrogenase, which acts on substrates with more than 12 carbon atoms in the acyl residues; medium-chain acyl-CoA dehydrogenase, which process those with 4 to 14 carbons; and short-chain acyl-CoA dehydrogenase for those with 4 to 6 carbons.

Genetic deficiencies of these enzymes most commonly mimic primary systemic carnitine deficiency (66,84). However, myopathic forms also exist. Long-chain acyl-CoA dehydrogenase deficiency can present in infancy or adulthood. Infants and children may develop muscle weakness and hypotonia, experience episodes of muscle pain and fatigue associated with high serum creatine kinase levels, and have attacks of myoglobulinuria (85). Adults present with weakness of the proximal, cervical, and masticatory muscles (86). Deficiencies of all three fatty acid acyl-CoA dehydrogenase activities (termed multiple acyl-CoA dehydrogenase deficiency) have been reported in a 38-year-old man who presented with a 2-year history of neck pain and proximal muscle weakness, elevated serum creatine kinase levels, myopathic changes on electromyography, and abnormal accumulation of lipid on muscle biopsy (87). Treatment with riboflavin resulted in normalization of muscle histology and improved strength. A trifunctional enzyme deficiency has been described in infants with findings similar to systemic carnitine deficiency and in children and adults with episodic muscle weakness and myoglobinuria associated with respiratory failure (88,89).

## Mitochondrial Myopathies

Mitochondria are the powerhouse of cells, functioning to provide the energy required for all biosynthetic and motor activities (see Chapter 2). They are the size of bacteria and composed of a two-layered membrane that encloses a matrix (Fig. 3). These organelles possess their own DNA, which is small, containing 16.5 kilobases (kb), compared with

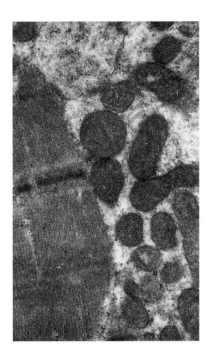

**FIG. 3.** Electron microscopy picture of mitochondria in normal skeletal muscle.

the 3 million kb of nuclear or DNA. Mitochondrial DNA encodes for 13 structural subunits of respiratory chain complexes, two ribosomal RNA molecules, and 22 transfer RNAs. Mitochondria are self-replicating, have limited lifespan, and maintain their numbers by a form of division that resembles the binary fusion of bacteria.

Mitochondrial myopathies are conditions that cause major morphologic abnormalities in mitochondrial number, size, and structure and result from disruption of the processes oxidative metabolism and energy transfer, specifically those of the respiratory chain and oxidative phosphorylation. Although the function of mitochondria is critical to every organ system, skeletal muscle and brain are often most affected by these disorders. Diseases that affect muscle are termed mitochondrial myopathies; those that involve multiple tissue, primarily brain and muscle, are called mitochondrial encephalomyopathies. These diseases can be characterized by genetic and biochemical criteria (90–92).

The most typical morphologic change in mitochondrial diseases is the ragged red fiber, a distorted-appearing fiber that contains large peripheral and intermyofibrillar aggregates of abnormal mitochondria (Fig. 4). These appear as red deposits with the modified Gomori trichome stain and are found primarily in type I and, to a lesser degree, in type IIA fibers. The presence of ragged red fibers is not specific for a mitochondrial myopathy. An occasional ragged red fiber may be seen in presumably normal muscle and as a consequence of aging (93). However, the presence of these fibers does indicate the possibility of one of those diseases. On the other hand, many diseases that result from mitochondrial defects do not manifest this change (94). Histochemical analysis often reveals an absence of staining for cytochrome oxidase and an increase in staining for succinate dehydrogenase (94,95). Additional changes, such as increased amounts of lipid or glycogen, intramitochondrial inclusions, or changes in mitochondrial size or shape, can be seen at the ultrastructural level (Fig. 5).

**TABLE 6.** *Clinical manifestations of mitochondrial encephalomyopathies*

| | |
|---|---|
| Muscle | Limb weakness |
| | Exercise intolerance |
| | Lack of muscle mass |
| | External ophthalmoplegia |
| Nervous system | Stroke-like episodes |
| | Seizures |
| | Myoclonus |
| | Optic neuropathy |
| | Optic atrophy |
| | Pigmentary retinopathy |
| | Sensorineural hearing loss |
| | Extrapyramidal signs |
| | Sensorimotor neuropathy |
| | Ataxia |
| | Leukodystrophy |
| | Mental retardation |
| | Dementia |
| | Migraine headache |
| Endocrine | Diabetes mellitus |
| | Hypothyroidism |
| | Growth hormone deficiency |
| | Delayed puberty |
| | Infertility |
| Cardiac | Conduction abnormalities |
| | Hypertrophic cardiomyopathy |
| Gastrointestinal | Dysmotility |
| | Intestinal pseudo-obstruction |
| | Hepatic failure |
| | Pancreatic exocrine failure |
| Renal | Bartter's-like syndrome |
| | Renal tubular acidosis |
| Dermatologic | Lipomas |
| | Hirsutism |
| | Purpura |
| Hematologic | Sideroblastic anemia |
| | Acanthocytosis |
| | Pancytopenia |
| Psychiatric | Depression |
| | Schizophrenic episodes |

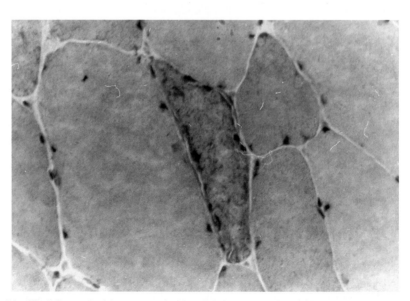

**FIG. 4.** Modified Gomori trichrome stain identifying a ragged red fiber, a characteristic histologic finding in many mitochondrial myopathies. The dark-appearing cell is the result of aggregates of mitochondria.

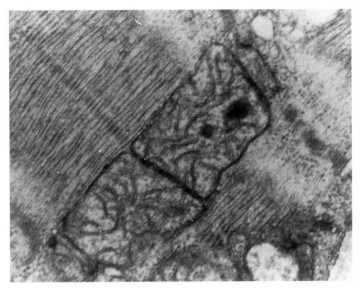

**FIG. 5.** Abnormal-shaped mitochondria in skeletal muscle from an adult with a mitochondrial myopathy.

Mitochondrial diseases are associated with a variety of clinical manifestations (Table 6). In general, they can be divided into syndromes that cause myopathy, with or without ophthalmoplegia, and those in which central nervous system manifestations predominate. The former primarily affect muscle, causing manifestations such as exercise intolerance, muscle weakness that may have a limb-girdle or fascioscapulohumeral distribution, or extraocular muscle dysfunction with or without bulbar and limb involvement. Hypermetabolism, salt craving, and peripheral neuropathy have been reported in other cases, indicating extreme heterogeneity. Although most of these diseases affect infants, some do not develop until later in life. Adult-onset mitochondrial myopathies most commonly cause exercise intolerance, proximal or generalized weakness, and rarely myoglobulinemia. Individuals may even present in their seventies (83). Serum creatine kinase levels may be normal or elevated, and electrophysiologic studies are not particularly distinctive.

The classification and characterization of mitochondrial myopathies on a genetic basis requires appreciation of the differences between mitochondrial DNA and nuclear DNA (Table 7). In contrast to nuclear DNA, mitochondrial DNA is circular and is derived totally from the mother's oocyte. Multiple mitochondria are present in every cell, and

**TABLE 7.** *Mitochondrial genetics*

| | |
|---|---|
| Maternal inheritance | Virtually all mtDNA is derived from the oocyte. Although sons and daughters can be affected, only the later can transmit the disease. |
| Polyplasmia | Each cell contains multiple mtDNA genomes. |
| Heteroplasmy | Not all mtDNA molecules are identical. |
| Threshold effect | The phenotypic expression is determined by the relative proportion of wild-type vs. mutant genomes per cell or per tissue. |
| Mitotic segregation | Mitochondria distribute randomly with cell division. This increases or decreases the proportion of mutant genomes. |
| Nuclear factors influence | Nuclear DNA factors can influence the expression of mtDNA mutations. |

each contains multiple genomes. Mitochondrial DNA is subject to frequent spontaneous mutations for two reasons. First, it is constantly exposed to oxygen free radicals leaked from the electron transport chain, and second it lacks a DNA repair system. In normal tissues all mitochondrial DNA molecules are identical, a state termed homoplasmy. In inherited disease, homoplasmy is maintained with the defect present in all mitochondrial DNA copies in all cells. If spontaneous mutations occur, different populations, mutant and wild types, exist within the same cells. This state is termed heteroplasmy. The phenotypic expression of a pathogenic mutation is largely determined by the relative properties of mutant versus wild types with one phenotype predominating. The term threshold effect is applied to that phenomenon. With heteroplasmy at cell division, the proportion of mutant mitochondrial genomes may shift, leading to phenotypic changes. Consequently, mitochondrial diseases can be inherited or develop later in life (90, 93,96,97).

A rational classification of the mitochondrial encephalomyopathies can be developed according to the type of genetic defects (Table 8) (91,92,94). These can be subclassified as to whether they result from defects in mitochondrial DNA, in nuclear DNA, or defective communication between the two (98–114).

Mitochondrial DNA mutations can result in single or multiple duplications or point mutations. The Kearns-Sayre syndrome consists of the triad of ophthalmoplegia, pigmentary retinopathy (retinitis pigmentosa), and an onset before age 20 years with cardiac conduction block, a cerebellar syndrome, or a cerebrospinal fluid protein greater than 100 mg/dL. Kearns-Sayre syndrome can result from larger scale deletions, duplications, or point mutations (98,109). Most cases of sporadic progressive external ophthalmoplegia, which can be associated with a variety of defects affecting all complexes of the respiratory chain, are attributed to large deletions of mitochondrial DNA (99), but some are the result of point mutations (108). Multiple deletions have been described in cases of familial myopathy and late-onset mitochondrial myopathy in the elderly (103–105). At least

---

**TABLE 8.** *Classification of mitochondrial encephalomyopathies based on genetic defect*

Mitochondrial DNA defects
Single deletions or duplications
    Kearns-Sayre syndrome (KSS) (98)
    Progressive external ophthalmoplegia (PEO) (99)
    Pearson's syndrome (100)
Multiple deletions
    Familial recurrent myoglobinuria (101)
    Dilated cardiomyopathy (102)
    Aging (93,103–105)
Point mutations
    Mitochondrial encephalopathy, lactic acidosis with stroke-like episodes (106)
    Myoclonus epilepsy with ragged red fibers (107)
    Myopathy-cardiomyopathy (108)
    KSS (108)
    PEO (108)
Nuclear DNA defects
  Autosomal dominant PEO (110,111)
  Fatal infantile myopathy with cytochrome *c* oxidase (COX) deficiency (112,113)
  Benign infantile myopathy with COX deficiency (112,113)
  Mitochondrial neuropathy, gastrointestinal encephalomyopathy or mitochondrial neuropathy, pseudo-
    obstruction, ophthalmoplegia, and polyneuropathy (114)
  Limb-girdle myopathy (94)
Intercommunication defects between nuclear and mitochondrial DNA
  Fatal infantile myopathy with mtDNA depletion (115)

three different point mutations have been identified in patients with the syndrome of mitochondrial encephalomyopathy, lactic acidosis, and stroke-like episodes (106).

Mutations in nuclear DNA, many of which remain to be defined, can cause a variety of syndromes (94,109–111). For example, nuclear DNA-encoded cytochrome *c* oxidase subunits are absent in individuals with both benign and fatal infantile myopathy (112). An autosomal dominant progressive external ophthalmoplegia is attributed to the absence of a *trans*-acting nuclear factor. These individuals experience facial and limb weakness, ptosis, dysphonia, dysphagia, exercise intolerance, and cataracts with onset between 24 and 30 years (111).

Acquired forms of mitochondrial myopathies are being recognized in association with the use of certain therapeutic agents and with other disease states. The use of zidovudine in the treatment of individuals infected with the human immunodeficiency virus can cause a ragged red fiber-positive mitochondrial myopathy (116). The drug has been shown to be incorporated into mitochondrial DNA and results in a reduction of mitochondrial DNA content (117). Abnormal mitochondria have been obscured on histology of muscle from patients with clofibrate myopathy (118). Rheumatic diseases associated with abnormal mitochondria or muscle tissue deficient for cytochrome *c* oxidase include polymyositis, inclusion body myositis, and polymyalgia rheumatica (119–122). Histologically abnormal mitochondria have also been seen in cases of Duchenne and myotonic muscular dystrophies, facioscapulohumeral and oculopharyngeal myopathies, Parkinson's disease, periodic paralysis, and malignant hyperthermia (123–128). Which of these associations with mitochondrial changes are related to the disease and which are secondary to an aging phenomenon, and therefore coincidental, is uncertain (129).

To date, the only approach to therapy of a mitochondrial myopathy is palliative. Results from each individual and each disease are variable. Although not always successful, therapeutic trials are warranted in every patient. Treatments include dietary supplementation and vitamins. L-Carnitine (50 to 200 mg/kg/day) and creatine monohydrate (5 g twice a day) have been helpful in some patients with mitochondrial myopathies (130,131). Riboflavin (30 to 400 mg/day) has been used in patients with complex I defects (132). Ascorbate (vitamin C, up to 4,000 mg/day) with or without menadione (vitamin $K_3$, 40 to 500 mg/day) has used to bypass defects in complex III (133). Coenzyme $Q_{10}$ (60 to 200 mg/day) has been used in the treatment of a familial mitochondrial myopathy from $Q_{10}$ deficiency and ill-defined defects involving multiple complexes (134). Whereas there may be a certain logic applied to the choice of a particular therapy, the decision is empiric and combinations of various agents should be considered.

## DISORDERED PURINE METABOLISM

### Myoadenylate Deaminase Deficiency

Myoadenylate deaminase, a distinct isoenzyme of adenylate deaminase found only in skeletal muscle, catalyzes the irreversible deamination of AMP to IMP and plays an important role in the purine nucleotide cycle (see Chapter 2). A deficiency of myoadenylate deaminase was first reported in 1978. The myoadenylate deaminase gene is located on the short arm of chromosome 1 (135). A single mutant allele appears to be responsible for most, if not all, cases of primary deficiency (136). This nonsense mutation in exon 2 results in normal abundance of myoadenylate deaminase transcripts but deficient (generally less than 2% of normal) enzyme protein. Some individuals with a primary deficiency complain of exercise intolerance due to fatigue with postexertional cramps and myalgias, but most are asymptomatic (137). Levels of serum enzymes such as creatine kinase and aldolase are usually normal, and electromyograms are normal or nonspecific. The measurement of venous lactate and ammonia concentrations after forearm ischemic exercise is effective for screening for myoadenylate deaminase deficiency (see Chapter 14). These patients experience increased levels of lactate but no change in levels of ammonia compared with baseline.

The secondary or acquired deficiencies have been reported and are associated with a wide variety of other neuromuscular diseases, including periodic paralysis, influenza-like illness, Kugelberg-Welander disease, amyotrophic lateral sclerosis, spinal muscular atrophy, facial and limb-girdle myopathies, polymyositis, dermatomyositis, systemic lupus erythematosus, systemic sclerosis, diabetes, hyperthyroidism, and gout (138). Higher residual activities of immunoreactive enzyme protein occur in the secondary deficiencies, and reductions occur in other muscle enzymes such as creatine kinase and adenylate kinase as well (137). Furthermore, the reduction in enzyme activity parallels a decrease in myoadenylate deaminase messenger RNA (139). The factors responsible for molecular changes underlying the secondary deficiency states are not understood.

The precise relationship between myoadenylate deaminase deficiency and disease manifestations is unknown. Approximately 2% of whites and African Americans are homozygous for the nonsense mutation, and although some deficient individuals report symptoms of myopathy, clearly most are asymptomatic. The disparity between the frequency of the mutant allele and the prevalence of symptoms suggests that either the deficiency is not the major cause of the myopathy in individuals with the inherited defect or some compensatory mechanisms protects from the harmful effects of the mutation.

A potential molecular explanation for amelioration of symptoms secondary to this nonsense mutation in exon 2 of the *AMPD1* gene has been proposed (140). The primary transcript of the *AMPD1* gene is subject to alternative splicing. If in that process the only exon alternatively removed is exon 2, then a fraction of the *AMPD1* transcripts would encode a functional peptide and the defect would be at least partially eliminated.

## PRIMARY DISORDERS INVOLVING ION CHANNELS AND ELECTROLYTE FLUX

The term channelopathy has been given to a group of conditions that cause periodic myotonia or muscle stiffness (Table 9) (141,142). Each of these diseases is characterized by a disturbance in the excitation of muscle fiber membranes resulting from disorders of voltage-gated sodium, chloride, or calcium channels. These diseases are believed to be either inherited by autosomal dominant transmission or the result of new mutations.

**TABLE 9.** *Channelopathies*

Sodium channel disorders
   Hyperkalemic periodic paralysis
   Paramyotonia congenita
   Normokalemic periodic paralysis
   Sodium channel myotonia
   Potassium-activated myotonia
Chloride channel disorders
   Thomsen's dominant myotonia congenita
   Becker's recessive myotonia congenita
Calcium channel disorders
   Hypokalemic periodic paralysis

## Disorders of Sodium Channels

### Hyperkalemic Periodic Paralysis

This disease usually begins with myotonia in infancy or episodic weakness in childhood. Attacks most commonly begin in the morning, last 15 minutes to 3 hours, and can be provoked by immobility, rest after exercise, emotional stress, or ingestion of potassium. Initially, affected individuals have normal strength between attacks but may develop persistent weakness over time (143). The frequency of attacks may decrease later in life.

Serum potassium levels are persistently elevated between attacks and may rise at the onset of weakness only to fall to normal or low levels during attacks. Serum creatine kinase levels are usually elevated. Myotonia is demonstrable with electromyography in some patients but absent in others (144).

Two distinct mutations have been identified in patients with well-characterized classic familial hyperkalemic periodic paralysis (145,146). These cause alterations in the membrane-spanning segments of the sodium channels and are linked to chromosome 17.

Management includes regular and frequent feedings, a low-potassium diet, and avoidance of strenuous exercise. Some attacks can be aborted by ingesting carbohydrate such as glucose at 2 g/kg, by using a thiazide diuretic or acetazolamide orally, or by inhalation of a β-adrenergic agent (147). Attacks may be prevented by the continuous use of a thiazide diuretic or acetazolamide (148,149).

### Paramyotonia Congenita

Paramyotonia congenita is characterized by myotonia that worsens with activity, in contrast to classic forms of myotonia that improve with exercise. Myotonia can also develop with cold exposure. Protracted exercise and cold exposure can also cause weakness. This form commonly involves the face, neck, and long muscles of the hands. Attacks begin at birth and occur throughout life with interattack weakness developing in some patients.

Although serum potassium levels are usually low during attacks, potassium loading can precipitate attacks. Serum creatine kinase levels may be elevated, and electromyography reveals cold-induced alterations in compound muscle action potential (CMAP) amplitudes (150,151). This condition, which can be attributed to a sodium channel mutation, may require no treatment. In those more symptomatic, acetazolamide or onexilitine can be used (150,152).

### Other Sodium Channel Diseases

Normokalemic periodic paralysis resembles hyperkalemic periodic paralysis but differs in that serum potassium levels are normal even during severe attacks (153). These patients improve with large doses of sodium. The term sodium channel myopathy is applied to patients with manifestations very similar to paramyotonia congenita but who only develop stiffness, and not weakness, with exercise or cold exposure (154). Patients with potassium-activated myotonia do not experience episodic paralysis but develop myotonia with potassium loading (152). Their myotonia is not temperature sensitive, and they improve with lowering potassium levels.

## Disorders of Chloride Channels

Two inherited forms of myotonia congenita have been described that result from defects in the chloride channel gene (141,142,155,156). Dominant myotonia congenita,

Thomsen's disease, is characterized by generalized myotonia that can begin shortly after birth or in the first or second decade of life. The myotonia is painless, is provoked by voluntary muscle contraction, but disappears with repeated contracture or warm up. Weakness is not a feature of this disease. In fact, some patients appear muscular and are quite strong. Lid lag and percussion blepharospasm myotonia are observed in some patients. Recessive myotonia congenita, Becker's myotonia, is quite similar to the dominant form but is more severe. It typically does not become apparent until age 10 to 14 years. These patients develop myotonia and weakness that resolve with warm up. Electromyography reveals typical myotonia, and patients respond to mexiletine if such therapy is necessary.

## Disorders of Calcium Channels and Calcium Distribution

### *Hypokalemic Periodic Paralysis*

Hypokalemic periodic paralysis is an autosomal dominant disorder that typically becomes symptomatic after age 6 but before age 30 years. Individuals are apparently normal only to develop episodes of painless paralysis associated with hypokalemia. Attacks often occur at night or with awakening and may follow ingestion of high-carbohydrate or sodium-containing meals (157,158). Weakness can be profound. The patient may not be able to walk and may develop quadriplegia. Attacks usually resolve over 2 to 4 hours but may persist up to 72 hours. They may occur once a day or once in a lifetime (159). Over time, the frequency of attacks decreases and progressive persistent weakness may develop.

During attacks, reflexes are hypoactive or absent but sensation is normal. Myotonia cannot be detected by electromyography. However, eyelid myotonia may be present, even between attacks. These symptoms, as with those observed in other forms of periodic paralysis, are due to a transient inexcitability of muscle fibers (160).

Serum potassium levels are normal except during attacks. Muscle biopsies reveal numerous vacuoles, especially during attacks. Although the exact mechanism is not understood, the disease has been linked to mutations in the dihydropyridine-sensitive calcium channel gene (161).

Treatment is designed to limit the severity and duration of acute attacks and decrease their frequency. Oral potassium at a dose of 25 mEq every 30 minutes is used during acute attacks. Intravenous therapy should be avoided if possible (142). To prevent attacks, patients are advised to take a low-carbohydrate low-sodium diet. In addition, a carbonic anhydrase inhibitor such as acetazolamide or dichlorphenamide may be used. Rarely do these agents actually worsen the condition. In that setting, triamterene or spironolactone may be substituted (142,162).

### *Malignant Hyperthermia*

Malignant hyperthermia is a hereditary disorder characterized by hypercatabolic reactions that can be induced by anesthetic agents or by emotional or physical stress (163,164). The hypercatabolic reactions are due to a sudden increase in the concentration of calcium in the sarcoplasm as a result of a defect in calcium release from the sarcoplasmic reticulum.

Malignant hyperthermia reactions may develop with the first exposure to general anesthesia or, in up to half of individuals, after 1 to as many as 13 previously uneventful inductions (165). The incidence of recognized reactions varies between 1:15,000 anesthetics in children and up to 1:200,000 anesthetics in all age groups. Reactions are more likely if a potent inhaled anesthetic is used with succinylcholine for a long period of time or if the anesthesia was preceded by vigorous exercise, extensive muscle trauma, or fever.

The hypercatabolic reactions include intense muscle rigidity associated with tachycardia and other arrhythmias, hypertension followed by hypotension, hyperventilation, fever, and a flushed appearance followed by a mottled cyanosis. Serum creatine kinase levels increase in proportion to the amount of rhabdomyolysis.

Susceptibility to malignant hyperthermia has an autosomal dominant inheritance with defects in more than one gene potentially responsible. In most individuals, the susceptibility results from a point mutation in the locus for the ryanodine receptor at chromosome 19q13.1 (166). Ryanodine receptors of the sarcoplasmic reticulum associate with dihydropyridine receptors of the transverse tubules coupling the two systems. Calcium release channels occupy the gap between the two receptors. In other families, the candidate appears to be the sodium channel gene located on the long arm of chromosome 17 (167).

The diagnosis is made at the time of anesthesia, but some patients have a history of muscle cramps and aches that develop spontaneously, after exertion, with infections, or with emotional stress. The prevalence of malignant hyperthermia is increased in individuals with Duchenne muscular dystrophy, central core disease, and myotonic dystrophy (168–170).

Serum creatine kinase levels may be normal on increased with no exposure to anesthetic agents in affected and unaffected family members. Electromyographic abnormalities are present in two thirds of individuals. The most common findings include increased numbers of polyphasic action potentials, short-duration action potentials, and fibrillation.

Histology of muscle tissue is usually normal, although fiber size variation, faintly basophilic angular fibers, hypertrophical fibers, and increased numbers of fibers with central nuclei may be observed. Mitochondrial changes can be seen with oxidation enzyme stains and with electron microscopy (165).

The caffeine halothane contracture test can be performed on skeletal muscle biopsy specimens (171,172). This requires meticulous attention to the biopsy itself and the transport and preparation of the tissue. Briefly, strips of muscle are secured by a clamp or suture to a plastic electrode frame immersed in an aerated bathing solution. The other end of each strip is sutured to a force displacement transducer. Muscle fascicles are then stimulated with a platinum plate or prong electrode at a constant rate. Contracture is measured over time in some strips with increasing doses of caffeine added to the bath. Caffeine is known to accelerate calcium release from the sarcoplasmic reticulum. Halothane, an agent known to induce malignant hyperthermia reactions, is added to other strips. The amplitudes of contractures observed are compared with values obtained using normal muscle.

Although malignant hyperthermia reactions can be fatal, survival is expected in over 97% of events. Dantrolene sodium is the agent of choice for the treatment and prevention of reactions (165,173). The actions of this agent inhibit twitch and resting tensions of muscle and in some unknown way prevent the release of calcium from the sarcoplasmic reticulum (174). An analogue of dantrolene, azumolene, can also be used (175).

## Sarcoplasmic Reticulum Calcium-ATPASE Deficiency

In 1969, Brody (176) reported a patient with impaired muscle relaxation that worsened during exercise associated with abnormal calcium flux in sarcoplasmic reticulum. Subsequently, additional cases have been reported, and the specific defect has been identified as a deficiency of sarcoplasmic reticulum calcium-ATPase (177,178).

Symptoms usually begin in childhood with exercise-induced stiffness, cramps, and difficulty with relaxation. Generally, symptoms begin within a few minutes of beginning to exercise. After a few seconds to minutes, exercises can be resumed; however, the time required for muscle relaxation increases. Myalgia at rest and muscle weakness may develop. Exertional rhabdomyolysis has also been reported.

Initially, limb muscles are affected. With time, the process also involves those of the trunk and face. Physical examination will show delayed opening of a clinched fist or delayed opening of closed eyes with furrowing of the brow when the eyes begin to open. Serum creatine kinase levels are normal or minimally elevated. Electromyography is normal with the finding of electrical silence in contracted muscles during the phase of delayed relaxation. Histology of muscles may be normal or show type II fiber atrophy.

The disease results from an absence of the fast-twitch isoform of sarcoplasmic reticulum calcium-ATPase (179). This enzyme is an integral membrane protein and serves to pump calcium out of the cytoplasm into the sarcoplasmic reticulum against a large concentration gradient. The disease is familial with autosomal dominant, autosomal recessive, and X-linked inheritance reported (176,177).

The diagnosis is made by biochemical or immunohistochemical analysis of muscle tissue (180,181). Therapeutic results with dantrolene and verapamil have been mixed (177).

## SECONDARY (OR ACQUIRED) METABOLIC MYOPATHIES

Myopathy can result from a variety of diseases involving the endocrine system, nutritional states, or electrolyte imbalance (Tables 10 and 11). This is easily understood because

**TABLE 10.** *Causes of secondary (acquired) metabolic myopathies*

Endocrine
  Acromegaly
  Hypothyroidism
  Hyperthyroidism
  Hypoparathyroidism
  Addison's disease
  Cushing's disease and syndrome
  Hyperaldosteronism
  Carcinoid syndrome
  Pheochromocytoma
  Diabetic neuromyopathy
Metabolic—nutritional
  Uremia
  Cirrhosis
  Malabsorption
  Vitamin D deficiency
  Vitamin E deficiency
  Lipid metabolism disorders
    Acquired carnitine deficiency
    HMG-CoA reduction inhibitor use
Electrolyte imbalance
  Hyponatremia
  Hypernatremia
  Hypokalemia
  Hyperkalemia
  Hypocalcemia
  Hypercalcemia
  Hypophosphatemia
  Hypomagnesemia

HMG-CoA, 3-hydroxy-3-methylglutaryl coenzyme A.

**TABLE 11.** *Symptoms of myopathy resulting from electrolyte abnormalities*

| Abnormalities | Weakness | Myalgia | Cramps |
|---|---|---|---|
| Hyponatremia | + | − | + |
| Hypernatremia | + | + | + |
| Hypokalemia | + | + | + |
| Hyperkalemia | + | − | − |
| Hypophosphatemia | + | + | + |
| Hypocalcemia | + | − | + |
| Hypercalcemia | + | + | − |
| Hypomagnesemia | + | + | + |

hormones play such an important role in energy metabolism and electrolytes are so crucial for the processes of nerve and muscle function (see Chapter 2). Myopathies are typically manifested by weakness, exercise intolerance resulting from fatigue and postexertional myalgias, cramps, and stiffness. The onset is usually insidious. In these cases, the myopathic changes almost always disappear with successful treatment of the underlying disorder. Some of these disorders, however, can cause rhabdomyolysis (see Chapter 13).

## Endocrine Diseases

### Acromegaly

Approximately half of patients with acromegaly have proximal muscle weakness, myalgia, and reduced exercise tolerance (182). The weakness and fatigue often seem out of proportion to the amount of muscle wasting observed. Weakness of the hands may result from carpal tunnel syndrome. Electromyography reveals myopathic changes, and muscle biopsy shows atrophy and hypertrophy of both type I and type II fibers, excess glycogen content, and increased number of satellite cells (182,183).

## Thyroid Diseases

Myopathic symptoms occur in about 40% of patients with hypothyroidism. These include weakness, fatigue, stiffness, myalgias, and cramps. The latter symptoms may be associated with exercise and aggravated by cold exposure (184). The most characteristic picture of myopathy in hypothyroidism is the combination of proximal weakness, slurring dysarthria, delay in relaxation phase of reflexes, and an elevated serum creatine kinase level (185). Other physical findings may be delayed muscle relaxation (pseudomyotonia) or myoedema, a sustained enlargement caused by a sustained electrically silent contraction that occurs after tapping the muscle with a reflex hammer. Elevations of serum creatine kinase levels may reach levels tenfold of normal, and electromyographic changes of fibrillation and positive waves may be seen (186).

Most patients with hyperthyroidism have objective muscle weakness (187). Commonly there is proximal weakness with variable atrophy. Also common are cramps, myalgias, and fasciculations. Reflexes demonstrate brisk return. Exophthalmos and extraocular muscle dysfunction may result from glycoprotein accumulation and inflammatory changes (188,189). Serum creatine kinase levels are most often normal or low (190) but may be very high when myonecrosis occurs in thyroid storm (191). Electromyography and muscle biopsy typically show nonspecific myopathic changes. A syndrome similar to hypokalemic periodic paralysis may occur in some patients with hyperthyroidism (192). There is an increase of myasthenia gravis in patients with either hypo- or hyperthyroidism (193).

## Disorders of Parathyroid Hormone

Both hypoparathyroidism (parathyroid hormone deficiency) and pseudohypoparathyroidism may be associated with muscle weakness and elevated serum creatine kinase levels (194,195). More commonly, however, patients experience tetany, cramps, and carpopedal spasm. Primary hyperparathyroidism may cause generalized proximal muscle weakness, tongue fasciculations, and hyperreflexia (196,197). Secondary hyperparathyroidism that develops in patients with chronic renal failure can be associated with a primarily lower extremity myopathy (198). That setting in chronic renal failure may be complicated by the coexistence of secondary carnitine deficiency (199).

## Adrenal Gland Disorders

Weakness is a characteristic complaint of patients with adrenal insufficiency whether it is the result of destruction of the gland (Addison's disease) or from the combination of adrenal suppression from corticosteroid usage and lack of adequate replacement therapy (199). The latter situation, sometimes referred to as iatrogenic Addison's disease, usually develops when corticosteroid therapy is withdrawn or in the setting of an infection where the dosage of corticosteroid is inadequate to allow appropriate response to the level of stress. In addition to becoming weak, patients develop gastric upset, diarrhea, and mental status changes, and the disease for which they are taking the corticosteroid flares or becomes more difficult to manage. They may become relatively hypotensive and hypoglycemic. However, in contrast to patients with true Addison's disease who become hyponatremic and hyperkalemic, patients with the idiopathic variety develop only hyponatremia. Serum potassium levels remain normal. The hyponatremia results from an inability to clear free water as a result of cortisol deficiency. Potassium balance is maintained, however, through the action of mineral corticoids.

Over three fourths of patients with Cushing's disease develop a proximal myopathy (200). Serum creatine kinase levels are usually normal, but electromyography may show myopathic changes. Type II fiber atrophy is typically observed on muscle histology (201,202). Similar change can develop in patients taking corticosteroids for treatment of asthma, inflammatory myopathy, or other autoimmune diseases. This may cause a confusing clinical situation in patients with polymyositis. If the patient gets weak or stops improving, is it because the disease is worse, indicating the need for more corticosteroid, or because of the development of steroid myopathy, which would necessitate decreasing the dosage. No diagnostic test is available to answer that question other than to empirically raise or lower the dose of corticosteroid and look for improvement.

An acute severe myopathy can develop within days of initiation of high-dose corticosteroid therapy. This has been termed the "acute necrotizing myopathy of intensive care" (203,204). This is more often seen with intravenous administration and may be triggered by factors related to the underlying disease, immobility, and neuromuscular blockage. It is more frequently encountered in patients requiring mechanical ventilation for treatment of asthma or sepsis. This may be seen in association with critical care polyneuropathy but is more commonly separate (205).

Conn's syndrome or primary aldosteronism is associated with both episodic and generalized weakness (206). These problems are thought to result from hypokalemia.

## Diabetes Mellitus

The more typical clinical picture of diabetic amyotrophy is the abrupt onset of generalized weakness of one extremity resulting from infarction of proximal major nerve trunks. Less commonly, diabetic patients may develop progressive weakness of proximal muscles. This is usually of insidious onset and may be associated with pronounced atrophy. This presentation is believed to result from a proximal intramuscular crural neuropathy (207). In both settings, muscle biopsies show arteriolar occlusions and muscle infarction with necrosis.

## REFERENCES

1. McArdle B. Myopathy due to a defect in muscle glycogen breakdown. *Clin Sci* 1951;24:13–35.
2. Mommaerts WFHM, Illingworth B, Pearson CM, et al. A functional disorder of muscle associated with the absence of phosphorylase. *Proc Natl Acad Sci USA* 1959;45:791–797.
3. Anderson S, Bankier AT, Barrel BG, et al. Sequence and organization of the human mitochondrial genome. *Nature* 1981;290:457–465.
4. Halley DJJ, Konings A, Hupkes P, Glaiard H. Regional mappings of the human gene for lysosomal α-glucosidase by in situ hybridization. *Hum Genet* 1984;67:326–328.
5. Martiniuk F, Bodkin M, Tzall S, Hirschhorn R. Isolation and partial characterization of the structural gene for human acid ψ glucosidase. *DNA Cell Biol* 1991;10:283–292.
6. Engel AG, Hirschorn R. Acid maltase deficiency. In: Engel DG, Franzini-Armstrong C, eds. *Myology*, 2nd ed. New York: McGraw-Hill, 1994:1533–1553.
7. Barohn RJ, McVey AL, DiMauro S. Adult acid maltase deficiency. *Muscle Nerve* 1993;16:672–676.
8. Cimiamon J, Slomin AE, Black KS, et al. Elevation of the lumbar spine in patients with glycogen storage disease: CT demonstrations of paraspinal muscle atrophy. *J Neuroradiol* 1991;12:1099–1103.
9. Kretzchmar HA, Wagner H, Hubner G, et al. Aneurysm and vacuolar degeneration of cerebral arteries in late onset acid maltase deficiency. *J Neurol Sci* 1990;98:169–183.
10. Margolis ML, Hills AR. Acid maltase deficiency in the adult. *Am Rev Respir Dis* 1986;134:328–331.
11. Mobentian S, Puntozzi RL, Daniele P, Fredman H. Treatment of acid maltase deficiency with a diet high in branched-chain aminoacids. *J Parent Ent Nutr* 1990;14:210–212.
12. Issacs H, Savage N, Badenhorst M, Whistle T. Acid maltase deficiency: a case study and review of the pathophysiological changes and proposed therapeutic measures. *J Neurol Neurosurg Psychiatry* 1986;49:1011–1018.
13. Tsujino S. Shanske S, DiMauro S. Molecular heterogeneity of myophosphorylase deficiency. *N Engl J Med* 1993;329:241–245.
14. Tsujino S, Shanske S, Nonaka I, et al. Three new mutations in patients with myophosphorylase deficiency. *Am J Hum Genet* 1994;54:44–52.
15. Tsujino S, Shanske S, Martinuzzi A, et al. Two novel missense mutations in Caucasian patients with myophosphorylase deficiency (McArdle's disease). *Hum Mutat* 1995;6:276–277.
16. Bartram C, Edwards R, Clague J, Beynon R. McArdle's disease a nonsense mutation in exon 1 of the muscle glycogen phosphorylase gene explains some but not all cases. *Hum Mol Genet* 1993;2:1291–1293,
17. Braakhakke JP, de Bruin MI, Stegeman DF, et al. The second wind phenomenon in McArdle's disease. *Brain* 1986;109:1087–1101.
18. Pernow BB, Havel RJ, Jennings DB. The second wind phenomenon in McArdle's syndrome. *Acta Med Scand* 1967;472[Suppl]:294–307.
19. De LaMaza M, Patten BM, Williams JC, Chambers JP. Myophosphorylase deficiency: a new cause of hypotonia simulating infantile muscular atrophy. *Neurology* 1980;30:402.
20. Cornelio F, Bresolin N, DiMauro S, et al. Congenital myopathy due to phosphorylase deficiency. *Neurology* 1983;33:1383–1385.
21. Felice KJ, Schneebaum AB, Royden Jones Jr H. McArdle's disease with late-onset symptoms: case report and review of the literature. *J Neurol Neurosurg Psychiatry* 1992;55:407–408.
22. Wortmann RL. Myositis or myopathy. *J Rheumatol* 1989;16:1525–1527.
23. Fleckenstein JL, Peshock RM, Lewis SF, Haller RG. Magnetic resonance imaging of muscle injury and atrophy in glycolytic myopathies. *Muscle Nerve* 1989;12:849–855.
24. Bendahan D, Confort-Gouncy S, Kozak-Ribbens C, Cozzone PJ. [31]P NMR characterization of the metabolic abnormalities associated with the lack of glycogen phosphorylase activity in human forearm muscle. *Bichoem Biophys Res Commun* 1992;185:16–21.
25. Sahlin K, Areskoa NH, Haller RG, et al. Impaired oxidative metabolism increases adenine nucleotide breakdown in McArdle's disease. *J Appl Physiol* 1990;69:1231–1235.
26. Haller RG, Lewis SF, Cook JD, Blomqvist CG. Myophosphorylase deficiency impairs muscle oxidative metabolism. *Ann Neurol* 1985;17:196–199.

27. Servidei S, Shanske S, Zeviani M, et al. McArdle's disease: biochemical and molecular genetic studies. *Ann Neurol* 1988;24:774–781.
28. Mineo I, Kono N, Hara N, et al. Myogenic hyperuricemia. A common pathophysiologic feature of glycogenosis types III, V, and VII. *N Engl J Med* 1987;317:75–80.
29. Valen PA, Nakayama DA, Veum J, et al. Myoadenylate deaminase deficiency and forearm ischemic exercise testing. *Arthritis Rheum* 1987;30:661–668.
30. DiMauro S, Arnold S, Miranda A, Rowlane P. McArdle's disease: the mystery of reappearing phosphorylase activity in muscle culture. A fetal isoenzyme. *Ann Neurol* 1978;3:60–66.
31. Martinuzzi A, Vergani L, Fanin M, et al. Muscle-type glycogen phosphorylase (M-GP) activity in innervated and non-innervated cultured muscle of McArdle's patients. *J Clin Invest* 1993;92:1774–1780.
32. Slonim A. Gloans P. Myopathy in McArdle's syndrome: improvement with high-protein diet. *N Engl J Med* 1985;312:355–359.
33. Jensen KE, Jakobsen J. Thomsen C, Henriksen O. Improved energy kinetics following high-protein diet in McArdle's syndrome: a 31P magnetic resonance spectroscopy study. *Acta Neurol Scand* 1990;81:499–503.
34. Beyon RJ, Bartram C, Hopkins P, et al. McArdle's disease: molecular genetics and metabolic consequences of the phenotype. *Muscle Nerve* 1995;3:S18–S22.
35. Sernella S, Riepe RE, Langston C, et al. Severe cardiomyopathy in branching enzyme deficiency. *J Pediatr* 1987;111:51–56.
36. Reusche E, Asku F, Goebel HH, et al. A mild juvenile variant of type IV glycogenosis. *Brain Dev* 1992;14:36–43.
37. Bruno C, Servdei S, Shanske S, et al. Glycogen branching enzyme deficiency in adult polyglucosan body disease. *Ann Neurol* 1993;33:88–93.
38. Yang-Feng TL, Zhena K, Yu J, et al. Assignment of the human glycogen debrancher gene to chromosome 1P21. *Genomics* 1992;13:931–934.
39. Coleman R, Winters H, Wolf B, Chen YT. Glycogen debranching enzyme deficiency: long-term study of serum enzyme activities and clinical features. *J Inherit Metab Dis* 1992;15:869–881.
40. Bruno C, Servidei S, Shanske S, et al. Glycogen branching enzyme deficiency in adult polyglucosan body disease. *Ann Neurol* 1993;33:88–93.
41. Huijing F, Fernandes J. X-chromosomal inheritance of live glycogenosis with phosphorylase kinase deficiency. *Am J Hum Genet* 1969;21:275–284.
42. Tonin P, Lewis P, Servidei S, DiMauro S. Metabolic causes of myoglobinuria. *Ann Neurol* 1990;27:181–185.
43. Eishi Y, Takemura T, Sone R, et al. Glycogen storage disease confined to the heart with deficiency activity of cardiac phosphorylase kinase: a new type of glycogen storage disease. *Hum Pathol* 1985;16:193–198.
44. Clemens P, Yamamoto M, Engel AG. Adult phosphorylase b kinase deficiency. *Ann Neurol* 1990;28:529–538.
45. Wilkinson D, Tonin P, Shanske S, et al. Clinical and bio-chemical features of 10 adult patients with muscle phosphorylase kinase deficiency. *Neurology* 1994;44:461–466.
46. Vora S, Miranda AF, Hernandez E, Francke U. Regional assignment of the human gene for platelet-type phosphofructokinase (PFKP) to chromosome 10p, a novel use of polyspecific rodent anti sera to localize human enzyme genes. *Hum Genet* 1993;63:374–379.
47. Sherman JB, Raben N, Nicastri C, et al. Common mutations in the phosphofructokinase-M gene A Ashkenazi: Jewish patients with glycogenosis VII (Tarui's disease) and their population frequency. *Am J Hum Genet* 1994;55:305–313.
48. Raben N, Nichols RC, Boerkoel C, et al. Various classes of mutations in patients with phosphofructokinase deficiency (Tarui's disease). *Muscle Nerve* 1995;3[Suppl]:S39–S44.
49. Sivakumar K, Vasconcelos O, Goldfarb L, Dalakas MC. Late-onset muscle weakness in partial phosphofructokinase deficiency: a unique myopathy with vacuolar, abnormal mitochondria, and an absence of the common exon 5/intron 5 junction point mutation. *Neurology* 1996;46:1337–1342.
50. Lewis SF, Vora S, Haller RG. Abnormal oxidative metabolism and $O_2$ transportion phosphofructokinase deficiency. *J Appl Physiol* 1991;70:391–398.
51. Haller RG, Lewis SF. Glucose-induced exertional fatigue in muscle phosphofructokinase deficiency. *N Engl J Med* 1991;324:364–369.
52. Bertocci LA, Haller RG, Lewis SF, et al. Abnormal high energy phosphate metabolism in human muscle phosphofructokinase deficiency. *J Appl Physiol* 1991;70:1201–1207.
53. Kono N, Mineo I, Shimizu T, et al. Increased plasma uric acid after exercise in muscle phosphofructokinase deficiency. *Neurology* 1986;36:106–108.
54. Mineo I, Tarui S. Myogenic hyperuricemia: what can we learn from metabolic myopathies? *Muscle Nerve* 1995;3[Suppl]:S75–S81.
55. Toyoda H, Nakase T, Tomeoku M, et al. Improvement of hemolysis in muscle phosphofructokinase deficiency by restriction of exercise. *Intern Med* 1996;335:222–226.
56. Tonin P. Shanske S, Miranda AF, et al. Phosphoglycerate kinase deficiency: biochemical and molecular genetic studies in a new myopathic variant (PGK Alberta). *Neurology* 1993;43:387–391.
57. DiMauro S, Dalakas M, Miranda AF. Phosphoglycerate kinase deficiency: a new cause of recurrent myoglobinuria. *Trans Am Neurol Assoc* 1989;106:202–205.
58. Tsujino S, Shanske S, Sakoda S, et al. The molecular genetic basis of muscle phosphoglycerate mutase (PGAM) deficiency. *Am J Hum Genet* 1993;54:472–477.

59. Kanno T, Mackawa M. Lactate dehydrogenase M-subunit deficiencies: clinical features, metabolic background, and genetic heterogeneities. *Muscle Nerve* 1995;3[Suppl]:S54–S60.

60. Bryan W, Lewis SSF, Bertocci L, et al. Muscle lactate dehydrogenase deficiency: a disorder of anaerobic glycogenolysis associated with exertional myoglobinuria. *Neurology* 1990;40:[Suppl]:203.

61. Engel AG, Angelini C. Carnitine deficiency of skeletal muscle associated with lipid storage myopathy: a new syndrome. *Science* 1973;179:899–902.

62. Karpati G, Carpenter S, Engel AG, et al. The syndrome of systemic carnitine deficiency: clinical, morphologic, biochemical and pathophysiologic features. *Neurology* 1975;25:16–24.

63. DiDonata S. Disorders of lipid metabolism affecting skeletal muscle: carnitine deficiency syndromes, defects in the catabolic pathway, and Chanarin disease. In: Engel AG, Franzini-Armstrong C, eds. *Myology*, 2nd ed. New York: McGraw-Hill, 1994:1587–1609.

64. Carrier HM, Berthillier G. Carnitine levels in normal children and adults and in patients with diseased muscle. *Muscle Nerve* 1990;3:326–334.

65. Rebouche CJ, Paulson DJ. Carnitine metabolism and function in humans. *Annu Rev Nutr* 1986;6:41–66.

66. Treem WR, Stanley CA, Finegold DN, et al. Primary carnitine deficiency due to a failure of carnitine transport in kidney, muscle, and fibroblasts. *N Engl J Med* 1998;319:1331–1336.

67. Row PC, Valle D, Brusilow SW. Inborn errors of metabolism referred with Reye's syndrome. A changing pattern. *JAMA* 1988;260:3167–3170.

68. Saudubray JM, Ogier H, Carpenter C. Neonatal management of organic acidurias: clinical update. *J Inherit Metab Dis* 1984;7[Suppl 1]:2–11.

69. Allen RJ, Wong P, Rothenberg SP, et al. Progressive neonatal leukoencephalopathy due to absent methylenetetra hydrofolate reductase, responsive to treatment. *Ann Neurol* 1980;8:211–214.

70. Holme E, Greter J, Jacobson CE. Carnitine deficiency induced by pivampicillin and pivmecillinam therapy. *Lancet* 1989;1:469–470.

71. Laub MC, Paetzke-Brunner I, Jaeger G. Serum carnitine during valproic acid therapy. *Epilepsia* 1986;27:559–562.

72. Cederblad G, Fahraeus L, Lindgren K. Plasma carnitine and renal-carnitine clearance during pregnancy. *Am J Clin Nutr* 1986;44:379–383.

73. Ahmed S, Robertson HT, Golper TA, et al. Multicenter trial of L-carnitine in maintenance hemodialysis patients. II. Clinical and biochemical effects. *Kidney Int* 1990;38:912–918.

74. Turnball DM, Shepherd IM, Ashworth B, et al. Lipid storage myopathy associated with low acyl-CoA dehydrogenase activities. *Brain* 1988;111:815–828.

75. Lindsley HB, Kepes JJ, Tekkanat KK, Wortmann RL. Treatment of carnitine palmityltransferase (CPT) deficiency with L-carnitine and riboflavin. *Arthritis Rheum* 1990;33[Suppl]:S70.

76. Bersen PL, Gabreels FJM, Ruitenbeck W, et al. Successful treatment of pure myopathy, associated with complex I deficiency, with riboflavin and carnitine. *Arch Neurol* 1991;48:334–338.

77. DiMauro S, Melis-DiMauro P. Muscle carnitine palmitoyltransferase deficiency and myoglobinuria. *Science* 1973;182:929–931.

78. Zierz S. Carnitine palmitoyltransferase deficiency. In: Engel AG, Franzini-Armstrong C, eds. *Myology*, 2nd ed. New York: McGraw-Hill, 1994:1577–1586.

79. Ross NS, Hoppel CL. Partial muscle carnitine palmitoyltransferase deficiency. Rhabdomyolysis associated with transiently decreased muscle carnitine content after ibuprofen therapy. *JAMA* 1987;257:62–65.

80. Kieval RI, Sotrel A, Weinblatt ME. Chronic myopathy with a partial deficiency of the carnitine palmitoyltransferase enzyme. *Arch Neurol* 1989;46:575–576.

81. Faigel HC. Carnitine palmitoyltransferase deficiency in a college athlete: a case report and literature review. *J Am Coll Health* 1995;44:51–54.

82. Videen JS, Haseler LJ, Karpinski N, Terkeltaub RA. Noninvasive evaluation of adult onset myopathy form of carnitine palmityltransferase II (CPT II) deficiency using proton magnetic resonance spectroscopy (MRS) of muscle. *J Rheumatol* 1999. (in press).

83. Carey MP, Poulton K, Hawkins C, Murphy RP. Carnitine palmitoyltransferase deficiency with an atypical presentation and ultrastructural mitochondrial abnormalities. *J Neurol Neurosurg Psychiatry* 1987;50: 1060–1070.

84. Stanley CA. New genetic defects in mitochondrial fatty acid oxidation and carnitine deficiency. *Adv Pediatr* 1987;34:59–88.

85. Hale DE, Batshaw ML, Coates PM, et al. Long-chain acyl-CoA dehydrogenase deficiency: an inherited cause of non-ketotic hypoglycemia. *Pediatr Res* 1985;19:666–671.

86. DiDonato S, Taroni F, Gellera C, et al. Long-chain acyl CoA dehydrogenase deficiency in muscle in an adult with lipid myopathy. *Neurology* 1988;38:269A–271A.

87. Turnbull DM, Shepherd IM, Ashworth B, et al. Lipid storage myopathy associated with low acyl-CoA dehydrogenase activities. *Brain* 1988;111:815–828.

88. Jackson S, Kler RS, Bartlett K, et al. Combined enzyme defect of mitochondrial fatty acid oxidation. *J Clin Invest* 1992;90:1219–1225.

89. Schaefer J, Jackson S, Trumball DM. Lipid storage myopathics and inborn errors of fatty acid oxidation. In: Lane RJM, ed. *Handbook of muscle disease*. New York: Marcel Dekker, 1996:431–442.

90. Morgan-Hughes JA. Mitochondrial diseases. In: Engel AG, Franzini-Armstrong C, eds. *Myology*, 2nd ed. New York: McGraw-Hill, 1994:1610–1660.

91. Shanske S, DiMauro S. Diagnosis of the mitochondrial encephalomyopathies. *Curr Opin Rheumatol* 1997;9: 496–503.
92. Zeviani M, Tiranti V, Piantadosi C. Mitochondrial disorders. *Medicine* 1998;77:59–72.
93. Rifai Z, Welle S, Kamp C, Thornton CA. Ragged red fibers in normal aging and inflammatory myopathy. *Ann Neurol* 1995;37:24–29.
94. Hirano M, DiMauro S. Clinical features of mitochondrial myopathies and encephalomyopathies. In Lane RJM, ed. *Handbook of muscle disease*. New York: Marcel Decker, 1996:479–504.
95. Shoubridge EA, Karpati G, Hastings KEM. Deletion mutants are functionally dominant over wild-type mitochondrial genomes in skeletal muscle fiber segments in mitochondrial disease. *Cell* 1990;62:43–49.
96. Linnane AW, Marzuki S, Ozawa T, Tanaka M. Mitochondrial DNA mutations is an important contributor to aging and degenerative diseases. *Lancet* 1989;1:642–645.
97. DiMauro S, Moraes CT. Mitochondrial encephalomyopathies. *Arch Neurol* 1993;50:1197–1207.
98. Moraes CT, DiMauro S, Zeviani M, et al. Mitochondrial DNA deletions in progressive external ophthalmoplegia and Kearns-Sayre syndrome. *N Engl J Med* 1989;320:1293–1299.
99. Holt IJ, Harding AE, Cooper JM, et al. Mitochondrial myopathies: clinical and biochemical features of 30 patients with major deletions of muscle mitochondrial DNA. *Ann Neurol* 1989;26:699–708.
100. McShane MA, Hammans SR, Sweeney M, et al. Pearson syndrome and mitochondrial encepholomyopathy in patients with a depletion of mtDNA. *Am J Hum Genet* 1991;48:39–42.
101. Ohno K, Tanaka M, Sahashi K, et al. Mitochondrial DNA deletions in inherited recurrent myoglobinuria. *Ann Neurol* 1991;29:364–369.
102. Hattori K, Tanaka M, Sugiyama S, et al. Age-dependent increase in deleted mitochondrial DNA in the human heart: possible contributory factor to cardiomyopathy. *Am Heart J* 1991;121:1735–1742.
103. Johhson W, Karpati G, Carpenter S, et al. Late-onset mitochondrial myopathy. *Ann Neurol* 1995;37:16–23.
104. Genge A, Karpati G, Arnold D, et al. Familial myopathy with conspicuous depletion of mitochondria in muscle fibers: a morphologically distinct disease. *Neuromusc Disord* 1995;5:139–144.
105. Kawashima S, Ohta S, Kagawa Y, et al. Widespread tissue distribution of multiple mitochondrial DNA deletions in familial mitochondrial myopathy. *Muscle Nerve* 1994;17:741–746.
106. Lertrit P, Noer A, Jean-Francois M, et al. A new disease-related mutation for mitochondrial encephalomyopathy, lactic acidosis and stroke-like episode (MELAS) syndrome affects the ND4 subunit of the respiratory complex I. *Am J Hum Genet* 1992;51:457–468.
107. Silvestri G, Moraes C, Shanske S, et al. A new mtDNA mutation in the tRNALys gene associated with myoclonic epilepsy and ragged-red fibers (MERRF). *Am J Hum Genet* 1992;51:1213–1217.
108. Zeviani M, Gallera C, Antozzi C, et al. Materially inherited myopathy and cardiomyopathy: associated with mutation in mitochondrial DNA tRNA$^{Leu(UUR)}$. *Lancet* 1991;338:143–147.
109. Silvestri G, Ciafaloni E, Santorelli F, et al. Clinical features associated with the A>G transition at nucleotide 8344 of rtDNA ("MERRF" mutation). *Neurology* 1993;43:1200–1206.
110. Zeviani M, Servidei S, Gallera C, et al. An autosomal dominant disorder with multiple deletions of mitochondrial DNA starting at the D-loop region. *Nature* 1989;339:309–311.
111. Servidei S, Zeviani M, Manfredi M, et al. Dominantly inherited mitochondrial myopathy with multiple deletions of mitochondrial DNA—clinical morphologic and biochemical studies. *Neurology* 1991;41:1053–1059.
112. DiMauro S, Hicano M, Bonilla E, et al. Cytodrome oxidase deficiency: progress and problems. In: Schapira AVH, DeMauro S, eds. *Mitochondrial disorders in neurology*. Boston: Butterworth-Heinemann, 1994:91–115.
113. Sciacco M, Gassparo-Rippe P, Vu TH, et al. Study of mitochondrial depletion in muscle by single-fiber polymerase chain reaction. *Muscle Nerve* 19998;21:1374–1381.
114. Hirano M, Silvestri G, Brake DM, et al. Mitochondrial neuropathy, gastrointestinal encephalomyopathy (MNGIE): clinical, biochemical and genetic features of an autosomal recessive mitochondrial disorder. *Neurology* 1994;44:721–727.
115. Tritschler H-J, Andreeta F, Moraes CT, et al. Mitochondrial myopathy in childhood associated with depletion of mitochondrial DNA. *Neurology* 1992;4:209–217.
116. Chariot P, Monnet I, Mouchet M, et al. Determination of the blood lactate: pyruvate ratio as a noninvasive test for the diagnosis of zidovudine myopathy. *Arthritis Rheum* 1994;37:583–586.
117. Simpson MV, Chin CD, Keilbaugh SA, et al. Studies on the inhibition of mitochondrial DNA replication by 3′azido-3′-deoxythymidine and other dideoxynucleoside analogs which inhibit HIV-I replication. *Biochem Pharm* 1989;38:1033–1036.
118. Bardosi A, Scheidt P, Goebel H. Mitochondrial myopathy: a result of clofibrate/etiofibrate treatment? *Acta Neuropathol (Berl)* 1985;68:164–168.
119. Oldfors A, Moselemi RA, Fyhr IM, et al. Mitochondrial DNA deletions in muscle fibers in inclusion body myositis. *J Neuropathol Exp Neurol* 1995;54:581–587.
120. Blume G, Peesstronk A, Frank B, Johns DR. Polymyositis with cytochrome oxidase negative muscle fibers: early quadriceps weakness and poor response to immunosuppressive therapy. *Brain* 1997;120:39–45.
121. Levine TD, Pestronk A. Inflammatory myopathy with cytochrome oxidase negative muscle fibers: methotrexate treatment. *Muscle Nerve* 1998;21:1724–1728.
122. Harle JR, Pellissier JF, Desnuelle C, et al. Polymyalgia rheumatica and mitochondrial myopathy: clinicopathologic and biochemical studies in five cases. *Am J Med* 1992;92:167–172.

123. Cullen MJ, Fulthorpe JJ. Stages in fiber breakdown in Duchenne muscular dystrophy: an electromicroscopy study. *J Neurol Sci* 1975;24:179–200.

124. Fardeau M. Ultrastructural decisions in progressive muscular dystrophies: a critical study of their specificity. In: Canal N, Scarlato G, Walton JN, eds. *Muscle diseases.* Amsterdam: Exerpta Medica, 1970:98–108.

125. Hudgson P, Bradley W, Jenkinson M. Familial mitochondrial myopathy. Part I. Clinical, electrophysiological and pathological findings. *J Neurol Sci* 1974;16:343–370.

126. Julien J, Vital C, Vallat J, et al. Oculopharyngeal muscular dystrophy: a case with abnormal mitochondrial and fingerprint inclusions. *J Neurol Sci* 1974;21:164–169.

127. Cooper J, Mann V, Kreig D, Schapira A. Human mitochondrial complex I dysfunction. *Biochem Biophys Acta* 1992;1601:1988–1203.

128. Guarino M, Tarateta A, DiStefano A. Mitochondrial cytopathy in familial periodic hypokalemic paralysis. *Lancet* 1984;2:49.

129. Harding HE. Growing old: the most common mitochondrial disease of all? *Nat Genet* 1992;2:251–252.

130. Campos Y, Huertas R, Lorenzo G, et al. Plasma carnitine insufficiency and effectiveness of L-carnitine therapy in patients with mitochondrial myopathy. *Muscle Nerve* 1993;16:150–153.

131. Tarnopolsky MA, Roy BD, MacDonald JR. A randomized, controlled trial of creatine monohydrate in patients with mitochondrial cytopathies. *Muscle Nerve* 1997;20:1502–1507.

132. Vianey-Liaud C, Divry P, Gregersen N, Mathieu M. The inborn errors of mitochondrial fatty acid oxidation. *J Inherit Metab Dis* 1987;10[Suppl 1]:159–198.

133. Bouzidi MF, Schagger H, Collombet JM, et al. Decreased expression of ubiquinol-cytochrome C reductase subunits in patients exhibiting mitochondrial myopathy with progressive exercise intolerance. *Neuromusc Disord* 1993;3:599–604.

134. Ogasahara S, Engel AG, Frens D, Mack D. Muscle coenzyme $Q_{10}$ deficiency in familial mitochondrial encephalopathy. *Proc Natl Acad Sci USA* 1989;86:2379–2387.

135. Sabina RL, Morisaki T, Clarke P, et al. Characterization of the human and rat myoadenylate deaminase genes. *J Biol Chem* 1990;265:9423–9433.

136. Morisaki T, Gross M, Morisaki H, et al. Molecular basis of AMP deaminase deficiency in skeletal muscle. *Proc Natl Acad Sci USA* 1992;89:6457–6461.

137. Fishbein WN. Myoadenylate deaminase deficiency: inherited and acquired forms. *Biochem Med* 1985;33:158–169.

138. Sabina RL, Holmes EW. Myoadenylate deaminase deficiency. In: Scriver CR, Beaudet AL, Sly WS, Valle D, eds. *The metabolic basis of inherited disease*, 7th ed. New York: McGraw-Hill, 1995:1769–1780.

139. Sabina RL, Sulaiman AR, Wortmann RL. Molecular analysis of acquired myoadenylate deaminase deficiency in polymyositis (idiopathic inflammatory myopathy). *Adv Exp Biol Med* 1991;309B:203–205.

140. Morisaki H, Morisaki T, Newby LK, Holmes EW. Alternative splicing: a mechanism for phenotypic rescue of a common inherited defect. *J Clin Invest* 1993;91:2275–2280.

141. Rüdel R, Lehmann-Horn F. Membrane changes in cells from myotonia patients. *Physiol Rev* 1985;65:310–356.

142. Ptáček L. The familial periodic paralysis and nondystrophic myotonias. *Am J Med* 1998;104:58–70.

143. Ptáček LJ, Johnson KJ, Griggs RC. Genetics and physiology of the myotonic muscle disorders. *N Engl J Med* 1993;328:482–489.

144. Ricker K, Camancho L, Grafe P, et al. Adynamia episodica hereditaria: what causes the weakness? *Muscle Nerve* 1989;10:883–891.

145. Ptáček LJ, George AL, Jr, Griggs RC, et al. Identification of a mutation in the skeletal muscle $Na^+$ channel alpha-subunit in hypokalemic periodic paralysis. *Cell* 1991;67:1021–1027.

146. Rojas CV, Wang JZ, Schwartz LS, et al. Met-to-Val mutation in the skeletal muscle $Na^+$ channel alpha-subunit in hyperkalemic periodic paralysis. *Nature* 1991;354:387–389.

147. Clausen T, Regulation of active $Na^+$-$K^+$ transport in skeletal muscle. *Physiol Rev* 1986;66:542–580.

148. Kicker K, Böhlen R, Rohkamm R. Different effectiveness of tocanide and hydrochlorothiazide in paramyotonia congenita with hyperkalemic episodic paralysis. *Neurology* 1983;33:1615–1618.

149. Carson MJ, Pearson CM. Familiar hyperkalemic periodic paralysis with myotonic features. *J Pediatr* 1964;64:853–865.

150. Jackson CE, Barohn RJ, Ptáček LJ. Paramyotonia congenita: abnormal short exercise test and improvement after mexiletine therapy. *Muscle Nerve* 1994;17:763–768.

151. deSilva SM, Kunel RW, Griffin JW, et al. Paramyotonia congenita or hyperkalemic periodic paralysis? Clinical and electrophysiological features of each entity in one family. *Muscle Nerve* 1990;13:21–26.

152. Trudell RG, Kaiser KK, Griggs RC. Acetazolamide-responsive myotonia congenita. *Neurology* 1987;37:488–491.

153. Poskanzer DC, Kerr DNS. A third type of periodic paralysis with normokalemia and favorable response to sodium chloride. *Am J Med* 1961;31:328–341.

154. Lerche H, Heine R, Pika U, et al. Human sodium channel myotonia: slowed channel inactivation due to substitution for a glycine within the III/IV linker. *J Physiol* 1993;470:13–23.

155. Abdalla JA, Casley WL, Cousin HK, et al. Linkage of Thomsen disease to the T-cell-receptor beta (TCRB) locus on chromosome 7q35. *Am J Hum Genet* 1992;51:579–584.

156. Koch MC, Steinmeyer K, Lorenz C, et al. The skeletal muscle chloride channel in dominant and recessive human myotonia. *Science* 1992;257:797–800.

157. Riggs JE. Periodic paralysis. *Clin Neuropharmacol* 1989;12:249–257.
158. Kantola IM, Tarssanen LT. Familial hypokalemic periodic paralysis in Finland. *J Neurol Neurosurg Psychiatry* 1992;55:322–324.
159. Gamstrop I. Disorders characterized by spontaneous attacks of weakness connected with changes of serum potassium. *Prog Clin Biol Res* 1989;306: 175–195.
160. Rüdel R, Ricker K. The periodic paralysis. *Trends Neurosci* 1985;8:467–470.
161. Fouad G, Dalakas M, Servedei S, et al. Genotype-phenotype correlations of DHP receptor alpha-1 gene mutations causing hypokalemic periodic paralysis. *Neuromusc Disord* 1997;7:33–38.
162. Torres CF, Griggs RC, Moxley RT, Bender AN. Hypokalemic periodic paralysis exacerbated by acetazolamide. *Neurology* 1981;31:1423–1428.
163. Gronert GA. Malignant hyperthermia. In: Engel AF, Franzini-Armstrong C, eds. *Myology*, 2nd ed. New York: McGraw-Hill, 1994:1661–1678.
164. Britt BA. Malignant hyperthermia. In: Lane RJM, ed. *Handbook of muscle disease*. New York: Marcel Dekker, 1996:451–471.
165. Britt BA. Malignant hyperthermia—a review. In: Schonbaum E, Lomax P, eds. *Thermoregulation: pathology, pharmacology and therapy*. New York: Pergamon Press, 1991:179–292.
166. Gillard EF, Otsu K, Fujii J, et al. A substitution of cysteine for arginine 614 in the ryanodine receptor is potentially causative of human malignant hyperthermia. *Genomics* 1991;11:1751–1757.
167. Okkers A, Meyers DA, Meyers S, et al. Adult muscle sodium channel α-subunit is a gene candidate for malignant hyperthermia susceptibility. *Genomics* 1992;14:829–831.
168. Harriman DGF, Ellis FR. Central core disease and malignant hyperthermia. *Br Med J* 1973;1:545.
169. Lehmann-Horn F, Iaizzo PA, Klein W. Neuromuscular diseases and the association to malignant hyperthermia. *J Neurol Sci* 1990;98:135.
170. Kansch K, Lehmann-Horn F, Janka M, et al. Evidence for linkage of the central core disease locus to the proximal arm of human chromosome 19. *Genomics* 1991;10:765–769.
171. European MH Group. A protocol for the investigation of malignant hyperthermia (MH) susceptibility. *Br J Anaesth* 1984;56:1267–1269.
172. Larach MG. Standardization of the caffeine halothane muscle contraction test. *Anesth Analg* 1989;69:511–515.
173. Britt BA, Scott E, Frodis W, et al. Dantrolene. In vivo studies in malignant hyperthermia susceptible (MHS) and normal muscle. *Can Anaesth Soc J* 1984;31:130–154.
174. Lopez JR, Lopez M, Allen P. Dantrolene reduces myoplasmic free $Ca^{2+}$ in patients with malignant hyperthermia. *Acta Cient Venezol* 1990;461:135–137.
175. Leslie GC, Part NJ. The effect of EU4093 (azumolene sodium) on the contraction of intrafusal muscle of the skeletal muscle of the anesthetized rat. *Br J Pharmacol* 1989;97:1151–1156.
176. Brody I. Muscle contracture induced by exercise: a syndrome attributed to decreased relaxing factor. *N Engl J Med* 1969;281:187–192.
177. Karpati G, Charuk J, Carpenter S, et al. Myopathy caused by a deficiency of $Ca^{2+}$ adenosine triphosphatase in sarcoplasmic reticulum (Brody's disease). *Ann Neurol* 1986;20:38–49.
178. Poels PJE, Wevers RA, Braakhekke JP, et al. Exertional rhabdomyolysis in a patient with Ca-ATPase deficiency. *J Neurol Neurosurg Psychiatry* 1993;56:823–826.
179. Brandl CJ, deLeon S, Martin DR, MacLennon DH. Adult forms of the $Ca^{2+}$ ATPase of sarcoplasmic reticulum: expression in developing skeletal muscle. *J Biol Chem* 1987;262: 3768–3774.
180. Benders AAGM, Timmermans JAH, Oosterhof A. Deficiency of $Na^{+}/K^{+}$-ATPase and SR Ca-ATPase in skeletal muscle and cultured muscle cells of myotonic dystrophy patients. *Biochem J* 1993;293:269–274.
181. Benders AAGM, Veerkamp JH, Oosterhof A, et al. $Ca^{2+}$ homeostasis in Brody's disease: a study in skeletal muscle and cultural muscle cells and the effects of dantrolene and verapamil. *J Clin Invest* 1994;94:741–748.
182. Khaleeli AA, Levy RD, Edwards RHT, et al. The neuromuscular features of acromegaly: a clinical and pathological study. *J Neurol Neurosurg Psychiatry* 1984;47:1009–1015.
183. Mastaglia FL. Pathological changes in skeletal muscle in acromegaly. *Acta Neuropathol* 1973;24:273–286.
184. Wilson J, Walton JN. Some muscular manifestations of hypothyroidism. *J Neurol Neurosurg Psychiatry* 1959; 22:320–324.
185. Wise MP, Blunt S, Lane RJM. Neurological presentations of hypothyroidism: the importance of slow relaxing reflexes. *J R Soc Med* 1995;88:272–274.
186. Venables GS, Bates D, Show DA. Hypothyroidism with true myotonia. *J Neurol Neurosurg Psychiatry* 1978; 41:1013–1015.
187. Ramsay ID. Muscle dysfunction in hyperthyroidism. *Lancet* 1966;2:931–934.
188. Kaminski HJ, Ruff RL. Endocrine myopathies (hyper- and hypofunction of adrenal, thyroid, pituitary, and parathyroid glands and iatrogenic corticosteroid myopathy). In: Engel AG, Franzini-Armstrong C, eds. *Myology*, 2nd ed. New York: McGraw-Hill, 1994:1726–1753.
189. Hallin E, Feldon SSE. Graves ophthalmopathy. II. Correlation of clinical signs with measures derived from computed tomography. *Br J Ophthalmol* 1998;72:678–682.
190. Docherty I, Harrop JS, Hine KR, et al. Myoglobin concentration, creatine kinase activity, and creatine kinase B subunit concentration in serum during thyroid disease. *Clin Chem* 1984;30:42–45.
191. Bennett WR, Huston DP. Rhabdomyolysis in thyroid storm. *Am J Med* 1984;77:733–735.
192. Satoyoshi E, Murakami K, Koine H, et al. Periodic paralysis in hyperthyroidism. *Neurology* 1963;13:746–752.

193. Kiessling WR, Pflughaupt KW, Ricker K, et al. Thyroid function and circulating antithyroid antibodies in myasthenia gravis. *Neurology* 1981;31:771–774.
194. Yamaguchi H, Okamoto K, Shooji M, et al. Muscle histology of hypocalcemic myopathy in hypoparathyroidism. *J Neurol Neurosurg Psychiatry* 1987;50:817–818.
195. Cape CA. Phosphorylase A deficiency in pseudohypoparathyroidism. *Neurology* 1969;19:167–172.
196. Patten BM, Bilezidian JP, Mallette LE, et al. Neuromuscular involvement in primary hyperparathyroidism. *Ann Intern Med* 1974;80:182–193.
197. Frame B, Heinze EG, Block MA, Manson GA. Myopathy in primary hyperthyroidism. *Ann Intern Med* 968;68: 1022–1027.
198. Floyd M, Ayyar DR, Barwick DD, et al. Myopathy in chronic renal failure. *Q J Med* 1974;43:509–524.
199. Mor F, Green P, Wysenbeek AJ. Myopathy in Addison's disease. *Ann Rheum Dis* 1987;46:81–83.
200. Rothstein JM, Delitto A, Sinacore DR, Rose SJ. Muscle function in rheumatic disease patients treated with corticosteroids. *Muscle Nerve* 1983;6:128–135.
201. Lacomis D, Chad DA, Aronin N, Smith TW. The myopathy of Cushing's syndrome. *Muscle Nerve* 1993;16: 880–881.
202. Rebuffe-Scrive M, Krotkiewshi M, Elfverson J, Bjorntorp P. Muscle adipose tissue morphology and metabolism in Cushing's syndrome. *J Clin Endocrinol Metab* 1988;67:1122–1128.
203. Ramsay DA, Zochondne DW, Robertson DM, et al. A syndrome of acute severe muscle necrosis in intensive care unit patients. *J Neurol* 1993;52:387–398.
204. Hanson P, Dive A, Brucher J-M, et al. Acute corticosteroid myopathy in intensive care patients. *Muscle Nerve* 1997;20:1371–1380.
205. Lacomis D, Petrella JT, Guiliani MJ. Causes of neuromuscular weakness in the intensive care unit: a study of ninety-two patients. *Muscle Nerve* 1998;21:610–617.
206. Conn JW, Knopf RF, Nesbit RM. Clinical characteristics of primary aldosteronism from analysis of 145 cases. *Am J Surg* 1964;107:159–172.
207. Barohn RJ, Kissel JT. Painful thigh mass in a young woman: diabetic muscle infarction. *Muscle Nerve* 1992; 15:850–855.

*Diseases of Skeletal Muscle,*
edited by Robert L. Wortmann.
Lippincott Williams & Wilkins, Philadelphia © 2000

# 10

# Congenital Myopathies

## Edward H. Bossen

*Department of Pathology, Duke University School of Medicine and Duke University
Medical Center, Durham, North Carolina 27710*

Congenital myopathies are present at birth and have distinctive morphologic findings. There are many such disorders, most extremely rare, but three are the best known and most widely discussed in the literature: central core disease, nemaline myopathy, and centronuclear (or myotubular) myopathy. Although called congenital myopathies, all three have been discovered to have forms that become evident later in life.

### CENTRAL CORE DISEASE

Shy and Magee (1) first described this disorder in 1956. In most individuals, central core disease is a mild nonprogressive congenital myopathy that presents with proximal weakness. It can begin early, however, with significant hypotonia ("floppy baby") or delayed development. In older individuals, the weakness can range from barely perceptible

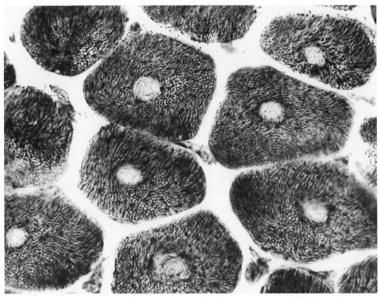

**FIG. 1.** Central core disease is characterized by a central area of decreased staining with oxidative enzyme stains nicotinamide adenine dinucleotide (reduced) tetrazolium reductase (NADH-TR) magnification ×520.

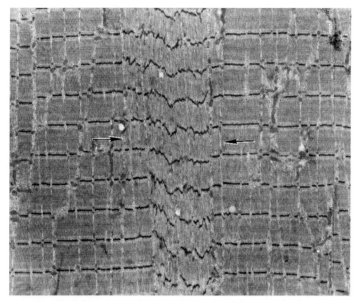

**FIG. 2.** Reasonably well-aligned myofibrils are seen in structured cores (between the arrows). Magnification ×5,250.

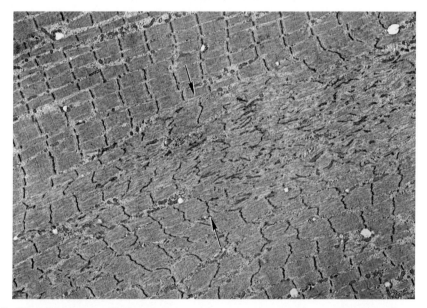

**FIG. 3.** Disorganized myofibrils are present in an unstructured core (between the arrows). Magnification ×5,250.

to mild facial weakness to generalized weakness (2). Other abnormalities include pes cavus, lumbar lordosis, kyphoscoliosis, and congenital hip dislocation (3,4). Muscle atrophy is usually mild. Tendon reflexes are usually normal but may be decreased or absent (2).

Central core disease may be associated with malignant hyperthermia (5,6). Even healthy family members of a central core disease patient may be susceptible to malignant hyperthermia (7). On the other hand, not all central core disease patients are susceptible to malignant hyperthermia, and certainly not all malignant hyperthermia patients have central core disease (8).

The genetic linkage is to the locus 19q13.1, which codes for the skeletal muscle ryanodine receptor RYR1 (9–12). The ryanodine receptor is located in the terminal cisternae of the sarcoplasmic reticulum disease (13) and transfers calcium from this site to the cytoplasm in response to depolarization (9). Four RYR1 mutations affecting amino acids between Cys 35 and Arg 614 or Arg 2162 and Arg 2458 have been described (14,15).

Morphologically, the muscle fibers show few changes on hemotoxylin and eosin stain other than a few hypertrophic and atrophic fibers with increased internal nuclei. Histochemical staining may reveal marked type I fiber predominance (16,17). An oxidative enzyme stain (e.g., NADH-TR) will reveal a central pale zone in the type I fibers (Fig. 1). They resemble target or targetoid fibers. Electron microscopic studies demonstrate two types of cores, structured and unstructured. The structured cores (Fig. 2) maintain cross striations, whereas the unstructured do not (Fig. 3) (16). Cores run the length of the fibers, whereas target and targetoid fibers involve limited numbers of sarcomeres (18).

## NEMALINE MYOPATHY

Nemaline myopathy was described and named in 1963 by Shy et al. (19). The term "nemaline" is derived from the Greek *nema*, or thread. Conen et al. (20) described the same findings as myogranules also in 1963. There are several forms of the disease: severe neonatal, classic benign congenital, adult, and human immunodeficiency virus (HIV)-associated. The neonatal form is usually fatal (21), primarily because of respiratory problems (22).

Most patients with congenital or infantile classic form have a mild nonprogressive myopathy. There may be feeding difficulty and delayed motor milestones (23). Kyphoscoliosis, pes cavus, high arch palate, an elongated face, and wasting of muscles, particularly paraspinal and proximal limb muscles, are seen (24). Extraocular muscles are not affected (23). Deep tendon reflexes may be absent (25). Hand tremors (mini-polymyoclonus) similar to that seen in spinal muscular atrophy have been described (26). Rarely, cardiac involvement is present (27).

The principal clinical findings in adult-onset nemaline myopathy are muscle weakness and wasting, particularly of the limb-girdle and proximal muscles. Neck extensors may be involved (28). Patients with adult onset may also have respiratory insufficiency, which could be the presenting manifestation (29). Immunologic disorders and dysphagia may develop (30). The creatine kinase may be normal or mildly elevated. Electromyography is generally myopathic (23).

Patients with an acquired HIV-associated nemaline myopathy are similar to other adult-onset patients. The myopathy may be the first sign of HIV infection or manifest latter as a component of acquired immunodeficiency syndrome (31).

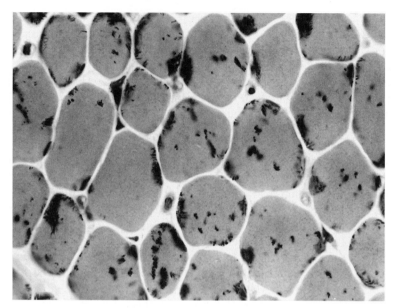

**FIG. 4.** Numerous dark rodlike bodies are present. Trichrome, magnification ×680.

Histologically, in classic cases one finds the muscle biopsy to have scattered or clustered rounded atrophic fibers with only mild fibrosis and, rarely, degenerating fibers. Atypical cases have been reported with loss or disarray of the myofibrils (21). Rod-shaped bodies, about 1 μm in diameter and a few microns long, are present within the cytoplasm of many fibers. These can be seen as dark red objects with the modified Gomori trichrome stain of frozen sections (Fig. 4). The rods are difficult to see in paraffin-embedded sections but can be demonstrated with the phosphotungstic acid hematoxylin stain (24). They are better demonstrated by electron microscopy (Fig. 5). Both type I and type II fibers may be affected, although the changes are primarily seen in type I fibers, which generally are predominant (23). Muscle spindle fibers (intrafusal fibers) may have rods (32). Intranuclear rods have been reported (33).

Electron microscopy demonstrates the rods to resemble Z-disk material, and frequently they are associated with the Z disk. Studies have demonstrated that the principal component is α-actinin (28), but desmin is also present (27). It has been suggested that the basic problem is the failure of a mechanism that restricts α-actinin to the Z disk (34). Some childhood-onset cases show an increase in the number of rods over time. The number of rods do not correlate with the severity of the disorder (35). Rarely, rods have been described in the heart (27,36). Smooth muscle is not affected (37).

Genetic studies have shown the disorder can be transmitted by autosomal recessive, autosomal dominant, or sporadic inheritance (38). The candidate gene for the adult form is located on chromosome 1p13-1q25 (39), but abnormalities of chromosome 2q have been demonstrated in some (40).

The HIV-associated nemaline myopathy (31,41) differs from the usual adult-onset nemaline myopathy in that it may demonstrate other abnormalities such as fiber necrosis and vacuoles. Also, the rods are smaller than seen in the standard nemaline myopathy (42). Loss of thick filmanets has also been reported (43).

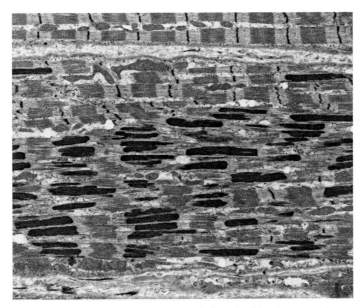

**FIG. 5.** Rectangular nemaline rods are obvious in this electron micrograph. Magnification ×7,500.

## CENTRONUCLEAR (MYOTUBULAR) MYOPATHY

Centronuclear myopathy, also known as myotubular myopathy, was first described as myotubular myopathy by Spiro et al. (44) and as centronuclear myopathy by Sher et al. (45). There are three forms of the disease, which vary in time of onset, severity, and genetic transmission: severe X-linked myotubular myopathy, infantile and early childhood centronuclear myopathy, and late childhood or adult-onset centronuclear myopathy.

Hypotonia, global weakness with a weak cry and feeding, delayed motor milestones, external ophthalmoplegia, and ptosis are common findings during infancy (46). The face is long and thin. Greater than normal body length and long digits are frequent (47). Atrophy and areflexia are common (48). Cardiomyopathy of uncertain origin has rarely been reported (49). Ninety percent of the X-linked myotubular myopathy patients will usually die of respiratory failure (50). In the other forms, the disease is slowly progressive or nonprogressive. Some adult-onset cases may have signs of the disease in childhood. The creatine kinase is usually normal but can be elevated. Electromyographic studies are myopathic, although some neuropathic features may be seen (48).

The diagnosis is established by muscle biopsy. The muscle biopsy demonstrates type I fiber predominance. The diagnostic feature is the presence of central nuclei in numerous muscle fibers (Fig. 6). The exact percentage required for the diagnosis has not been established, but it is reasonable to expect at least 30% to 50% of the fibers on cross-section to demonstrate internal nuclei. When the muscle fibers are examined longitudinally, one sees the internal nuclei separated by internuclear space (Fig. 7). Because a cross-section of the muscle will necessarily transect some fibers at the level of nuclei and some at the level of the intranuclear space, internal nuclei will not be seen in all muscle fibers in a given cross-section. Internal nuclei in skeletal muscle are to be expected during the developmental stages, up to approximately 16 weeks of gestational age. After that time,

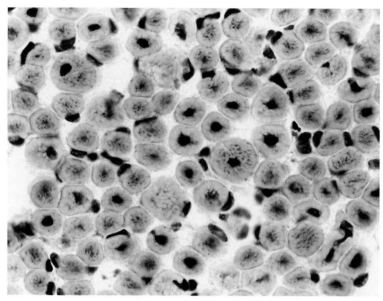

**FIG. 6.** Muscle cross-section of an infant with centronuclear myopathy demonstrating a high percentage of internal nuclei. Central nuclei are not seen in some fibers in the cross-section because the plane of section is through the internuclear space (see longitudinal section, Fig. 7). Hemotoxylin & eosin, magnification ×680.

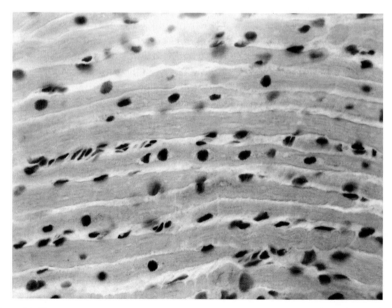

**FIG. 7.** Longitudinal section of muscle of a patient with centronuclear myopathy. Hemotoxylin & eosin, magnification ×680.

most nuclei will be at the periphery of the muscle fiber. Myotonic dystrophy should be considered in the differential diagnosis because selected muscles, particularly the muscles of respiration, may have a high percentage of internal nuclei (51).

Genetic studies indicate that the severe congenital form is X-linked and has been localized to Xq28. More specifically, the gene has been demonstrated to normally produce a protein referred to as myotubularin (52,53). The more benign infantile, childhood, and adult forms may be either autosomal dominant or recessive. In addition, sporadic cases are reported (54). The cause of this disorder is unclear, although some suspect that at least the X-linked form represents delayed muscle maturation (1).

## REFERENCES

1. Shy GM, Magee KR. A new congenital non-progressive myopathy. *Brain* 1956;79:610–621.
2. Ramsey PL, Hensinger RN. Congenital dislocation of the hip associated with central core disease. *J Bone Joint Surg* 1975;57A:648–651.
3. Shuaib A, Paasuke RT, Brownell AKW. Central core disease. Clinical features in 13 patients. *Medicine* 1987;66:389–396.
4. Armstrong RM, Koenigsberger R, Mellinger J, Lovelace RE. Central core disease with congenital hip dislocation: study of two families. *Neurology* 1971;21:369–376.
5. Denborough MA, Dennett X, Anderson RM. Central-core disease and malignant hyperpyrexia. *Br Med J* 1973; 1:272–273.
6. Loke J, MacLennan DH. Malignant hyperthermia and central core disease: disorders of $Ca^2$ release channels. *Am J Med* 1998;104:470–486.
7. Islander G, Henriksson K-G, Ranklev-Twetman E. Malignant hyperthermia susceptibility without central core disease (CCD) in a family where CCD is diagnosed. *Neuromusc Disord* 1995;5:125–127.
8. Halsall PJ, Bridges LR, Ellis FR, Hopkins PM. Should patients with central core disease be screened for malignant hyperthermia? *J Neurol Neurosurg Psychiatry* 1996;61:119–121.
9. Greenberg DA. Calcium channels in neurological disease. *Ann Neurol* 1997;42:275–282.
10. Mulley JC, Kozman HM, Phillips HA, et al. Refined genetic localization for central core disease. *Am J Hum Genet* 1993;52:398–405.
11. MacLennan DH, Duff C, Zorzato F, et al. Ryanodine receptor gene is a candidate for predisposition to malignant hyperthermia. *Nature* 1990;343:559–561.
12. Kausch K, Lehmann-Horn F, Janka M, et al. Evidence for linkage of the central core disease locus to the proximal long arm of human chromosome 19. *Genomics* 1991;10:765–769.
13. Phillips MS, Fujii J, Khanna VK, et al. The structural organization of the human skeletal muscle ryanodine receptor (RYR1) gene. *Genomics* 1996;34:24–41.
14. Zhang Y, Chen HS, Khanna VK, et al. A mutation in the human ryanodine receptor gene associated with central core disease. *Nat Genet* 1993;5:46–50.
15. Otsu K, Nishida K, Kimura Y, et al. The point mutation $Arg^{615} \rightarrow$ Cys in the $Ca^{2+}$ release channel of skeletal sarcoplasmic reticulum is responsible for hypersensitivity to caffeine and halothane in malignant hyperthermia. *J Biol Chem* 1994;269:9413–9415.
16. Gonatas NK, Perez MC, Shy GM, Evangelista I. Central core disease of skeletal muscle. Ultrastructural and cytochemical observations in two cases. *Am J Pathol* 1965;47:503–524.
17. Dubowitz V, Roy S. Central core disease of muscle: clinical, histochemical and electron microscopic studies of an affected mother and child. *Brain* 1970;93:133–146.
18. Carpenter S and Karpati G. Central core disease. In: *Pathology of skeletal muscle*. New York: Churchill Livingstone, 1984:435–441.
19. Shy GM, Engel WK, Somers JE, Wanko T. Nemaline myopathy. A new congenital myopathy. *Brain* 1963;86: 793–821.
20. Conen PE, Murphy EG, Donohue WL. Light and electron microscopic studies of myogranules in a child with hypotonia and muscle weakness. *Can Med Assoc J* 1963;89:983–986.
21. Schmalbruch H, Kamieniecka Z, Arrœ M. Early fatal nemaline myopathy: case report and review. *Dev Med Child Neurol* 1987;29:800–804.
22. Sasaki M, Takeda M, Kobayashi K, Nonaka I. Respiratory failure in nemaline myopathy. *Pediatr Neurol* 1997; 16:344–346.
23. North KN, Laing NG, Wallgren-Pettersson C, ENMC International Consortium on Nemaline Myopathy. Nemaline myopathy: current concepts. *J Med Genet* 1997;34:705–713.
24. Engel WK, Wanko T, Fenichel GM. Nemaline myopathy. A second case. *Arch Neurol* 1964;11:22–39.
25. Hudgson P, Gardner-Medwin D, Fulthorpe JJ, Walton JN. Nemaline myopathy. *Neurology* 1967;17:1125–1142.
26. Colamaria V, Zanetti R, Simeone M, et al. Minipolymyoclonus in congenital nemaline myopathy: a nonspecific clinical marker of neurogenic dysfunction. *Brain Dev* 1991;13:358–362.

27. Ishibashi-Ueda H, Imakita M, Yutani C, et al. Congenital nemaline myopathy with dilated cardiomyopathy: an autopsy study. *Hum Pathol* 1990;21:77–82.
28. Engel WK, Oberc MA. Abundant nuclear rods in adult-onset rod disease. *J Neuropathol Exp Neurol* 1975;34: 119–132.
29. Falgà-Tirado C, Pérez-Pemán P, Ordi-Ros J, et al. Adult onset of nemaline myopathy presenting as respiratory insufficiency. *Respiration* 1995;62:353–354.
30. Gyure KA, Prayson RA, Estes ML. Adult-onset nemaline myopathy. A case report and review of the literature. *Arch Pathol Lab Med* 1997;121:1210–1213.
31. Cabello A, Martínez-Martín P, Gutiérrez-Rivas E, Madero S. Myopathy with nemaline structures associated with HIV infection. *J Neurol* 1990;237:64–66.
32. Karpati G, Carpenter S, Andermann F. A new concept of childhood nemaline myopathy. *Arch Neurol* 1971;24: 291–304.
33. Goebel HH, Warlo I. Nemaline myopathy with intranuclear rods-intranuclear rod myopathy. *Neuromusc Disord* 1997;7:13–19.
34. Morris EP, Nneji G, Squire JM. The three-dimensional structure of the nemaline rod Z-band. *J Cell Biol* 1990; 111:2961–2978.
35. Wallgren-Pettersson C, Rapola J, Donner M. Pathology of congenital nemaline myopathy. A follow-up study. *J Neurol Sci* 1988;83:243–257.
36. Meier C, Gertsch M, Zimmerman A, et al. Nemaline myopathy presenting as cardiomyopathy. *N Engl J Med* 1983;308:1536–1537.
37. Matsuo T, Tashiro T, Ideka T, et al. Fatal neonatal nemaline myopathy. *Acta Pathol Jpn* 1982;32:907–916.
38. Wallgren-Pettersson C, Laing N. 40th ENMC Sponsored International Workshop: nemaline myopathy. *Neuromusc Disord* 1996;6:389–391.
39. Laing NG, Majda BT, Akkari PA, et al. Assignment of a gene (NEM1) for autosomal dominant nemaline myopathy to chromosome 1. *Am J Hum Genet* 1992;50:576–583.
40. Wallgren-Pettersson C, Avela K, Marchand S, et al. A gene for autosomal recessive nemaline myopathy assigned to chromosome 2q by linkage analysis. *Neuromusc Disord* 1995;6:441–443.
41. Dalakas MC, Pezeshkpour GH, Flaherty M. Progressive nemaline (rod) myopathy associated with HIV infection. *N Engl J Med* 1987;317:1602–1603.
42. Feinberg DM, Spiro AJ, Weidenheim KM. Distinct light microscopic changes in human immunodeficiency virus-associated nemaline myopathy. *Neurology* 1998;50:529–531.
43. Gonzales MF, Olney RK, So YT, et al. Subacute structural myopathy associated with human immunodeficiency virus infection. *Arch Neurol* 1988;45:585–587.
44. Spiro AJ, Shy GM, Gonatas NK. Myotubular myopathy. *Arch Neurol* 1966;14:1–14.
45. Sher JH, Rimalovski AB, Athanassiades TJ, Aronson SM. Familial centronuclear myopathy: a clinical and pathological study. *Neurology* 1967;17:727–742.
46. Heckmatt JZ, Sewry CA, Hodes D, Dubowitz V. Congenital centronuclear (myotubular) myopathy. A clinical, pathological and genetic study in eight children. *Brain* 1985;108:941–964.
47. Joseph M, Pai GS, Holden KR, Herman G. X-linked myotubular myopathy: clinical observation in ten additional cases. *Am J Med Genet* 1995;59:168–173.
48. Zanoteli E, Oliveira ASB, Schmidt B, Gabbai AA. Centronuclear myopathy: clinical aspects of ten Brazilian patients with childhood onset. *J Neurol Sci* 1998;158:76–82.
49. Verhiest W, Brucher JM, Goddeeris P, et al. Familial centronuclear myopathy associated with "cardiomyopathy." *Br Heart J* 1976;38:504–509.
50. De Angelis MS, Palmucci L, Leone M, Doriguzzi C. Centronuclear myopathy: clinical, morphological and genetic characters. A review of 288 cases. *J Neurol Sci* 1991;103:2–9.
51. Bossen EH, Shelburne JD, Verkaut BS. Respiratory involvement in infantile myotonic dystrophy. *Arch Pathol* 1974;97:259–262.
52. de Gouyon BM, Zhao W, Laporte J, et al. Characterization of mutations in the myotubularin gene in twenty six patients with X-linked myotubular myopathy. *Hum Mol Genet* 1997;6:1499–1504.
53. Laporte J, Guiraud-Chaumeil C, Vincent M-C, et al. Mutations in the MTM1 gene implicated in X-linked myotubular myopathy. *Hum Mol Genet* 1997;6:1505–1511.
54. Wallgren-Pettersson C, Clarke A, Samson F, et al. The myotubular myopathies: differential diagnosis of the X- linked recessive, autosomal dominant, and autosomal recessive forms and present state of DNA studies. *J Med Genet* 1995;32:673–679.

Diseases of Skeletal Muscle,
edited by Robert L. Wortmann.
Lippincott Williams & Wilkins, Philadelphia © 2000

# 11

# Neuropathic Disorders and Muscular Dystrophies

## David Lacomis

*Departments of Neurology and Pathology, University of Pittsburgh School of Medicine;
University of Pittsburgh Medical Center Health System, Presbyterian University Hospital,
Pittsburgh, Pennsylvania 15213*

A variety of conditions that cause proximal muscle weakness are not myopathies, and some of these, in fact, can simulate an inflammatory myopathy. These noninflammatory causes of proximal weakness include disorders typically considered to be neuropathic. In addition, adult-onset muscular dystrophies can also stimulate an inflammtory myopathy (Table 1). The neuropathic causes of proximal muscle weakness can be classified according to the anatomic site of the causal pathology. Although disorders of the central nervous system can cause proximal weakness, more causes are the result of diseases affecting the peripheral nervous system. The functional component of the peripheral nervous system is the motor unit. Each motor unit consists of an anterior horn cell or cranial nerve motor nucleus, its axon and neuromuscular junction, plus all its innervated muscle fibers. Each of these anatomic locations must be considered when evaluating a patient with proximal weakness because pathology within any component of the motor unit can cause that presentation.

The initial step in working with patients with weakness should be to determine if the problem is neurogenic or myopathic. In neurogenic disorders, certain clinical features implicate involvement of a particular component of the motor unit. For example, anterior horn cell disorders are usually associated with fasciculations (random contractions of muscle fibers within a motor unit), muscle atrophy, and cramps. Peripheral neuropathies affecting sensory and motor fibers usually present with paresthesias in addition to weakness and hyporeflexia. Autonomic symptoms, such as light-headedness, decreased sweating, and impotence, may also occur. Defects in neuromuscular junction transmission may lead to fatigue and a diurnal variation in findings such that symptoms worsen late in the day. In both neuromuscular junction and anterior horn cell disorders, cranial muscles may also be affected, leading to facial weakness, dysphagia, and dysarthria. Ocular muscles may be weak in disorders that affect neuromuscular junction transmission but not in those that involve anterior horn cell. In contrast, myopathies usually present with proximal weakness with or without myalgias. Muscle atrophy and loss of tendon reflexes only occur late in the course, and there is no sensory loss or fasciculations.

The most useful laboratory test in the evaluation of muscle weakness is determination of the serum creatine kinase. The level of this enzyme is often elevated in inflammatory or necrotizing myopathies and most muscular dystrophies. It is elevated in some metabolic myopathies but not in neuromuscular junction disorders or in most congenital myopathies and neuropathies. However, creatine kinase may be elevated in anterior horn cell

**TABLE 1.** *Differential diagnosis of proximal weakness with diagnostic features*

| Disorder | Weakness | | | Sensory disturbance | Loss DTR early | Increased CK | NCS/EMG | Biopsy | Other |
|---|---|---|---|---|---|---|---|---|---|
| | Proximal | Distal | Ocular or bulbar | | | | | | |
| Anterior horn cell | | | | | | | | | |
| Amyotrophic lateral sclerosis | +++ | +++ | +++ | 0 | ++[a] | + | Neurogenic (motor); fasciculations | Neurogenic atrophy (muscle) | Upper motor neuron signs Fasciculations |
| Chronic spinal muscular atrophy | +++ | + | + | 0 | +++ | + | Neurogenic (motor); fasciculations | Neurogenic atrophy (muscle) | Fasciculations |
| Spinobulbar muscular atrophy | ++ | ++ | +++ | 0[b] | ++ | + | Neurogenic (motor); fasciculations | Neurogenic atrophy (muscle) | Gynecomastia fasciculations |
| Polyradiculopathies | | | | | | | | | |
| C5-6 | ++ | 0 | 0 | + | + | 0 | Focal neurogenic (root) | — | Neck pain (usually) |
| L-4 | ++ | 0 | 0 | + | + | 0 | Focal neurogenic (root) | — | Low back pain (usually) |
| Brachial plexopathy | | | | | | | | | |
| Upper trunk | +++ | 0 | 0 | ++ | ++ | 0 | Neurogenic: motor and sensory | — | Usually painful |
| Polyneuropathy | | | | | | | | | |
| CIDP | +++ | +++ | + | +++ | +++ | 0 | Demyelination and axon loss (sensorimotor) | Neuropathy variable[c] | Rare pure motor variant |
| Neuromuscular junction | | | | | | | | | |
| Myasthenia gravis | ++ | + | +++ | 0 | 0 | 0 | Decrement with RNS and abnormal SFEMG | Normal or type 2 fiber atrophy (muscle) | Diurnal variation |
| Lambert-Eaton myasthenic syndrome | +++ | + | + | 0 | +++ | 0 | Low motor amplitudes; incremental[c] response | Normal or type 2 fiber atrophy (muscle) | Autonomic symptoms |
| Myopathies | | | | | | | | | |
| Muscular dystrophies | +++ | + | + | 0 | 0 | +++ | Myopathy with fibrillation potentials | Chronic myopathy | Multiple types[c] |
| Congenital myopathies | +++ | ++ | ++ | 0 | 0 | +/0 | Mildly myopathic | Rods, cores[c] central nuclei, etc. | Dysmorphic features |
| Acid maltase deficiency | +++ | + | + | 0 | 0 | ++ | Myopathic with CRDs/myotonia | Vacuolar myopathy; glycogen | Respiratory involvement |

[a]DTR may also be increased.
[b]Low sensory amplitudes on NCS.
[c]See text for descriptions.
0, absent; +, occasionally; ++, common; +++, usually; DTR, deep tendon reflexes; CK, creatine kinase; NCS/EMG, nerve conduction studies/electromyogram; RNS, repetitive nerve stimulation; SFEMG, single-fiber EMG; CRDs, complex repetitive discharges; CIDP, chronic inflammatory demyelinating polyneuropathy.

disorders and in some other chronic neurogenic processes that affect motor axons, possibly due to "secondary" changes in muscle fibers. Thus, an elevated serum creatine kinase level is a very nonspecific finding.

Localizing the cause of weakness to a component of the motor unit can be readily accomplished with an electromyogram and nerve conduction studies. Histopathologic examination of muscle and, less often, nerve biopsy specimens may also be necessary for making a definitive diagnosis.

## ANTERIOR HORN CELL DISORDERS

### Amyotrophic Lateral Sclerosis

Amyotrophic lateral sclerosis is the most common adult-onset anterior horn cell disease, with an incidence of 1 in 100,000. Males are slightly more commonly affected than females. Amyotrophic lateral sclerosis generally presents between the ages of 55 and 75 years, but younger or older adults may be affected (1). Approximately 10% of patients have a familial (autosomal dominant) disorder, and a small percentage of these patients are known to harbor a mutation in the gene coding for superoxide dismutase 1 (2,3). Most other cases are sporadic and of uncertain cause. Rarely, there is an associated malignancy such as a lymphoma (4,5).

Patients usually present with weakness, less commonly with fasciculations, and rarely with respiratory failure (1,6). Weakness can involve any limb often in combination with oropharyngeal, facial, or respiratory musculature and manifest as dysphagia, dysarthria, facial weakness, or dyspnea. Although onset with unilateral limb weakness is common, patients may present with bilateral progressive proximal weakness. A key feature distinguishing an anterior horn cell disorder from myopathy is the presence of fasciculations. These only occur in the setting of anterior horn cell or motor axon diseases and do not occur in myopathies unless there is an associated neurogenic component. In addition to fasciculations and weakness, muscle atrophy is commonly seen in anterior horn cell disorders (Fig. 1). Sometime during the course of amyotrophic lateral sclerosis and sometimes initially, patients develop upper motor neuron signs including spasticity, brisk deep tendon reflexes, and often Babinski signs or other "pathologic" reflexes. None of those changes are expected in a myopathy. In fact, the combination of hyperreflexia in a weak fasciculating limb is nearly pathognomonic for amyotrophic lateral sclerosis.

More than one half of patients with amyotrophic lateral sclerosis have mild to moderate elevations in serum creatine kinase that may contribute to an erroneous diagnosis of myopathy (6). Electrodiagnostically, however, the needle examination should eventually reveal widespread evidence of denervation (fibrillation potentials or positive sharp waves) along with fasciculations and chronic neurogenic changes, including high-amplitude long-duration polyphasic motor unit potentials that fire in decreased numbers at a normal or rapid rate (7) (Fig. 2). Nerve conductions reveal normal sensory responses with low or normal motor amplitudes. Although a muscle biopsy is not usually obtained for diagnosis of amyotrophic lateral sclerosis, such a specimen should reveal classic changes of neurogenic atrophy (Fig. 3). Autopsy studies reveal degeneration of ventral spinal roots, anterior horn cells, corticospinal tracts, and pyramidal neurons.

Treatment for amyotrophic lateral sclerosis is largely supportive. The glutamate antagonist riluzole has been used (8). The use of antioxidants, other glutamate antagonists, and neurotrophic growth factors is experimental.

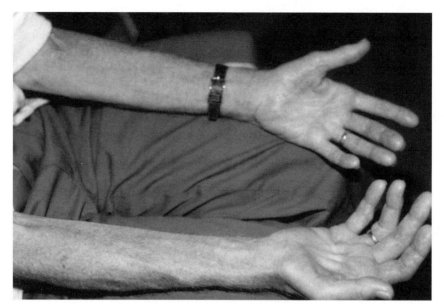

**FIG. 1.** Intrinsic hand muscle and forearm atrophy is seen in a patient with amyotrophic lateral sclerosis.

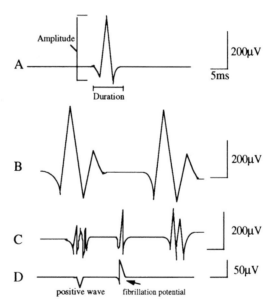

**FIG. 2.** Motor unit potentials detected via an electromyogram (EMG). **A:** Normal motor unit potential (MUP). **B:** MUPs from a patient with a neurogenic disorder such as a motor neuron disease. The MUPs are long in duration and higher in amplitude than normal and fire at rapid rates. Therefore, two of the same MUPs are seen adjacent to each other. **C:** MUPs typical of myopathy. The MUPs are short in duration, somewhat low in amplitude, and may be polyphasic, meaning that there are four or more crossings of the baseline as seen in the first and third MUPs. The MUPs shown in A, B, and C are all obtained during voluntary muscle contraction. **D:** A muscle at rest exhibits a positive wave and fibrillation potential, indicative of disconnection of the motor axon from its muscle that can occur in neurogenic processes or in processes in which there is muscle necrosis, inflammation, or alterations in sarcolemmal membrane integrity.

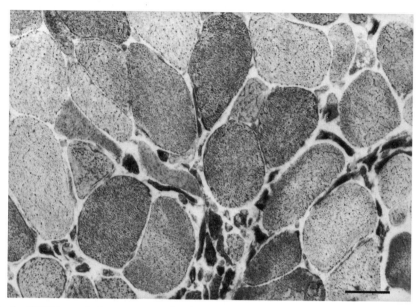

**FIG. 3.** An NADH-reacted cryostat section from a patient with amyotrophic lateral sclerosis reveals classic features of neurogenic atrophy, namely darkly staining angulated atrophic fibers that are either randomly distributed (acute denervation) or occur in groups (more long-standing disease). Bar, 50 μm.

## Spinal Muscular Atrophy

A mild form of chronic spinal muscular atrophy, either Kugelberg-Welander disease (spinal muscular atrophy type III) or spinal muscular atrophy type IV, is occasionally seen in adults (9,10). These disorders are uncommon, autosomal recessive in inheritance, and usually associated with a deletion in the survival motor neuron gene on chromosome 5q13 (11,12). Spinal muscular atrophy type III typically presents in childhood or adolescence, whereas spinal muscular atrophy type IV presents in adulthood. Affected patients have symmetric, progressive, proximal (especially lower extremity) weakness and are occasionally misdiagnosed with a muscular dystrophy. They may even have calf pseudohypertrophy, which is characteristically seen in Duchenne muscular dystrophy. Fasciculations may or may not be visible, and muscle atrophy and reduced tendon reflexes are common. Facial and bulbar (oropharyngeal) muscles are only occasionally affected, and upper motor neuron signs do not occur. The disorder progresses slowly, and life expectancy is nearly normal.

As in amyotrophic lateral sclerosis, the creatine kinase values are variable and may occasionally be elevated to very high levels. The electromyogram findings are similar to those seen in amyotrophic lateral sclerosis but with less fibrillation potential or spontaneous activity and with more chronic motor unit potential changes. Likewise, the histopathology of muscle is similar, revealing changes of neurogenic atrophy (10).

## Spinobulbar Muscular Atrophy

Spinobulbar muscular atrophy, or Kennedy's syndrome, is another rare slowly progressing form of anterior horn cell disease that can present with proximal weakness

(13,14). This X-linked disorder typically affects males with focal proximal or distal weakness that develops in their early to middle adult years. Bulbar muscles are commonly affected, leading to dysarthria and difficulty in swallowing. A postural tremor and quivering of the chin may be present, and fasciculations often occur in the limb muscles and tongue. There are no upper motor neuron signs. Gynecomastia and sometimes infertility result from associated androgen insensitivity.

Most electrodiagnostic findings are similar to those seen with amyotrophic lateral sclerosis. In contrast, however, the sensory nerve amplitudes are often reduced in Kennedy's syndrome due to degenerative changes in sensory ganglia that are usually asymptomatic (15,16). Kennedy's disease is a triplet repeat disorder involving the androgen receptor gene (17). Patients may benefit from treatment with androgens.

A recently reported form of proximal hereditary motor and sensory neuropathy with autosomal dominant inheritance and linkage to chromosome 3 has some features similar to Kennedy's syndrome, including an elevated serum creatine kinase level, proximal weakness, muscle atrophy, and fasciculations. However, sensory involvement is obvious, and there is no gynecomastia (18).

## POLYRADICULOPATHIES

Although most radiculopathies present with focal unilateral limb symptoms of pain or weakness, some polyradiculopathies can be diffuse or symmetric. Proximal leg weakness may be due to compression of the L-4 roots (or less likely the L-2 and L-3 roots). Proximal upper extremity weakness can occur from involvement of bilateral C-5 and C-6 roots. Patients with radiculopathies frequently, but not always, also have back or neck pain that may radiate down a limb in a dermatomal distribution. Compression on the nerve roots can lead to loss of the knee jerk (L2-4), biceps jerk (C5-6), or brachioradialis reflex (C5-6). Dermatomal sensory loss may be present. Cervical spinal cord compression, if present, tends to cause hyperreflexia and spasticity in the lower extremities, with occasional bowel and bladder dysfunction. Structural spine disease is the usual cause of radiculopathies. Specifically, central herniated disks with lateral extensions or narrowing of the neural foramina bilaterally due to bony degenerative changes could cause bilateral symptoms and signs. It would be most unusual for mass lesions other than herniated discs to cause bilateral symmetric weakness.

Radiographic investigations should disclose evidence of structural spine disease by using magnetic resonance imaging or computed tomographic myelography. Electromyography may also reveal findings of radiculopathy.

Polyradiculopathies can also result from inflammatory processes or other causes of leptomeningeal infiltration, such as Lyme disease, sarcoidosis, and viral infections (cytomegalovirus, Epstein-Barr virus, varicella-zoster, and others). Carcinomatous meningitis may affect nerve roots bilaterally. Those patients frequently have headaches, confusion, or cranial nerve palsies. They may not, however, have a prior diagnosis of malignancy (19). Vasculitis usually causes distal polyneuropathy or multiple mononeuropathies, but polyradiculopathy can be seen. Patients with any of the above-mentioned inflammatory or infiltrative disorders usually have abnormal spinal fluid with an elevation in protein and often a pleocytosis.

Polyradiculopathy also occurs in patients with type II diabetes generally over age 50. The degree of diabetes can range from mild to severe. This proximal polyradiculoneuropathy (also called diabetic amyotrophy or proximal diabetic neuropathy) usually presents with weight loss and unilateral thigh or buttock pain followed by proximal leg weakness with or without distal weakness (20). Serum creatine kinase levels are elevated in some patients with this disorder, and the spinal fluid protein is usually increased. The presence of asymmetric significant muscle atrophy, loss of the knee and ankle jerks, and pain without marked proximal sensory loss in the setting of diabetes (usually type II) are the classic features of the diagnosis. Electrophysiologic studies reveal polyradiculopathy often with a distal symmetric polyneuropathy or variable severity.

Although diabetic polyradiculopathy is self-limited and likely ischemic in origin, inflammatory nerve lesions have been noted in a number of patients raising the possibility of an immune-mediated disturbance (21).

## BRACHIAL PLEXOPATHIES

Brachial plexopathies usually present with shoulder or arm pain followed by weakness (22). Upper trunk brachial plexus involvement leads to proximal weakness in C5-6 innervated muscles such as the shoulder abductors, biceps, and brachioradialis and a reduction in the biceps and brachioradialis tendon reflexes. Sensory loss may be present in the lateral arm. Occasionally, brachial plexopathies occur bilaterally (usually in stages). Frequently, the cause of brachial plexopathy is unknown. The terms idiopathic brachial plexus neuropathy, neuralgic amyotrophy, or Parsonage-Turner syndrome have been applied to these disorders (23). In some cases, the condition follows an immunization, viral infection, or surgery. They can also be caused by trauma, infiltrative processes such as tumor, inflammatory diseases such as Lyme disease, and by genetic mechanisms (24). These disturbances tend to resolve over time, but improvement may take months.

Electromyography classically reveals evidence of denervation (fibrillation potentials or positive waves) and chronic neurogenic changes (polyphasic motor unit potentials of long duration), but fibrillation potentials are not found in the first 2 to 3 weeks. The chronic neurogenic changes develop over a longer period of time. Sensory and motor amplitudes are low in the representative regions of the brachial plexus. For example, there may be a reduction in the medial cutaneous sensory responses with a lower trunk lesion.

## POLYNEUROPATHY

Distal muscle weakness is the hallmark feature of most polyneuropathies. Such length-dependent axonal neuropathies tend to begin distally, proceed proximally, usually affect sensory and motor fibers, and sometimes involve autonomic fibers. However, some neuropathic processes affect proximal muscles and may simulate a myopathy. One such disorder is the primarily demyelinating process chronic inflammatory demyelinating polyneuropathy. Patients with chronic inflammatory demyelinating polyneuropathy may present with symmetric proximal weakness in legs more than the arms. Weakness usually develops in distal muscles, depending on which nerve segments are affected. Other features of chronic inflammatory demyelinating polyneuropathy include hyporeflexia or areflexia, distal sensory loss, and, uncommonly, cranial nerve involvement (25–27).

Analysis of spinal fluid is indicated when chronic inflammatory demyelinating polyneuropathy is considered. The protein is usually elevated, and there should be an absence or sparse number of inflammatory cells. This combination is sometimes termed albuminocytologic dissociation. Nerve conduction studies reveal demyelination and axon loss. Findings of demyelination include prolongation of distal latencies, a significant drop in the proximal motor amplitude (conduction block), prolongation of F waves, and significant slowing of the conduction velocities. Nerve biopsy specimens reveal endoneurial or epineurial inflammation in less than a third of patients (Fig. 4). Features of demyelination and remyelination, such as onion bulbs and thinly myelinated axons, are usually present, but occasionally only changes of axonal degeneration are noted.

Most patients with chronic inflammatory demyelinating polyneuropathy improve with intravenous gammaglobulin, plasmapheresis, or corticosteroid therapy.

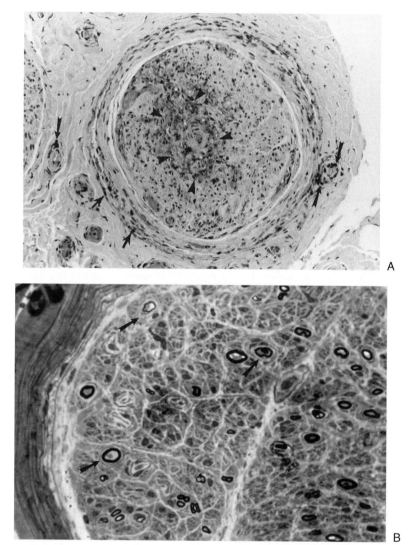

A

B

**FIG. 4. A:** Chronic inflammatory demyelinating polyneuropathy. In this leukocyte common antigen immunostained paraffin section, a region of endoneurial inflammation is outlined by the arrowheads. The inflammatory cell nuclei stain very darkly, and the cytoplasm is moderately dark. There are also dark-staining perivascular lymphocytes seen in the epineurial connective tissue (*long arrows*), and occasional inflammatory cells are seen in the perineurium (*short arrows*) (original magnification, ×250). **B:** A 1-μm-thick toluidine blue-stained plastic section of a nerve biopsy specimen from a patient with chronic inflammatory demyelinating polyneuropathy reveals a moderately severe drop-out in myelinated axons and occasional thinly myelinated axons surrounded by redundant Schwann cell cytoplasm termed onion bulbs arrows (original magnification, ×750).

The Guillain-Barré syndrome, also called acute inflammatory demyelinating polyneuropathy, can also present with proximal weakness, but the clinical course is more acute and should only rarely be confused with a typical subacute myopathy. The Guillain-Barré syndrome may follow a viral infection, influenza vaccine, or diarrheal illness from *Campylobacter jejuni* (28). There is usually rapid loss of tendon reflexes, mild sensory symptoms, an elevation in spinal fluid protein, and features of demyelination on nerve conduction studies (29).

The porphyric neuropathies may also present with subacute-onset proximal weakness. Of the neurovisceral porphyrias, acute intermittent porphyria is most common followed by hereditary coproporphyria, variegate porphyria, and aminolevulinic acid-dehydratase deficiency (30). The neurologic symptoms are similar in all three disorders. Attacks, precipitated by fasting, drugs, hormones, or alcohol, usually begin before puberty but may not develop until later. Concurrent abdominal symptoms are common, and central nervous system features can include seizures and cognitive changes. The neuropathy primarily affects proximal motor fibers and bulbar and facial nerve-innervated muscles. Wrist and finger extensor muscle weakness may occur. Although sensory symptoms are less common, when present they affect the trunk more than distal limbs.

The electrophysiologic findings disclose a primarily axonal neuropathy, although some features of demyelination may be present. Screening for porphyria is dependent on identifying elevated urinary δ-aminolevulinic acid and porphobilinogen levels. More specific tests measuring components of the heme pathway in urine, feces, and serum are required to make a definitive diagnosis (31). For example, in acute intermittent porphyria, the stool porphyrins are usually normal or slightly increased, and the erythrocyte porphobilinogen deaminase is reduced. In variegate porphyria, the predominant stool porphyrin is protoporphyrin. Finally, in hereditary coproporphyria, the predominant stool porphyrin is coproporphyrin. The treatment of porphyria includes use of pain medications and intravenous glucose. Heme therapy has been tried, but its effectiveness is debated (31).

## NEUROMUSCULAR JUNCTION DISORDERS

### Myasthenia Gravis

Myasthenia gravis is a postsynaptic disorder of neuromuscular junction transmission usually caused by immune-mediated destruction of acetylcholine receptors. Other inherited forms of myasthenia that are non–immune-mediated exist but are rare.

The prevalence of myasthenia gravis is approximately 14 per 100,000 in the United States (32). It is more prevalent in young women in their second and third decades, whereas males predominate over the age of 60. Two thirds of patients present with ptosis and diplopia. Rarely, when the disorder remains confined to ocular muscles, it is termed ocular myasthenia. Involvement of the oropharyngeal and limb muscles occurs initially in some patients but often develops later. Weakness in nonocular cranial nerve-innervated muscles can cause facial weakness, dysarthria, dysphagia, or difficulty chewing. Some patients also develop life-threatening respiratory muscle involvement (33). An occasional patient presents with primarily proximal weakness, so-called limb-girdle myasthenia (34). Patients with myasthenia gravis tend to have a diurnal variation in symptoms that become weaker later in the day and tend to feel strongest upon awakening (35,36).

Approximately 20% of patients with myasthenia gravis have a thymoma detected by chest computed tomography (Fig. 5), whereas most others have thymic hyperplasia. Edrophonium, an acetylcholinesterase inhibitor, may be administered intravenously as

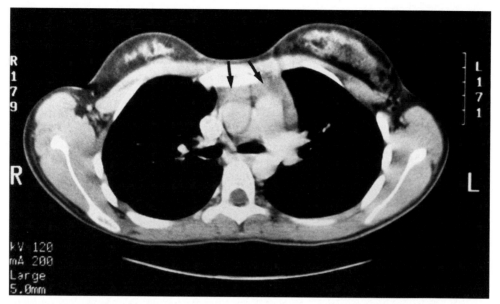

**FIG. 5.** A computed tomography of the chest from a woman with myasthenia gravis reveals a thymoma seen in the retrosternal region (*arrows*). The thymoma was not invasive and was surgically removed without any complications.

a diagnostic test for myasthenia gravis. However, a positive response is not specific for the disease. The finding of acetylcholine receptor-binding antibodies in the serum is more specific. These are present in at least 90% of patients with generalized myasthenia gravis and up to 71% with ocular myasthenia (37). Some patients who do not have binding antibodies have acetylcholine receptor-modulating antibodies. Anti-striated muscle antibodies may also be present and are a marker of thymoma in some patients; however, this is not a sensitive or very specific test because false-positive results occur, especially in the elderly.

Electrophysiologic testing is very useful in diagnosing myasthenia gravis. Repetitive motor nerve stimulation at low rates of 2 to 3 Hz often leads to an abnormal decremental response of at least 10% between the first and fifth responses (Fig. 6). The yield is higher in generalized myasthenia gravis and when proximal nerves, such as the spinal accessory or facial motor nerves, are assessed. Single-fiber electromyography is a more sophisticated test. This technique measures jitter, the variation in time intervals of neuromuscular junction transmission between successive muscle fiber action potentials. It is the most sensitive test of neuromuscular junction transmission and is abnormal in the vast majority of patients with myasthenia gravis. However, it must be interpreted with caution because it is not specific. Other neuromuscular disorders associated with axonal degenerative or affecting neuromuscular transmission can cause abnormalities on single-fiber electromyography.

Other autoimmune processes can occur in patients with myasthenia gravis. One must consider such disorders, especially thyroid disease, in the diagnostic evaluation.

Treatment for myasthenia gravis is usually quite successful. Cholinesterase inhibitors, such as pyridostigmine, may improve the symptoms of myasthenia, but immunosuppression is usually required to alter the course of the disease. Options for im-

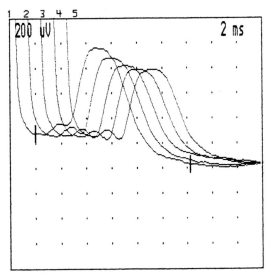

**FIG. 6.** This photograph depicts 3-Hz repetitive stimulation of the ulnar nerve recording at the abductor digiti minimi muscle in a patient with myasthenia gravis. There is a 20% drop (decrement) in amplitude (baseline to peak) and a 23% decrement in area (area under the curve) between the first and fifth responses. The abnormal decrement was significantly reduced after 1 minute of exercise but recurred minutes after exercise.

munosuppression include prednisone, azathioprine, and, occasionally, cyclosporine. In patients with "myasthenic crisis," either plasma exchange or intravenous gammaglobulin may be beneficial (35). Thymectomy is recommended for all patients with thymomas and for most with generalized myasthenia gravis under the age of 60 years (38). It remains controversial whether or not thymectomy should be performed in older myasthenics and whether or not a transsternal versus a transcervical approach should be undertaken.

### Lambert-Eaton Myasthenic Syndrome

Lambert-Eaton myasthenic syndrome is a rare disorder of presynaptic neuromuscular junction transmission caused by antibodies directed against voltage-gated calcium channels. The disorder is either paraneoplastic and most commonly associated with a small cell carcinoma of the lung or is immune-mediated without associated tumor (36).

Patients with this syndrome typically present with symmetric proximal weakness affecting the lower extremities more than the upper extremities. Mild abnormalities of cranial muscles may develop, including ptosis. Autonomic symptoms include a dry mouth. In addition, the deep tendon reflexes are reduced. Occasionally, the deep tendon reflex responses actually increase after 10 seconds of exercise (39).

Laboratory studies usually disclose antibodies against P/Q or N type (or both) voltage-gated calcium channels (37,40). The serum creatine kinase level is generally normal. Light microscopy of skeletal muscle is normal or may reveal only type II fiber atrophy. Nerve conduction studies are very useful and typically reveal low motor amplitudes with normal sensory responses. The motor amplitude, however, increases

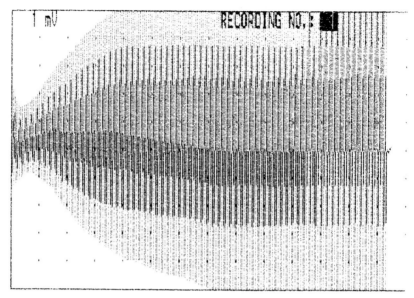

**FIG. 7.** In this patient with Lambert-Eaton myasthenic syndrome, 30-Hz repetitive stimulation of the ulnar nerve produced a 100% increment in amplitude by the 50th response after an initial decrement of 34% measured at the 10th response. (The horizontal graduations are 500 ms per division.)

dramatically after either 10 seconds of exercise or with repetitive stimulation at 30 to 40 Hz (Fig. 7). Exercise is believed to facilitate calcium and, subsequently, acetylcholine release.

Treatment options include removal of a tumor if present, immunosuppression with prednisone or other medications, plasma exchange, intravenous gammaglobulin, or pyridostigmine. Experimental use of 3,4-diaminopyridine has proven useful for treatment of Lambert-Eaton myasthenic syndrome, but this medication is not approved by the U.S. Food and Drug Administration (41).

## MYOPATHY

Myopathy is the most common cause of progressive proximal muscle weakness. The metabolic myopathies are discussed in Chapter 9. Inherited disorders that are usually mildly progressive or static are called congenital myopathies (see Chapter 10). The term muscular dystropy is applied to the largest group of inherited myopathies. The term dystrophy implies a progressive degenerative disorder of muscle.

### Muscular Dystrophies

#### *Dystrophinopathies*

Deficiencies in the cytoskeletal protein dystrophin lead to the most common form of childhood muscular dystrophy, Duchenne muscular dystrophy (42). Duchenne muscular dystrophy is an X-linked disorder that affects 20 to 30 males per 100,000. One third of the cases arise from spontaneous mutations. The disorder presents in early childhood and is progressive, leading to the death of affected males in their early twenties (43–45).

A more benign form of dystrophinopathy, termed Becker's muscular dystrophy, usually presents in mid-childhood to mid-adolescence but may be first detected in adults. The incidence of Becker's muscular dystrophy is 3 to 6 per 100,000 male births. Becker's muscular dystrophy is an allelic variant of Duchenne muscular dystrophy. In contrast to patients with Duchenne muscular dystrophy, in which less than 3% of the normal amount of dystrophin is present, patients with Becker's muscular dystrophy usually have 3% to 20%, or even more, of the normal amount of dystrophin. Becker's muscular dystrophy usually results from an in-frame deletion in the gene encoding for dystrophin (46).

Patients with either dystrophinopathy usually present with progressive proximal weakness that is more prominent in the legs than arms and an associated pseudohypertrophy of the calves. Neck flexors are less weak in Becker's muscular dystrophy than in Duchenne muscular dystrophy patients. Accordingly, affected Becker's muscular dystrophy children usually lack the head lag sign when pulled up from a supine position, a finding common in Duchenne. In addition, there may be a history of delayed motor development. In general, patients with Becker's muscular dystrophy can walk until they are at least 16 years of age. Some can walk past age 27. The average age of death in Becker's muscular dystrophy is 42 years and is often the result of respiratory or cardiac complications.

Laboratory features include a markedly elevated serum creatine kinase level, with values usually more than ten times normal. Typical myopathic changes with fibrillation potentials are seen with electromyography. Muscle biopsy specimens reveal hyaline fibers, groups of regenerating myofibers, endomysial fibrosis, occasional inflammatory infiltrates, and a deficiency in dystrophin by immunohistochemical staining (Fig. 8) (47). Western blot can be used to quantitate dystrophin, and DNA studies may identify a specific mutation in about 60% of patients. Assessment of cardiac function is essential because cardiomyopathy may occur in both Becker's muscular dystrophy and Duchenne muscular dystrophy (48).

Prednisone has been shown to be useful in improving strength and slowing the progression of muscle weakness. However, side effects can be a problem (49). Research of the use of gene therapy for dystrophinopathies is ongoing.

### Emery-Dreifuss Muscular Dystrophy

Emery-Dreifuss muscular dystrophy is a rare X-linked disorder with the abnormal gene located at Xq28. The protein deficiency is muscle emerin. This protein may also be reduced in skin (50). Affected males present in childhood with slowly progressive weakness in the anterior compartment of the distal lower extremities and in the upper arms followed by flexion contractures of the elbows and tightening of the Achilles tendons (Fig. 9) (51). Patients often hold their neck in extension and present with a rigid spine. Cardiac conduction abnormalities are common and may require pacemaker placement to prevent sudden death (52). The serum creatine kinase level is usually elevated but less so compared with the dystrophinopathies. Electromyogram and muscle biopsy show nonspecific chronic myopathic features (Fig. 10).

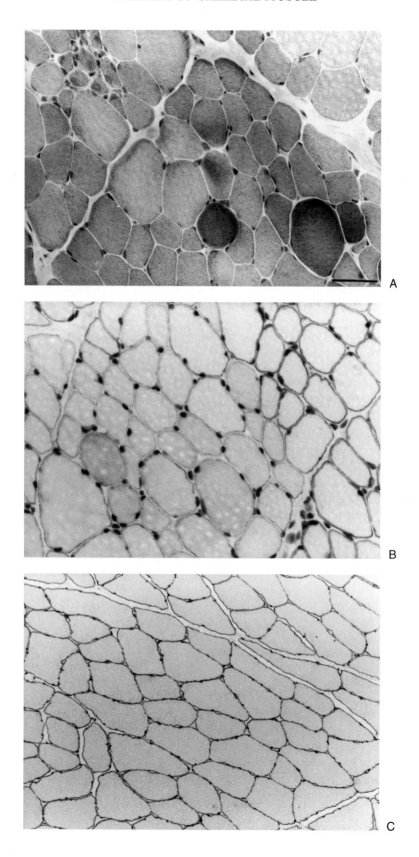

**FIG. 8.** Becker's muscular dystrophy. **A:** A Gomori trichrome-stained cryostat section reveals an abnormal variation in myofiber sizes with several dark staining (hyalinized) fibers and a focus of atrophic regenerating fibers that have plump nuclei (*upper left*). On hemotoxylin and eosin-stained sections, the regenerating fibers had a basophilic appearance. **B:** Immunohistochemical staining against the carboxy terminus of the dystrophin molecule produces generally reduced staining in this patient with Becker's muscular dystrophy. Some of the muscle fibers in the upper right corner have nearly normal staining and may be revertant fibers. **C:** In comparison, a normal control muscle reacted with the same antibody exhibits normal, dark, homogenous subsarcolemmal staining. Bar, 50 μm.

### Limb-Girdle Muscular Dystrophies

Historically, muscular dystrophy patients with proximal weakness without features of Duchenne muscular dystrophy were placed in the category of limb-girdle muscular dystrophy. In the early molecular era, some patients diagnosed with limb-girdle muscular dystrophy were found to have Becker's muscular dystrophy. Subsequently, genetic advances have begun to identify specific mutations in about 10% of other limb-girdle muscular dystrophy kindreds. Most are autosomal recessive (Table 2). Defects in dystrophin-associated glycoproteins such as sarcoglycan and laminin have been reported (Fig. 11). A deficiency in calpain, which is involved with calcium-mediated proteolysis, may also lead to limb-girdle muscular dystrophy. A complete description of these disorders is beyond the scope of this textbook, but comprehensive references are available (53–58).

In general, patients with limb-girdle muscular dystrophy present with slowly progressive proximal upper and lower extremity weakness. Onset can occur in childhood or adult

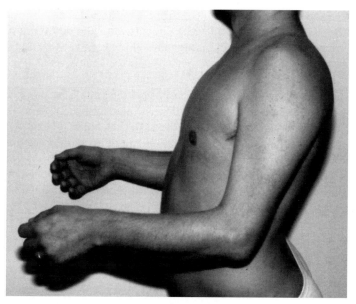

**FIG. 9.** Emery-Dreifuss muscular dystrophy. In this photograph, the patient is trying to extend his arms at the elbows but cannot do so because of flexion contractures. Atrophy in the humeral region and hyperlordotic posture is also noted.

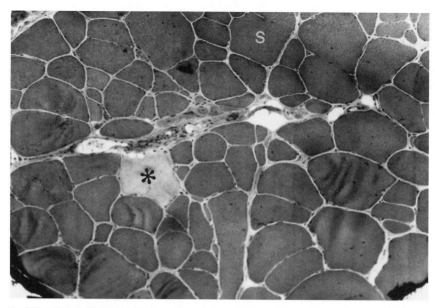

**FIG. 10.** This Gomori trichrome-stained cryostat section of a muscle biopsy specimen from a patient with Emery-Dreifuss muscular dystrophy reveals an abnormal variation in myofiber sizes, excess of internalized nuclei, increase in endomysial connective tissue, a necrotic fiber (*asterisk*), and a fiber that is splitting (*S*) (original magnification, ×250).

years. Most patients do not have an affected family member, which is consistent with the autosomal recessive inheritance.

Scapular muscles may be weakened, and some patients may have large calves. Exercise intolerance is noted rarely. The serum creatine kinase level is usually elevated but can decline with the use of prednisone in some patients. The electromyogram findings are similar to those with any dystrophy or chronic inflammatory myopathy. In fact, some may be misdiagnosed with inflammatory myopathy.

Muscle histopathology generally reveals nonspecific myopathic changes (similar to those shown in Fig. 10) without inflammatory cell infiltrates. A review of 97 muscle biopsies from 81 individuals with limb-girdle muscular dystrophy showed a dystrophic pattern in 80% and myopathic changes in the rest. Seventeen percent had neurogenic changes as well (59). Inflammatory cell infiltrates can be seen on occasion, but invasion of nonnecrotic fibers by lymphocytes is generally not present. However, even invasion of nonnecrotic fibers would not necessarily exclude limb-girdle muscle dystrophy because it has been reported in other dystrophies, namely the dystrophinopathies.

**TABLE 2.** *Limb-girdle muscular dystrophies (LGMD) and genetic aspects*

| Type | Inheritance | Deficiency | Mutation |
| --- | --- | --- | --- |
| LGMD 1 | AD | Unknown | Chromosome 5 (linkage only) |
| LGMD 2A | AR | Calpain III | Chromosome 15q15 |
| LGMD 2B | AR | Unknown | Chromosome 2p13-p16 |
| LGMD 2C | AR | τ-Sarcoglycan | Chrosme 13q12 |
| LGMD 2D | AR | α-Sarcoglycan (adhalin) | Chromosome 17q21 |
| LGMD 2E | AR | β-Sarcoglycan | Chromosome 4q12 |
| LGMD 2F | AR | δ-Sarcoglycan | Chromosome 5q33-q34 |

AR, autosomal recessive; AD, autosomal dominant.

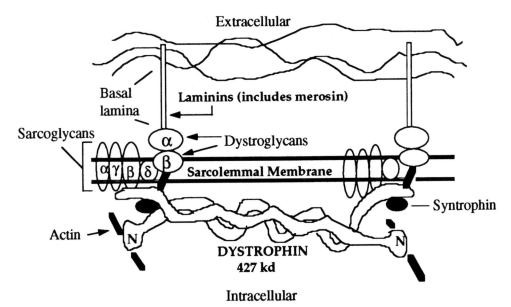

**FIG. 11.** Dystrophin and dystrophin-associated glycoproteins. Dystrophin is shown as the 427-kDa molecule that is anchored to the sarcolemmal membrane and is also attached to actin thin filaments. At the sarcolemmal membrane, dystrophin is associated with syntrophin and α- and β-dystroglycans. Adjacent to the dystroglycans are four sarcoglycans. The dystroglycans are then attached to laminins in the basal lamina region.

Features that suggest the diagnosis of limb-girdle muscular dystrophy rather than inflammatory myopathy include a slower disease progression and lack of response to immunosuppressive therapy. However, corticosteroid therapy may be useful in some (60,61). The identification of a mutation is the most useful in differentiating an inflammatory myopathy from limb-girdle muscle dystrophy. A preliminary histopathologic study has shown cell surface membrane attack expression in limb-girdle muscle dystrophy and not in inflammatory myopathies (62). If confirmed, this finding may also help differentiate the disorders.

### *Myotonic Dystrophy*

Myotonic dystrophy is the most common adult form of muscular dystrophy. It is an autosomal dominant multisystem disorder that results from the abnormal expansion of an unstable CTG trinucleotide repeat located on the untranslated end of chromosome 19. The incidence is 1 in 8,000 (63,64).

Because patients generally present with distal weakness, they are usually not confused with other myopathies. However, proximal weakness does occur later in the course. Other common clinical features include abnormal facies with atrophy (Fig. 12), frontal balding in men (and rarely women), ptosis, dysphagia, and nasal speech. Myotonia, an impairment in muscle relaxation, can often be demonstrated as a delay in release of grip or as a delay in relaxation after percussion of the thenar or hypothenar eminences. Patients may also complain of muscle cramping due to myotonia. Cataracts, cardiac conduction defects, gastrointestinal disorders, and insulin resistance are possible coincidental manifestations (65).

The serum creatine kinase level is usually mildly elevated but may be normal. The presence of myotonia on an electromyogram is the hallmark feature (Fig. 13). Myopathic

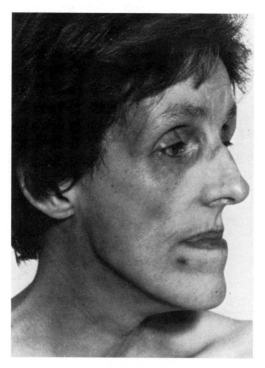

**FIG. 12.** Myotonic dystrophy. The patient has ptosis and a narrow face with weakness of the jaw and other facial muscles. (From Harper PS, Rüdel R. Myotonic dystrophy. In: Engel AG, Franzini-Armstrong C, eds. *Myology*, 2nd ed. New York: McGraw-Hill, 1994:1194, with permission.)

(short-duration, low-amplitude, polyphasic) motor unit potentials are also noted. Histologically, there are nonspecific findings, including an excess of internalized nuclei, ring fibers, nuclear clumps, and atrophic and hypertrophic fibers (Fig. 14) (59). Definitive diagnosis is made by genetic testing that reveals the abnormal trinucleotide expansion. Compared with their affected parent, affected children tend to have longer repeat segments and a more severe phenotype (66).

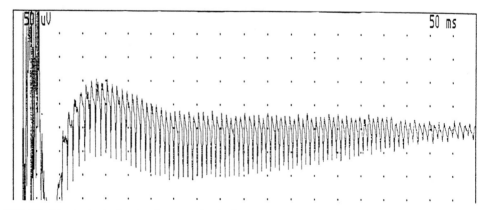

**FIG. 13.** Myotonic dystrophy. A myotonic discharge is depicted after needle insertion during an electromyogram study. This particular discharge had a waning character due to the reduction in both the amplitude and frequency of firing. Other myotonic discharges may wax and wane.

Symptomatic treatment for myotonia includes phenytoin. Orthotics and other conservative treatments such as physical therapy are also used (65,67). Patients and their physicians should also be aware of an increased risk of perioperative, mainly pulmonary, complications (68).

Proximal myotonic myopathy is a more recently identified form of myotonic myopathy (69,70). This disorder does present with progressive proximal muscle weakness beginning in adulthood and, sometimes, in childhood. Distal muscles are strong. Unless affected family members are identified, it can easily be confused with an acquired myopathy. The dis-

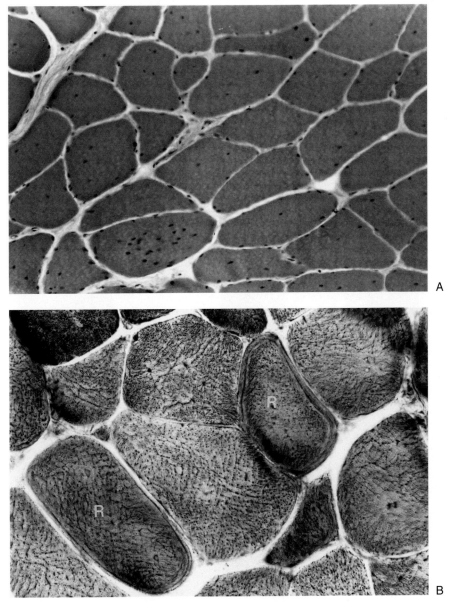

**FIG. 14.** Myotonic dystrophy. **A:** This hemotoxylin and eosin-stained cryostat section reveals characteristic but nonspecific histopathologic features, including a significant excess of internalized nuclei and a variation of myofiber sizes (original magnification, ×250). **B:** An NADH-TR reacted section shown at higher magnification reveals several ring fibers (*R*) (×500).

order is of unknown etiology but has autosomal dominant inheritance. It is not associated with the same gene locus as myotonic dystrophy, and the known mutations in sodium and chloride channels associated with other myotonic disorders are not present in these patients.

Patients usually have cataracts and at least electrophysiologic evidence of myotonia with occasional percussion myotonia and difficulty with grip release. Leg stiffness and significant, often ill-defined, pain in various muscles also occur. In addition to revealing myotonic discharges, an electromyogram may show myopathic motor unit potentials. The serum creatine kinase levels may be elevated, but not substantially. Muscle histology reveals nonspecific changes similar to those seen in myotonic dystrophy. Abnormalities of the cerebral periventricular white matter are seen with magnetic resonance imaging in some patients, but the clinical significance of these findings is unknown (71). Therapy may include phenytoin for myotonia and tricyclic antidepressants for pain.

### *Facioscapulohumeral Dystrophy*

Facioscapulohumeral dystrophy is an autosomal dominant form of muscular dystrophy. It is associated with an incompletely elucidated abnormality on chromosome 4q35. There is strong penetrance but varying expression. The incidence is 1 per 20,000 with a 10% mutation frequency. Patients present with facial weakness and weakness in scapular stabilizers that leads to scapular "winging" (Fig. 15). Hip-girdle and distal leg weakness can occur later. Weakness may be asymmetric, with the deltoid muscles typically spared (72,73). Additionally, systemic features include mild scoliosis, pectus excavatum, high-frequency sensorineural hearing loss, and retinal vasculopathy.

The serum creatine kinase level may be elevated, and an electromyogram demonstrates nonspecific myopathic findings. Histopathology is variable, with changes ranging from only

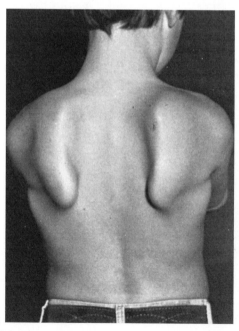
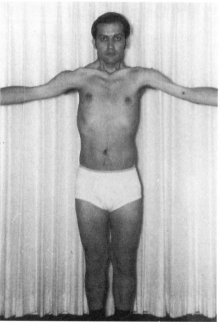

A                                                                                      B

**FIG. 15.** Facioscapulohumeral dystrophy. **A:** This boy exhibits "scapular winging." **B:** This patient has straightening of the clavicles, biceps atrophy, and bifacial weakness. (From Munsat TL. Facioscapulohumeral disease and the scapuloperoneal syndrome. In: Engel AG, Franzini-Armstrong C, eds. *Myology*, 2nd ed. New York: McGraw-Hill, 1994:1224–1228, with permission.)

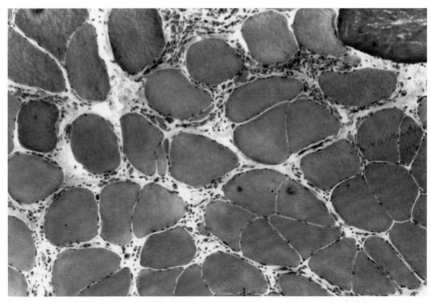

**FIG. 16.** Facioscapulohumeral dystrophy. This hemotoxylin and eosin-stained cryostat section reveals a significant variation in myofiber sizes with scattered atrophic, sometimes angulated, fibers. There is an increase in endomysial connective tissue, and scattered mononuclear inflammatory cells are also noted (original magnification, ×125).

occasionally atrophic fibers to more severe myopathic changes with inflammatory infiltrates (Fig. 16). Genetic testing may reveal an abnormal DNA fragment on chromosome 4.

The disease is usually progresses slowly, but approximately 20% of patients eventually require a wheelchair. There is no remittive treatment.

### Adult-onset Dystrophies

Two relatively rare adult-onset muscular dystrophies include oculopharyngeal muscular dystrophy and distal dystrophy of Welander. They are usually not confused with other myopathic processes because proximal weakness is uncommon. Oculopharyngeal muscular dystrophy is an autosomal dominant disorder of unknown etiology affecting French-Canadians more often than other ethnic groups. The disorder is linked to chromosome 14q11.2-q13 (74,75). Patients present with progressive ptosis and dysphagia usually during the fifth and sixth decades. Mild proximal weakness may occur later in the course. Histopathologically, rimmed vacuoles are noted in skeletal muscles, and intranuclear filamentous inclusions may be identified ultrastructurally (76,77). Histologically, these abnormalities are similar to those seen in inclusion body myositis.

Distal dystrophy of Welander is another late-life–onset muscular dystrophy that has primarily autosomal dominant inheritance. Although one family has been reported with an abnormal gene localized to chromosome 14, the precise genetic defect is not resolved (78). Onset is usually between ages 40 and 60 years, and patients develop slowly progressive weakness of intrinsic hand and later tibialis anterior muscles with or without calf pseudohypertrophy (79,80).

### REFERENCES

1. Mitsumoto H, Chad DA, Pioro EP. *Amyotrophic lateral sclerosis.* Philadelphia: FA Davis, 1998.
2. Siddique T, Figlewicz PA, Pericak-Vance MA, et al. Linkage of a gene causing familial amyotrophic lateral sclerosis to chromosome 21 and evidence of genetic locus heterogeneity. *N Engl J Med* 1991;324:1381–1384.

3. Wiedan-Pazos M, Goto TJ, Rabizadeh S, et al. Altered reactivity of superoxide dismutase in familial amyotrophic lateral sclerosis. *Science* 1996;271:515–518.
4. Rowland LP. Paraneoplastic primary lateral sclerosis and amyotrophic lateral sclerosis. *Ann Neurol* 1997; 4:703–705.
5. Younger DS, Rowland LP, Laton N, Hays AP. Lymphoma, motor neuron diseases and amyotrophic lateral sclerosis. *Ann Neurol* 1991;29:78–86.
6. Tandan R, Bradley WG. Amyotrophic lateral sclerosis. Part 1. Clinical features, pathology, and ethical issues in management. *Ann Neurol* 1985;18:271–280.
7. Daube JR. *American Association of Electrodiagnostic Medicine (AAEE) Minimonograph 18: EMG in motor neuron diseases*. Rochester, MN: AAEE, 1980.
8. Bensimom G, Lacomblez L, Meninger V, and the ALS/Rizole Study Group. A controlled trial of riluzole in amyotrophic lateral sclerosis. *N Engl J Med* 1994;330:585–591.
9. Kugelberg E, Welander L. Heredofamilial juvenile muscular atrophy simulating muscular dystrophy. *Arch Neurol Psychiatr* 1956;75:500–509.
10. Gardner-Medwin D, Hudgson P, Walton JN. Benign spinal muscular atrophy arising in childhood and adolescence. *J Neurol Sci* 1967;5:121–158.
11. Lefebrve S, Bürglen L, Reboullet S, et al. Identification and characterization of a spinal muscular atrophy-determining gene. *Cell* 1995;80:155–165.
12. Melki J, Abdelhak S, Sheth P, et al. Gene for chronic spinal muscular atrophies maps to chromosome 5q. *Nature* 1990;344:767–768.
13. Kennedy WR, Alter M, Sung JH. Progressive proximal spinal and bulbar muscular atrophy of late onset. *Neurology* 1968;18:671–680.
14. Olney RK, Aminoff MJ, So YT. Clinical and electrodiagnostic features of X-linked recessive bulbospinal neuropathy. *Neurology* 1991;41:823–828.
15. Ferrante MA, Wilbourn AJ. The characteristic electrodiagnostic features of Kennedy's disease. *Muscle Nerve* 1997;20:323–329.
16. Li M, Sobue G, Doyu M, et al. Primary sensory neurons in X-linked recessive bulbospinal neuronopathy: histopathology and androgen receptor gene expression. *Muscle Nerve* 1995;18:301–308.
17. Igarashi S, Tanno Y, Onodera O, et al. Strong correlation between the number of CAG repeats in androgen receptor genes and the clinical onset of features of spinal and bulbar muscular atrophy. *Neurology* 1992;42:2300–2302.
18. Takashima H, Nakagawa M, Nakahara K, et al. A new type of hereditary motor and sensory neuropathy linked to chromosome 3. *Ann Neurol* 1997;41:771–780.
19. Freilich RJ, Krol G, DeAngelis LM. Neuroimaging and cerebrospinal fluid cytology in the diagnosis of leptomeningeal metastasis. *Ann Neurol* 1995;38:51–57.
20. Barohn RJ, Sahenk Z, Warmolts JR, Mendell JT. The Bruns-Garland syndrome (diabetic amyotrophy). Revisited 100 years later. *Arch Neurol* 1991;48:1130–1135.
21. Said G, Elgrably F, Lacroix C, et al. Painful proximal diabetic neuropathy: inflammatory nerve lesions and spontaneous favorable outcome. *Ann Neurol* 1997;14:762–770.
22. Beghi E, Kurland LT, Mulder DW, Nicolosi A. Brachial plexus neuropathy in the population of Rochester, Minnesota. *Ann Neurol* 1985;18:320–323.
23. Parsonage MJ, Turner JWA. Neuralgic amyotrophy. The shoulder-girdle syndrome. *Lancet* 1948;1:973–978.
24. Pellegrino JE, Rebbeck TR, Brown MJ, Bird TD, Chance PF. Mapping of hereditary neuralgic amyotrophy (familial brachial plexus neuropathy) to distal chromosome 17q. *Neurology* 1996;46:1128–1132.
25. Barohn RJ, Kissel JT, Warmolts JR, Mendell JR. Chronic inflammatory demyelinating polyradiculoneuropathy. Clinical characteristics, course, and recommendations for diagnostic criteria. *Arch Neurol* 1989;46:878–884.
26. McCombe PA, Pollard JD, McLeod JG. Chronic inflammatory demyelinating polyradiculopathy. A clinical and electrophysiological study of 92 cases. *Brain* 1987;110:1617–1630.
27. Bouchard C, Lacroix C, Planté V, et al. Clinicopathologic findings and prognosis of chronic inflammatory demyelinating polyneuropathy. *Neurology* 1999;52:498–503Ω.
28. Lasky T, Terracciano GJ, Magder L, et al. The Guillain-Barrè syndrome and the 1992–1993 and 1993–1994 influenza vaccines. *N Engl J Med* 1998;339:1797–1802.
29. Ropper AH, Wijdis EFM, Truax BT (eds). *Guillain-Barrè syndrome*. Philadelphia: FA Davis, 1991.
30. Barohn RJ, Sanchez JA, Anderson KE. Acute peripheral neuropathy due to hereditary coproporphyria. *Muscle Nerve* 1994;17:793–799.
31. Tefferi A, Solberg LA, Ellefson RD. Porphyrias: clinical evaluation and interpretation of laboratory tests. *Mayo Clin Proc* 1994;69:289–290.
32. Phillips LH, Torner JC. Epidemiologic evidence for a changing natural history of myasthenia gravis. *Neurology* 1996;46:1233–1238.
33. Maher J, Grand Maison F, Nicolle MW, et al. Diagnostic difficulties in myasthenia gravis. *Muscle Nerve* 1998;21:577–583.
34. Oh SJ, Kuruoglu R. Chronic limb-girdle myasthenia gravis. *Neurology* 1992;42:1153–1156.
35. Drachman DB. Myasthenia gravis. *N Engl J Med* 1994;330:1797–1810.
36. Engel AG. Myasthenia gravis and myasthenic syndromes. *Ann Neurol* 1984;16:519–534.
37. Lennon VA. Serologic profile of myasthenia gravis and differentiation from the Lambert-Eaton myasthenic syndrome. *Neurology* 1997;48[Suppl 5]:S23–S27.

38. Verma P, Oger J. Treatment of acquired autoimmune myasthenia gravis: a topic review. *Can J Neurol Sci* 1992; 19:360–375.
39. O Neill JH, Murray NM, Newson-Davis J. The Lambert-Eaton syndrome. A review of 50 cases. *Brain* 1988;111:577–596.
40. Lennon VA, Kryzer TJ, Grienn GE, et al. Calcium-channel antibodies in the Lambert-Eaton syndrome and other paraneoplastic syndromes. *N Engl J Med* 1995;332:1467–1474.
41. McEvoy KM, Windebank AJ, Daube JR, Low PA. 3,4-Diaminopyridine in the treatment of Lambert-Eaton myasthenic syndrome. *N Engl J Med* 1989;321:1567–1571.
42. Hoffman EP, Fischbeck KH, Brown RH, et al. Characterization of dystrophin in muscle biopsy specimens from patients with Duchenne's or Becker's muscular dystrophy. *N Engl J Med* 1988;38:1363–1368.
43. Rowland LP. Clinical concepts of Duchenne muscular dystrophy. *Brain* 1988;111:479–495.
44. Brooke MH. *A clinician's view of neuromuscular diseases*, 2nd edition. Baltimore: Williams & Wilkins, 1986: 191–205.
45. Specht LA, Kunkel LM. Duchenne and Becker muscular dystrophies. In: Rosenberg RN, Pruisner SB, DiMauro S, Barchi RL, Kunkel LM, eds. *The molecular and genetic basis of neurological disease*. Boston: Butterworth-Heinemann, 1993:613–631.
46. Beggs AH, Hoffman EP, Snyder JR, et al. Exploring the molecular basis for variability among patients with Becker muscular dystrophy: dystrophin gene and protein studies. *Am J Hum Genet* 1991;49:54–67.
47. Kaido M, Arahata K, Hoffman EP, Nonaka I, Sugita H. Muscle histology in Becker muscular dystrophy. *Muscle Nerve* 1991;14:1067–1073.
48. de Visser M, de Voogt WG, la Riviere GV. The heart in Becker muscular dystrophy, facioscapulohumeral dystrophy, and Bethlem myopathy. *Muscle Nerve* 1992;15:591–596.
49. Mendell JR, Moxley RT, Griggs RC, et al. Randomized, double blind six-month trial of prednisone in Duchenne's muscular dystrophy. *N Engl J Med* 1989;24:1592–1597.
50. Mora M, Cartegni L, DiBlasi C, et al. X-linked Emery-Dreifuss muscular dystrophy can be diagnosed from skin biopsy or blood sample. *Ann Neurol* 1997;42:249–259.
51. Emery AEH, Dreifuss FE. Unusual type of benign X-linked muscular dystrophy. *J Neurol Neurosurg Psychiatry* 1966;29:338–342.
52. Merlini L, Granata C, Dominici P, Bonfiglioli S. Emery-Dreifuss muscular dystrophy: report of five cases in a family and review of the literature. *Muscle Nerve* 1986;9:481–485.
53. Duggan DJ, Gorospe JR, Fanin M, Hoffman EP, Angelini C. Mutations in the sarcoglycan genes in patients with myopathy. *N Engl J Med* 1997;336:618–624.
54. Dincer P, Leturcq F, Richard I, et al. A biochemical, genetic, and clinical survey of autosomal recessive limb girdle muscular dystrophies in Turkey. *Ann Neurol* 1997;42:222–229.
55. Eymard B, Romero NB, Leturcq F, Piccolo F, et al. Primary adhalinopathy (alpha-sarcoglycanopathy): clinical, pathologic, and genetic correlation in 20 patients with autosomal recessive muscular dystrophy. *Neurology* 1997; 48:1227–1234.
56. Campbell KP. Adhalin gene mutations and autosomal recessive limb-girdle muscular dystrophy. *Ann Neurol* 1995;38:353–354.
57. Angelini C, Fanin M, Freda MP, et al. The clinical spectrum of sarcoglycanopathies. *Muscle Nerve* 1999;52: 176–179.
58. Li M, Dickson DW, Spiro AJ. Abnormal expression of laminin β1 chain in skeletal muscle of adult-onset limb-girdle muscular dystrophy. *Arch Neurol* 1997;54:1457–1461.
59. van der Kool AJ, Ginjaar HB, Busch KMF, et al. Limb-girdle muscular dystrophy: a pathological and immunohistochemical reevaluation. *Muscle Nerve* 1998;21:584–590.
60. Angelini C, Fanin M, Menegazzo E, et al. Homozygans α-sarcoglycan mutation in two siblings; one asymptomatic and one steroid-responsive mild limb girdle muscular dystrophy patient. *Muscle Nerve* 1998; 21:769–775.
61. Connolly AM, Pestronk A, Mehta S, Al-Lozi M. Primary α-sarcoglycan deficiency responsive to immunosuppression over three years. *Muscle Nerve* 1998;21:1549–1553.
62. Spuler S, Engel AG. Unexpected sarcolemmal complement membrane attack complex deposits on nonnecrotic muscle fibers in muscular dystrophies. *Neurology* 1998;50:41–46.
63. Brook JD, McCurrah ME, Harley HG, et al. Molecular basis of myotonic dystrophy: expansion of a trinucleotide (CTG) repeat at the 3 end of a transcript encoding a protein kinase family member. *Cell* 1992;68:799–808.
64. Harley HG, Brook JD, Rundle SA, et al. Expansion of an unstable DNA region and phenotypic variation in myotonic dystrophy. *Nature* 1992;355:545–546.
65. Harper PS. *Myotonic dystrophy*, 2nd ed. Philadelphia: W.B. Saunders, 1989.
66. Ashizawa T, Dunne CJ, Dubel JR, et al. Anticipation in myotonic dystrophy. I. Statistical verification based on clinical and haplotype findings. *Neurology* 1992;42:1871–1877.
67. Munsat TL. Therapy of myotonia. A double-blind evaluation of diphenylhydantoin, procainamide and placebo. *Neurology* 1967;17:359–367.
68. Mathieu J, Allard P, Gobeil G, et al. Anesthetic and surgical complications in 219 cases of myotonic dystrophy. *Neurology* 1997;49:1646–1650.
69. Rier K, Koch MC, Lehmann-Horn F, et al. Proximal myotonic myopathy: a new dominant disorder with myotonia, muscle weakness, and cataracts. *Neurology* 1994;44:1448–1459.

70. Rier K, Koch MC, Lehmann-Horn F, et al. Proximal myotonic myopathy: clinical features of a multisystem disorder similar to myotonic dystrophy. *Arch Neurol* 1995;52:25–31.
71. Hund E, Jansen O, Koch MC, et al. Proximal myotonic myopathy with MRI white matter abnormalities of the brain. *Neurology* 1997;48:33–37.
72. Wimenga C, Padberg GW, Moerer P, et al. Mapping of facioscapulohumeral muscular dystrophy to chromosome 4q35-qter by multipoint linkage analysis and in situ hybridization. *Genomics* 1991;5:570–575.
73. The FSH-DY Group. A prospective, quantitative study of the natural history of facioscapulohumeral muscular dystrophy (FSHD): implications for therapeutic triamyotrophic lateral sclerosis. *Neurology* 1997;48:38–46.
74. Brais B, Xie Y-G, Sanson M, et al. The oculopharyngeal muscular dystrophy locus maps to the region of the cardiac and myosin heavy chain genes on chromosome 14q11.2-q13. *Hum Mol Genet* 1995;4:429–434.
75. Stajich JM, Gilchrist JM, Lennon F, et al. Confirmation of linkage of oculopharyngeal muscular dystrophy to chromosome 14q11.2-q13. *Ann Neurol* 1996;40:801–804.
76. Victor M, Hayes R, Adams RD. Oculopharyngeal muscular dystrophy. A familial disease of late life characterized by dysphagia and progressive ptosis of the eyelids. *N Engl J Med* 1962;267:1267–1272.
77. Barbeau A. The syndrome of hereditary late-onset ptosis and dysphagia in French-Canada. In: Kuhn E, ed. *Progressive muskeldystrophie, myotonie, myasthenie*. Berlin: Springer-Verlag, 1966:102–109.
78. Laing NG, Laing BA, Meredith C, et al. Autosomal dominant distal myopathy: linkage to chromosome 14. *Am J Hum Genet* 1995;56:422–427.
79. Welander L. Myopathia distalis tarda heredetaria: 249 examined cases in 72 pedigrees. *Acta Med Scand* 1951;264[Suppl]:1–124.
80. Barohn RJ. Distal myopathies and dystrophies. Semin Neurol 1993;13:247–255.

*Diseases of Skeletal Muscle,*
edited by Robert L. Wortmann.
Lippincott Williams & Wilkins, Philadelphia © 2000

# 12

# Fibromyalgia and Asthenic Syndromes

## Robert W. Simms

*Department of Medicine, Section of Rheumatology, Boston University Arthritis Center,
Boston, Massachusetts 02118*

Fatigue is a common symptom experienced by everyone at some time. It also represents one of the more challenging complaints for physicians to deal with in many patients. At the present, fatigue can be subclassified among at least four types: objective, subjective, systemic, and asthenia (Table 1) (1,2). Each of these can occur in healthy people as the consequence of a disease. Objective fatigue, the inability to sustain a specified force or work rate during exercise, can develop in normal people during exercise or in diseases such as myophosphorylase deficiency or myasthenia gravis. Subjective fatigue, which limits exercise because unpleasant sensations have developed, may occur in normal individuals because of the build up of lactic acid, anemia, or an electrolyte abnormality. Systemic fatigue typically develops after prolonged activity and results from hypovolemia, hypertension, or hypoglycemia.

In contrast to those fatigue states is asthenia. Individuals with asthenia are unable to perform ordinary daily activities because of the sensation of generalized weakness, tiredness, and exhaustion. These may be present at rest or develop after minor exertion and are associated with a reluctance to undertake physical or mental activity. The term asthenia can appropriately be used to describe the symptoms that develop in a systemic or debilitating illness such as a severe infection, cancer, or connective tissue disease. However, it can also be applied to patients in whom no neuromuscular, endocrine, vascular, or cardiopulmonary abnormality can be identified. Those patients have normal physical examinations and laboratory results but seem to lack pep and energy. It is difficult to classify patients with asthenia because of the paucity of markers and discriminating features.

Two syndromes have been described that allow categorization of at least some patients with asthenia: fibromyalgia syndrome and chronic fatigue syndrome. The significance of these syndromes is debated by many. They certainly overlap in some ways and are not in-

**TABLE 1.** *Categories of fatigue*

| | Symptoms |
|---|---|
| Objective fatigue | Inability to sustain a specified force or work rate |
| Subjective fatigue | Exercise limited by unpleasant sensations such as myalgia, dyspnea, or tachycardia |
| Systemic fatigue | Collapse after prolonged exercise from exhaustion due to hypovolemia, hypothermia, or hypoglycemia |
| Asthenia | Complaint of general weakness, tiredness, and exhaustion after no or minor exertion and a reluctance to undertake physical or mental activity |

clusive by any means. Nevertheless, they represent significant advances in defining the nature of this perplexing problem.

## FIBROMYALGIA

Fibromyalgia is a controversial chronic syndrome that manifests with muscle and joint pain, stiffness, and fatigue (3–5). Original descriptions of the condition may be traced back as far as the 18th century. The term was given at the turn of this century by Stockman, who described inflammation in fibrous intermuscular septa. The term fibromyalgia has replaced fibrositis because subsequent investigators have been unable to verify Stockman's findings (6). The diagnosis is considered a psychosomatic disorder by many, and several studies have demonstrated links to psychiatric disturbances (7–10). In the early 1950s a number of investigators became interested in the hypothesis that the condition was a muscle disorder (6). The absence of objective findings on physical examination and the lack of laboratory abnormalities associated with fibromyalgia have continued to fuel debate. More recently, the diagnosis has also come under attack with its application in the medicolegal and disability arenas (11–18).

### Epidemiology

The development of the American College of Rheumatology classification criteria for fibromyalgia in 1990 facilitated subsequent population-based studies of fibromyalgia (19). These simple criteria were developed using methodology similar to that developed for rheumatoid arthritis and systemic lupus erythematosus. In brief, investigators from many different sites identified patients who were believed to have fibromyalgia a priori and control subjects with conditions such as low back pain or tendonitis syndromes who could be potentially confused with fibromyalgia. These subjects were then subjected to a blinded standardized assessment. The simple criteria of widespread pain for 3 months' duration and mild or greater tenderness in greater than or equal to 11 of 18 tender points yielded a sensitivity of 88% and a specificity of 81% (Table 2).

Original estimates of the prevalence of fibromyalgia approximated 10% among general medical patients and up to 20% among rheumatology clinic attendees (20,21). A large population-based survey of approximately 3,000 individuals in Wichita, Kansas, characterized

**TABLE 2.** *American college of rheumatology criteria for the classification of fibromyalgia*

History of widespread pain
  Definition: Pain on each side of the body above and below the waist and in an axial location
    (neck, anterior chest, or thoracic spine or low back) for at least 3 months duration.
Pain in 11 of 18 tender point sites on digital palpation
  Definition: Pain, on digital palpation, must be present in at least 11 of the following
    18 tender point sites:
      Occiput
      Low cervical
      Trapezius
      Supraspinatus
      Second rib
      Lateral epicondyle
      Gluteal
      Greater trochanter
      Knee

From Ref. 19, with permission.

**TABLE 3.** *Pain groups in the community (n = 3, 0006)*

| Pain group | Percent in group | 95% Confidence interval |
| --- | --- | --- |
| No pain | 62.4 | 60.7, 64.1 |
| Transient pain | 5.0 | 4.2, 5.8 |
| Chronic regional pain | 20.1 | 18.7, 21.5 |
| Chronic widespread pain | 10.6 | 9.5, 11.7 |
| Nonmusculoskeletal pain | 1.8 | 1.3, 2.3 |

From Ref. 22, with permission.

individuals according to pain categories: no pain, nonwidespread pain, and widespread pain (22). Chronic widespread pain occurred in 10.6% of the sample (Table 3). A sample of 391 persons, including 193 with widespread pain, were examined and interviewed in detail. The prevalence of fibromyalgia was 3.4% for women and 0.5% for men. The prevalence of the syndrome increased with age in women, with the highest prevalence between ages 60 and 79 (Fig. 1). A cross-sectional postal survey of 2,034 adults in northern England showed a prevalence of 11.2% for chronic widespread pain (23), results very similar to those in the United States. In contrast, however, the prevalence of widespread pain in women was similar across age categories from 45 to 75 years, approximating 20%. Both studies found that the presence of widespread pain was strongly associated with other somatic complaints and with measures of depression and anxiety.

Both studies also found that tenderness was distributed as a continuum in the general population (22–24). In the Kansas study, tender point counts were distributed as a continuum in both men and women (Fig. 2) (25). In England there was a trend between the number of sites of pain and the number of tender points in the general population (24). These studies taken together suggest both pain and tenderness are distributed as a continuum in the general population. Fibromyalgia may represent a somewhat arbitrary designation of one end of this continuum.

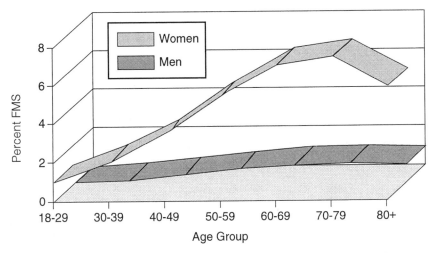

**FIG. 1.** Age-specific prevalence of fibromyalgia in the general population. FMS, fibromyalgia syndrome. (From ref. 22, with permission.)

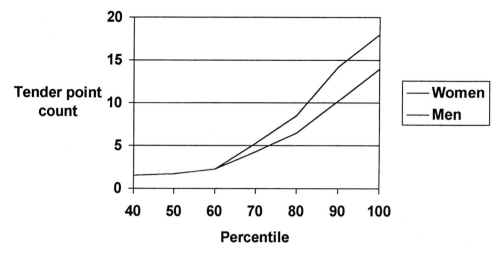

**FIG. 2.** Tender point counts in the general population. (From Ref. 22, with permission.)

## Outcome, Natural History, and Disability

There are no long-term, prospective, population-based data on outcome in fibromyalgia; however, available clinic-based studies suggest with one exception that chronic persistent symptoms are the rule (26–28). The longest follow-up study to date surveyed patients 10 years after their participation in a therapeutic trial (29). Moderate to severe pain or stiffness was reported in 55% of 28 patients. However, most reported global symptom severity at levels lower than those of 10 years earlier. The authors concluded that most patients appeared to have adapted to or coped with their condition. Noteworthy and concerning was that two patients had committed suicide, highlighting the importance of identifying and treating major depression in patients with fibromyalgia.

The issue of disability and fibromyalgia syndrome is one of the most contested controversies (17,30–33). In the largest population-based survey that assessed functional disability in the United States, high rates of self-reported functional disability were associated with the diagnosis (22). The prevalence of work disability among patients attending specialty clinics also appears to be high, with almost 15% of patients receiving Social Security disability payments compared with 2.2% of the U.S. population and to 28.9% of patients with rheumatoid arthritis (4). Because the assessment of severity as a measure of disability is based entirely on self-reported symptoms, concern regarding potential exaggeration or falsification has been voiced, particularly in the setting of compensation (30,31,34). Others have suggested that these concerns have been exaggerated, and the potential harm of denying justifiable disability is greater (35). One small study found that monetary awards for disability associated with posttraumatic fibromyalgia had no positive influence on symptoms (36).

## Diagnosis

The American College of Rheumatology criteria has become the de facto standard for diagnosis in the clinic, despite their primary intended function as classification criteria for investigations. Critics have argued that these criteria are tautologic because there is no independent "gold standard" by which to measure the performance of the criteria (31,37). The methodology of the study, however, was similar to that of other studies that generated criteria for systemic lupus erythematosus, rheumatoid arthritis, and various forms of vasculitis, all conditions for which there is no gold standard (38–40).

Although the criteria appear to be generally adequate in the clinic setting, they have not been validated in the medicolegal or compensation setting. For this reason, the Vancouver Consensus Report (a consensus conference of experts regarding the issues of fibromyalgia and disability) recommended that the diagnosis of fibromyalgia is "best made in the context of longitudinal observation, after recording and considering associated symptoms and their severity, and after considering, as well, concurrent medical and psychiatric symptoms" (17). No laboratory test or imaging procedure is of diagnostic or prognostic value.

Critics of the concept of fibromyalgia argue that applying the diagnosis is "unnecessary iatrogenic labeling" that only promotes illness behavior (31,32,41). Unfortunately, many patients with fibromyalgia undergo unnecessary diagnostic tests and in some cases surgical procedures before the diagnosis is considered (42). Applying the "label" earlier may actually protect patients from iatrogenic misadventures.

### Tender Points

Early studies of fibromyalgia emphasized the specific anatomic location of tenderness in patients with fibromyalgia (20,21). Furthermore, these studies suggested that "control sites" existed that were not tender, arguing that fibromyalgia patients were not "tender all over." It has become clear that patients with fibromyalgia are in fact more tender than control subjects at classic "tender points" and also at control sites, indicating a general lowering of pain threshold (43–45). Tender points, therefore, may be no more than convenient locations to assess a low pain threshold.

Given the observation that pain threshold and the number of tender points in the general population appear to be distributed as a continuum, the Vancouver Consensus Report recommended that patients who have fewer than the required number of tender points may also be diagnosed as having fibromyalgia, provided they have other characteristic symptoms, and tenderness at sites not specified by the American College of Rheumatology criteria does not exclude the diagnosis (17).

### Associated Disorders

Fibromyalgia has been associated with a number of conditions, including regional pain syndromes, other rheumatic conditions such as systemic lupus erythematosus, and a variety of infectious disorders (3,46–56). Myofascial pain syndrome and fibromyalgia syndrome appear to be closely related chronic musculoskeletal pain conditions.

Myofascial pain syndromes are localized musculoskeletal pain disorders, without evidence of intrinsic muscle, nerve, or joint pathology and most frequently involve the neck and shoulder girdle (3,47,48,57). Myofascial pain syndromes were thought to be accompanied by localized muscle tenderness that produced radiating symptoms or "trigger points," a local "twitch" response, and palpable "taut bands" (58). These examination features were thought to distinguish myofascial pain from fibromyalgia. However, the existence of these findings and their diagnostic specificity has been challenged (48). Myofascial pain syndrome, like fibromyalgia syndrome, has also been found to be associated with symptoms such as fatigue, sleep disturbance, and depression (3,59). Both fibromyalgia and myofascial pain syndromes are characterized by chronic pain as the predominant symptom. The pain is frequently accompanied by radiating numbness and tingling, although neurologic findings are normal. It appears that myofascial pain may evolve into fibromyalgia syndrome, and probably both diagnoses represent points on the continuum of chronic pain and tenderness (57).

Fibromyalgia has been linked to a variety of infectious conditions, including viruses such as coxsackievirus, parvovirus B19, human immunodeficiency virus (HIV), and most recently hepatitis C (54–56,60,62). Fibromyalgia has also been reported after treatment for Lyme disease (54,63). Many patients with suspected chronic Lyme disease may, in fact, have fibromyalgia with a false-positive or clinically insignificant Lyme serology (53,64). The association of fibromyalgia with infections of any type is at best tenuous, because the prevalence of fibromyalgia even in relatively large surveys of patients with infectious disorders is between 10% and 15%, virtually the same proportion as that seen in any general medical population (60–62). In the case of HIV-associated fibromyalgia, the presence of depressive symptoms appears to be a strong risk factor for the development of fibromyalgia (60).

Fibromyalgia syndrome may be quite common in systemic lupus erythematosus, with a prevalence between 20% and 40% (49,50). In one study of 102 patients with lupus, 22% met criteria for fibromyalgia (50). Lupus patients with fibromyalgia were more likely to be unable to perform daily activities, less likely to be employed, more likely to be divorced, and more likely to be receiving welfare or medical disability benefits. Interestingly, patients with fibromyalgia did not differ from their nonfibromyalgia lupus counterparts with measures of disease activity, such as serum complement levels, erythrocyte sedimentation rates, or the presence of double-stranded DNA. They did, however, have higher systemic lupus activity measure (SLAM) scores (50). Measures of activity of systemic lupus such as the SLAM index may therefore be confounded by the presence of fibromyalgia, although this does not appear to be the case with another activity index, the systemic lupus erythematosus activity index (49).

The association with trauma and fibromyalgia has been particularly contentious (34,65–69). In the largest study to date of this association, the prevalence of fibromyalgia syndrome was assessed in patients in Israel treated at a regional occupational clinic for neck injury or lower extremity fracture (66). Fibromyalgia was diagnosed in 21.6% of those with neck injury versus 1.7% of control subjects with lower extremity fractures. Although fibromyalgia syndrome was 13 times more frequent after neck injury than after lower extremity injury, it is not clear that all patients with neck injury were "captured" in this study's design. A referral bias may have been more likely to occur among those reporting neck injury in favor of enriching this group with fibromyalgia or chronic pain patients. In any case, the Vancouver Consensus Conference concluded that there are insufficient data to establish a causal relationship between fibromyalgia and trauma (17).

## Pathophysiology

Investigators have studied diverse potential mechanisms in fibromyalgia syndrome (Table 4). These studies have included those of muscle structure and biochemistry, sleep physiology, neurohormonal function, and psychological status. Although the pathophysiology of fibromyalgia remains unknown, the weight of evidence suggests that central or more specifically psychological factors play a prominent and probably a crucial role.

**TABLE 4.** *Studies of muscle in fibromyalgia syndrome*

| Study type | Author | Year | Findings |
|---|---|---|---|
| Histologic studies | | | |
| | Brendstrup | 1957 | Metachromatic substance in intrafibrillar tissue |
| | Awad | 1973 | Mucoid substance, giant myofilaments |
| | Fassbender | 1975 | Abnormal mitochondria |
| | Henriksson | 1985 | Moth-eaten type I fibers, ragged red fibers |
| | Bartels | 1986 | Reticular network, rubber band constrictions |
| | Bengtsson | 1986 | Ragged red, moth-eaten fibers |
| Metabolic studies | | | |
| | Bengtsson | 1986 | Low ATP, ADP, AMP, PCr at tender points |
| | Lund | 1986 | Low tissue $PO_2$ |
| | Mather | 1988 | Low PCr/ADP, PCr/Pi, pH |
| | DeBlecourt | 1991 | Normal at rest |
| | Jacobsen | 1992 | Rest Pi/PCr normal, high PCr during exercise |
| | Simms | 1994 | Normal PCr/Pi and pH at rest, during exercise, at tender and nontender sites |
| | Jubrias | 1994 | Normal Pi, PCr, increased PDE |
| | Simms | 1995 | Normal PDE |
| Strength studies | | | |
| | Jacobsen | 1987 | Low maximum isokinetic and isometric strength |
| | Lindh | 1994 | Low but submaximal isokinetic voluntary contraction |
| | Elert | 1992 | Normal |
| | Simms | 1994 | Normal maximal voluntary contraction at trapezius and tibialis anterior |

In aggregate, these studies have failed to demonstrate that muscles are abnormal in patients with fibromyalgia.
ATP, adenosine triphosphate; ADP, adenosine diphosphate; AMP, adenosine monophosphate; PCr, creatine phosphate; Pi, inorganic phosphorous; PDE, phosphodiesters.

## Muscle Studies

Given that patients with fibromyalgia complain of diffuse pain, especially in muscles, it is natural that the origin of the condition resides in muscle tissue. With the advent of the electron microscope, morphologic abnormalities were reported on muscle biopsy (6). Abnormalities described included "ragged red fibers" (70) and "rubber band morphology" (71). These studies, however, were uncontrolled and, in the absence of adequate and uniformly applied diagnostic criteria, are difficult to interpret (6). Nevertheless, these early morphologic studies suggested the possibility of a metabolic abnormality in muscles of fibromyalgia patients.

The suggestion that muscle metabolism was abnormal was made in the mid-1980s (72,73). Bengtsson et al. (74) measured high-energy phosphate metabolite concentrations in biopsy specimens from tender points in the trapezius muscles of 15 patients, from the nonpainful anterior tibialis muscle from 6 patients, and from the trapezius muscles of 8 healthy control subjects. All patients met clinical criteria proposed by Yunus et al. (20) for the diagnosis of fibromyalgia. Levels of ATP, ADP, AMP, and creatine phosphate were measured and were found to be lower in the trapezius specimens in patients than in those from the control group and lower than those from their own tibialis anterior muscles.

With the hypothesis that localized muscle ischemia could alter metabolism and cause muscle pain and tenderness, Lund et al. (73) attempted to determine the level of oxygenation in muscle directly by using an oxygen electrode. Ten patients meeting the Yunus criteria and eight healthy control subjects were studied. Multiple measures at each site were used to generate a "tissue oxygen pressure field histogram," which in normal subjects has a Gaussian shape. Abnormal histograms were found in the deep muscle tissue of the trapezius and brachioradialis sites in patients but not in control subjects, despite the fact that mean tissue oxygen tensions were identical. The authors concluded that abnormal tissue oxygenation in muscle and subcutaneous tissue occurs at trigger-point sites in fibromyalgia patients and that these abnormalities were responsible for an "energy crisis" that produced muscular pain in the condition.

Muscle detraining results in decreases in the concentration of high-energy muscle compounds such as ATP and creatine phosphate, lowered activities of anaerobic oxidative enzymes, and decreased capillary density (75). Because the studies of Bengtsson, Lund, and colleagues used healthy control subjects, it is possible that the findings of each were the result of localized muscle deconditioning or detraining. The importance of this point was underscored by the findings of Bennett et al. (76) in 1989 when they performed a standardized aerobic fitness measurement and found that over 80% of patients with fibromyalgia were substantially below the average level of aerobic fitness. These data suggest that generalized or localized muscle detraining could account for the metabolic "abnormalities" identified in earlier studies.

$^{31}$P-magnetic resonance spectroscopy is especially useful for the study of muscle energy metabolism because it is noninvasive, involves no ionizing radiation or labeling agents, and can be used to study subjects at rest and with exercise. The ability to study muscle under conditions of exercise is particularly useful in the study of suspected metabolic muscle disorders, because muscle may be energetically normal in the rest state and only display abnormalities when stressed (77,78).

Early studies using magnetic resonance spectroscopy reported conflicting results and were problematic because they were not performed under dynamic conditions. One controlled study performed under dynamic conditions found no difference between patients and control subjects at rest and during recovery after exercise, but patients with fibromyalgia were found to tolerate only half of the workload of the control subjects and showed smaller changes levels of inorganic phosphorus and creatine phosphate and in pH (79). It appeared that these differences, however, were the result of failure of the patients to fully fatigue their calf muscles compared with the control group. Additionally, the level of aerobic fitness was not accounted for. Park et al. (80) compared absolute values of creatine phosphate and ATP levels in the quadriceps muscles of 12 patients and normal control subjects at standardized levels of exercise. At rest and during exercise, creatine phosphate and ATP levels were 15% lower in patients than in the normal control subjects ($p < 0.001$ and $<0.03$, respectively). This study identified differences in the energetics of muscles in patients with fibromyalgia compared with control subjects, but the cause of these differences and the contribution of detraining or deconditioning are still uncertain (26).

Only one study has most fully accounted for the possible effects of deconditioning on muscle in fibromyalgia syndrome and has simultaneously studied two muscle sites under dynamic conditions (81). In this study, Simms et al. selected sedentary control subjects who had similar levels of aerobic fitness (determined by $Vo_2$max measurements) to compare with a group of patients with fibromyalgia syndrome. Furthermore, the maximal voluntary contraction of the studied muscles, namely the upper trapezius and the tibialis anterior, were similar in both groups, indicating that both groups could generate virtually identical muscle workloads. Magnetic resonance spectroscopy was performed in both groups at rest and during and after submaximal exercise protocol. When controlling for $Vo_2$max and maximum voluntary contraction, measurements of the principle high-energy phosphate metabolites and intracellular pH were not significantly different in the patients with fibromyalgia compared with the sedentary control subjects. Furthermore, there was no correlation between overall pain or local pain severity and the levels of creatine phosphate. These data, therefore, provided strong evidence that muscle energy metabolism at sites of muscle symptoms was not different than that in sedentary control subjects and that the findings of prior studies suggesting abnormal muscle energetics were confounded by muscle deconditioning.

A report by Jubrias et al. (82) raised the possibility that phosphodiesters could be abnormal in patients with fibromyalgia. Phosphodiesters result from the hydrolysis products of membrane phospholipids by phospholipase. The principle phosphodiesters are *sr*-glycerol-3-phosphorylcholine and *sn*-glyceral-3-phosphorylethanolamine and are detected frequently in $^{31}$P-magnetic resonance spectroscopy in a small peak between inorganic phosphorous and creatine phosphate (83,84). Spectroscopy was performed in the forearms of 11 patients with fibromyalgia syndrome and in 10 healthy control subjects before and after concentric and eccentric exercise in both dominant and nondominant forearms. No differences in inorganic phosphorous or creatine phosphate levels were found between patients and control subjects. An increased occurrence of phosphodiester peaks was observed in the nondominant forearms of patients when compared with control subjects, although this occurred in only 3 of 11 patients. These investigators postulated that the increased presence of phosphodiester peaks in fibromyalgia patients resulted from activity-induced disruption of the muscle membrane that is not repaired normally. This disruption could result in muscle pain. The difficulty with this hypothesis, however, is that phosphodiester levels were not quantitated. The presence or absence of detectable phosphodiester peaks may depend on factors other than the concentration of those compounds present in the sample. Moreover, defining the simple presence or absence of phosphodiester peaks does not adequately describe the potential biologic significance of the finding.

Finally, Simms and Hrovat (85) reexamined their data from the initial study and quantitated phosphodiesters in spectra of the tibialis anterior of 11 patients and 13 sedentary control subjects with similar levels of aerobic conditioning. Phosphodiester levels at rest, during exercise, and in recovery were found to be no different in patients compared with control subjects using both univariate and multivariate analyses. These data indicate that phosphodiesters are not increased in patients with fibromyalgia and therefore cannot be considered a marker of abnormal membrane disruption.

Other studies in fibromyalgia have examined muscle strength. An early study of this type suggested that patients with fibromyalgia had low isokinetic and isometric strength when compared with control subjects (86). Although the authors proposed that a metabolic defect might account for these results, lower extremity pain could have also produced these same findings. Subsequent studies that combined strength measurements with electrical stimulation of muscles suggested that lower maximal voluntary contraction was the result of submaximal force application in patients with fibromyalgia when compared with normal control subjects (81,87,88). These data suggest that intrinsic muscle strength in patients with fibromyalgia is not abnormal but that voluntary contractions, either maximal or submaximal, may be influenced by pain or muscle conditioning.

A popular theory of the genesis of pain in fibromyalgia was that excessive muscle tension led to increased excitability of nociceptors in muscle, in turn leading to "muscle hypertension" and chronic pain (89,90). Furthermore, defective sympathetic control was proposed to result in disturbed microcirculation and nociceptor excitation, based largely on the observation that selective sympathetic blockade reduced pain and the number of tender points (91). This theory invokes amplification of peripheral nocireceptor function through sensitization of the relevant dorsal horn pain transmission neurons (92). Through this mechanism, input from nocireceptors and mechanoreceptors, which otherwise would be subclinical, leads to the symptoms of pain and, through reflex mechanisms, to other features such as muscle tightness, dermatographia, and allodynia. However, studies using electromyographic techniques show no clear evidence of excessive muscle tension (6), and studies of muscle sympathetic function similarly show no evidence of sympathetic overactivity (93).

Others have hypothesized that many of the signs of fibromyalgia may be related to vertebral and sacroiliac dysfunction (94). This hypothesis holds that functional dysfunctions represent areas of altered spinal biomechanics, which with general or regional pain amplification results in heightened spinal reflex activity, causing muscle tightness, tender points, and myalgias.

A number of studies have examined the role of tender points in fibromyalgia syndrome. Initially, investigators proposed that patients with fibromyalgia were abnormally tender only at specific tender point sites and not at other control sites (21). In fact, detailed work to determine tenderness with a pressure gauge at both tender point sites and control sites has indicated that patients with fibromyalgia are more tender than normal control subjects everywhere and not simply at tender point sites (43–45). These data suggest that patients with fibromyalgia have a central basis for their pain syndrome, that fibromyalgia syndrome is literally a disorder of lowered pain threshold. Wolfe et al. (25) found that decreased pain threshold as measured by the tender point count (additive number of tender points) correlates with all the symptoms of fibromyalgia, suggesting that decreased pain threshold is an intrinsic aspect of patient distress.

### Sleep Physiology and Serotonin

Most patients with fibromyalgia complain of poor sleep. They report difficulty getting to sleep, frequent awakening, and early morning awakening. Early studies of fibromyalgia documented distinctive abnormalities in stage 4 sleep, consisting of alpha wave intrusion into the normal delta wave rhythm (95). Introduction of this sleep abnormality in healthy volunteers by triggering a subliminal buzzer as they entered stage 4 sleep produced a transient fibromyalgia-like syndrome (96). Subsequent studies have shown that the alpha-delta sleep abnormality is not specific to fibromyalgia but has also been reported in post-accident pain, depression, and rheumatoid arthritis. Furthermore, some maintain the "alpha wave intrusion" to be artifactual.

Moldofsky proposed that serotonin deficiency formed the basis of sleep abnormality in fibromyalgia because serotonin was involved in both pain modulation and maintenance of stage 4 sleep (95,96). Several studies have attempted to test the serotonin hypothesis. Two studies found low serum levels of serotonin in patients with fibromyalgia, apparently due to low levels of serotonin in platelets (97,98). Others, however, found no significant differences between plasma serotonin in patients with fibromyalgia compared with control subjects (99).

Substance P, a neuropeptide involved in pain transmission from the periphery to the central nervous system, which seems to inversely correlated with serotonin, was found to be significantly elevated in the cerebrospinal fluid of patients with fibromyalgia (100). Whether these and other unconfirmed findings indicating abnormalities in cerebrospinal fluid biogenic amines, serum somatomedin C, or prolactin levels are cause or effect remain to be determined (101–103).

## Studies of Regional Cerebral Blood Flow

Much evidence suggests that alterations in brain function may occur in response to painful stimuli. In healthy persons, for example, mild pain produced by electrical or heat stimulation of a finger produced significant increases in regional blood flow of the contralateral cortex, including the cingulate cortex and thalamus (104,105). Chronic pain, in contrast, appears to result in regional decreases in cerebral blood flow (106,107). Advanced cancer pain, for example, was found to decrease thalamic blood flow, with return to normal levels after cordotomy and relief of pain.

Investigators have examined brain function by measuring cerebral blood flow in fibromyalgia (108). Mountz et al. (108) performed single photon emission computed tomography of the brain of ten patients with fibromyalgia and seven control subjects. Low regional blood flow was found in the caudate and hemithalamus in patients compared with control subjects and correlated with pain threshold but not with psychological status. This study points to possible disturbances in brain function in patients with fibromyalgia, although the possible confounding effects of medication, the influence of depression, sex differences in regional blood flow, and the small numbers of patients and control subjects studied warrant cautious interpretation and further evaluation.

## Hypothalamic-Pituitary-Adrenal Axis Function

The hypothalamic-pituitary-adrenal (HPA) axis is thought to play a crucial role in the physiologic response to physical and emotional stress (109) and has been examined in conditions such as fibromyalgia. Despite the clinical similarity of fibromyalgia and chronic fatigue syndrome to depression, there appear to be differences in the HPA axis profiles (Table 5). The overall pattern of HPA axis function in fibromyalgia and chronic fatigue syndrome appears similar in that basal urinary cortisol is low compared with healthy control subjects, although there are differences in adrenocorticotropin and cortisol responses to corticotropin-releasing hormone. In contrast, the HPA axis profile of major depression appears to reflect hyperfunction (109). It appears that nonmelancholic forms of depression may have a HPA axis profile similar to both fibromyalgia and chronic fatigue syndrome with reduced activation of the axis. A characteristic profile of HPA dysfunction in fibromyalgia has yet to emerge, and it is unclear to what extent de-

**TABLE 5.** *Summary of HPA axis function in patients with fibromyalgia, chronic fatigue syndrome, and depression*

| Hormone measures | Fibromyalgia syndrome | Chronic fatigue syndrome | Major depression |
|---|---|---|---|
| **Stimulated hormone levels** | | | |
| oCRH stimulus | | | |
|   Cortisol response | Normal/increased | Decreased | Decreased |
| Low ACTH stimulus | Decreased | Normal | Normal |
|   Cortisol response | NR | Increased | Normal |
| High ACTH stimulus | | | |
|   Cortisol response | Normal | Decreased | Increased |
| **Basal levels** | | | |
| Urinary free cortisol | Decreased | Decreased | Increased |
| Plasma cortisol | NR | Decreased | Increased |

HPA, hypothalamic-pituitary-adrenal; oCRH, ovine corticotropin-releasing hormone; ACTH, adrenocorticotropic hormone; NR, not reported.
From Ref. 5, with permission.

pression confounds the reported observations. It is also worth noting that a controlled trial of low-dose corticosteroids provided no benefit in relieving the symptoms of fibromyalgia (110).

### Studies of Psychological Disturbance

Fibromyalgia has been frequently linked to psychological disturbance, although whether depression is an intrinsic component of fibromyalgia or whether it is caused by fibromyalgia is debated. Initial studies purporting the association of fibromyalgia with major depression using the Minnesota Multiphasic Personality Inventory (MMPI) were criticized because the presence of symptoms such as fatigue and widespread pain automatically increased scores for depression and hypochondriasis (111–114). Subsequent controlled studies using structured psychiatric interviews have found consistently high lifetime rates of major depression, which range from 34% to 71% (7,10,115).

The high association of fibromyalgia with depression is thought to be confounded by selection bias. Patients attending clinics specializing in fibromyalgia are more likely to possess higher rates of psychiatric distress, because they have more severe symptoms. Clarke et al. (110) found no significant differences between nonreferral patients with fibromyalgia and general medical outpatients with respect to the prevalence of depression. Wolfe et al. (22) examined psychological distress in a population-based study and compared the levels of psychological distress in this group with patients with fibromyalgia attending a clinic specializing in the treatment of the syndrome, finding high levels of psychiatric distress in both groups. These data suggest that psychiatric distress is inherent to the syndrome rather than a feature of health care-seeking behavior.

Aaron et al. (116) recently argued that psychological disorders are not intrinsically related to fibromyalgia, because "nonpatients" (people who meet the criteria for fibromyalgia but who have never sought medical care for their symptoms) were found to have a similar number of lifetime psychiatric diagnoses as healthy control subjects. These authors suggested on this basis that psychiatric disorders were not intrinsically related to fibromyalgia but that "psychiatric disorders contribute to the decision to seek medical care." This study should be viewed with caution because the severity of depression (as measured by the Trait Anxiety Inventory and Center for Epidemiological Studies Depression Scale) was significantly higher among nonpatients than control subjects although not as high as among patients. This finding suggests that level of distress, not the number of psychiatric diagnoses, leads to health care-seeking behavior among patients with fibromyalgia syndrome. Others have found that the level of psychological distress in fibromyalgia is highly correlated with pain threshold and other symptoms (22,25,117–119). It appears that changes in levels of psychological distress correlate closely with fluctuations in pain threshold (120).

If depression preceded the onset of fibromyalgia, this would constitute strong evidence favoring a causal role for depression in fibromyalgia. In an evaluation of 31 patients with fibromyalgia and 14 patients with rheumatoid arthritis, both the rate of a major affective disorder and the familial prevalence of major affective disorder were significantly higher in the patients with fibromyalgia than those with rheumatoid arthritis (8). In addition, depression was found to antedate the symptoms of fibromyalgia (8). The retrospective nature of this assessment, however, is subject to potential recall bias, and firm conclusions regarding the temporal relationship with depression and fibromyalgia cannot be drawn from this study alone.

Silman et al. (121) studied the association between psychological disorders and fibromyalgia in a large cohort by having almost 2,000 adults complete a variety of psychological assessments (including the General Health Questionnarie, Somatic Symptom Checklist, and the Self-Care Assessment Schedule) at the onset of the study and 1 year later. Subjects free of chronic widespread pain were found to be significantly at increased risk of chronic widespread pain if they possessed high levels of psychological distress, including depression. This study provides the first population-based prospective evidence for a link between psychological distress and depression and the development of fibromyalgia syndrome.

Other evidence for a relationship with depression has been the frequent association of fibromyalgia with other conditions that are themselves associated with depression, such as migraine headaches, irritable bowel syndrome, and panic disorder (115). It has been postulated that fibromyalgia, migraine, headache, sinusitis, irritable bowel syndrome, chronic fatigue syndrome, major depression, and panic disorder represent an affective spectrum of disorders that share a common physiologic and possibly heritable abnormality (122). The hypothesis that there is a common biologic link between fibromyalgia and depression has been strengthened by the finding that patients with fibromyalgia possess the same serotonin transporter gene genotype as those with major depression (123). The association of childhood sexual abuse with a high prevalence of depression and ethanol abuse among first-degree relatives of patients with fibromyalgia further supports the concept that fibromyalgia is a component of the "affective spectrum" (124,125).

## CHRONIC FATIGUE SYNDROME

The term chronic fatigue syndrome is used to represent a heterogeneous disorder at the more severe end of the spectrum of asthenic disorders. The syndrome has probably affected people throughout history but only recently has become more recognized as an entity. In the 1980s, several reports appeared linking a chronic disabling illness with elevated antibody titers to Epstein-Barr virus (126–128). In addition, an outbreak of a severe fatiguing illness was reported in Nevada, resulting in involvement by the Centers for Disease Control and Prevention (CDC) (129). Analysis of these cases and others led to the CDC sponsoring the development of a case definition of chronic fatigue syndrome in 1988 (130). Another group was assembled in 1993 to revise the definition (131).

The current most widely accepted definition of chronic fatigue syndrome states that it is an idiopathic process that causes self-reported persistent relapsing fatigue lasting greater than 6 consecutive months. In addition, four or more of the following symptoms must be present: impaired memory or concentration, sore throat, tender cervical or axillary lymph nodes, muscle pain, multi-joint pain, new headaches, unrefreshing sleep, and postexercise malaise. This definition, as were the criteria for fibromyalgia syndrome, is limited because it was developed from the personal experience of many individuals rather than from a defined data set. Similarly, it was established to facilitate research efforts as opposed to a clinical tool (132).

The prevalence of chronic fatigue syndrome is difficult to determine. Self-reporting surveys are anything but exact measures. The proportion of patients in a primary care practice who report chronic fatigue lasting 6 or more months ranges between 10% and 20% (133,134). In community surveys, approximately 1% to 3% report fatigue of that duration (135,136). Various applications of the CDC criteria for chronic fatigue syndrome have provided estimates ranging between 10 and 2,600 cases per 100,000 population (137). Regardless of its prevalence, it appears to affect women more than men, people of most races, and those of all socioeconomic groups.

Many consider the chronic fatigue syndrome to represent a post-infective state. Indeed, there have been historical associations made with infective agents such as Epstein-Barr virus, other viral infections, and brucellosis. Many patients report the onset of thin fatigue with a "flu-like" illness. To date, the only prospective study examining the association between viral infections and chronic fatigue syndrome provides clear evidence against the association (136). Furthermore, there is no evidence that chronic fatigue syndrome has ever been transmitted from one person to another (138).

Stress is the other frequently associated trigger for chronic fatigue syndrome. There exists a large amount of literature documenting the adverse effects of stress on the immune system and susceptibility to viral infection (139,140). Perhaps more important is the relationship between stress and psychological or psychiatric illness. A significant number of patients with chronic fatigue syndrome have a history of a previous or ongoing psychiatric diagnosis (141,142). It is also easy to recognize similarities between the afflictions of chronic fatigue syndrome with those of major depression. Fatigue, sleep disturbance, psychomotor changes, cognitive impairment, and mood changes are characteristic of each. However, to label chronic fatigue syndrome as simply a psychological disorder would be inappropriate (Table 5). As with fibromyalgia, these are individuals with diagnosed psychiatric disease, those that become depressed because of their chronic poorly understood condition, and those with no evidence of a psychological disorder (133–136,143).

### Overlap with Fibromyalgia

Although initially described as separate entities, increasingly fibromyalgia and chronic fatigue syndrome have been linked as the same disorder (3,26,115,144–146). Although the CDC criteria for chronic fatigue syndrome differ from the American College of Rheumatology criteria for fibromyalgia, the differences appear to reflect which symptoms patients regard as primary, that is, whether patients complain primarily of fatigue or of pain. Many studies have documented the strikingly similar demographic and clinical features of severe fatigue, sleep disturbance, musculoskeletal pain, and self-reported impairment in concentration and short-term memory (3,144,146). Furthermore, both conditions are also strongly linked to affective disorders, including major depression that often predates the other condition (115,147,148). Neither chronic fatigue syndrome nor fibromyalgia syndrome possess pathognomonic signs or diagnostic tests that have been validated in scientific studies. There remains no convincing evidence to date that either chronic fatigue syndrome or fibromyalgia syndrome are the result of chronic infection, viral or otherwise. It seems logical based on the current state of knowledge to group both fibromyalgia and chronic fatigue syndrome together.

### MANAGEMENT

### Therapeutic Agents

Tertiary amine tricyclics such as amitriptyline, imipramine, clomipramine, and doxepin inhibit neuronal reuptake of serotonin more than the secondary amine demethylated metabolites such as desipramine and nortriptyline. Because fibromyalgia syndrome was initially believed to be a disorder of sleep and pain, serotonin was implicated as a possible mediator. Tricyclics, as inhibitors of serotonin reuptake, were therefore logical choices for use in those patients.

Uncontrolled reports initially suggested that amitriptyline was useful. At low doses, amitriptyline appeared to cause rapid eye movement (REM) suppression and prolongation of stages 3 and 4 non-REM sleep (149). Low doses have generally been used by investigators to avoid the antidepressant effect of high doses and the increased frequency of side effects.

Four controlled trials have evaluated the efficacy of amitriptyline in fibromyalgia with trial duration ranging from 2 to 24 weeks and dose ranging from 10 to 50 mg/day (150–153). Three of these four trials indicated that amitriptyline compared favorably with placebo. However, the longest term trial showed no benefit when compared with placebo (154). Furthermore, the overall degree of benefit appears to be relatively small in relevant outcomes such as lessening of pain, fatigue, and sleep disturbance. Few patients achieved clinically important improvement. In clinical practice, attempts to increase doses of amitriptyline are generally limited by anticholinergic side effects such as dry mouth and drowsiness. In fact, as many as half of patients experience these troublesome side effects even at low doses, forcing discontinuation in perhaps one third.

Cyclobenzaprine is a tricyclic agent with similar chemical structure to amitriptyline that has been marketed as a muscle relaxant based on its ability to reduce brainstem noradrenergic function and motor neuron efferent activity. Several trials have examined the efficacy of this agent in fibromyalgia syndrome because it was thought to potentially offer some of the benefits of amitriptyline without its troubling side effects. In general, however, only modest or no efficacy has been demonstrated in short-term trials (155). In the only long-term trial comparing both amitriptyline and cyclobenzaprine with placebo, cyclobenzaprine fared no better than amitriptyline when compared with placebo in efficacy. Furthermore, more patients withdrew from the cyclobenzaprine treatment arm of the study (154).

To circumvent some of the difficulties encountered with amitriptyline and other agents, investigators have begun to study a new class of antidepressants that has demonstrated efficacy in the treatment of depression without many of the troublesome side effects of the tricyclic agents. These agents include fluoxetine, sertraline, paroxetine, and fluvoxamine. They are structurally unrelated but share the ability to selectively and potently block reuptake of serotonin. In the treatment of depression, there is currently no data to suggest that any one of the selective serotonergic receptor inhibitors is superior, and approximately 50% of patients who fail while taking one will improve when switched to another. These agents are not devoid of side effects, however, and central nervous system activation manifested by anxiety and insomnia is not uncommon (156).

In the treatment of fibromyalgia, a particularly attractive approach has been the use of combination therapy, using a selective serotonergic receptor inhibitor and a low-dose tricyclic agent. This approach has the advantage of using full-dose antidepressant therapy with the addition of a small dose of a relatively sedating tricyclic. The latter has the advantage of having a favorable effect on sleep. A recent study evaluated the efficacy of a combination approach using both fluoxetine 20 mg daily and amitriptyline 10 mg at bedtime versus either agent alone and placebo (133). In this trial, the combination worked better when compared with either agent alone (152). No increase in side effects was observed in the patients treated with the combination.

Alprazolam is a triazolobenzodiazipine approved for the treatment of anxiety and depression. Because its antidepressant and antianxiety effects may be comparable with tricyclic agents and because it may be better tolerated, several clinical trials have assessed its efficacy in patients with fibromyalgia. In the largest trial of 6 weeks' duration, no clear benefit was seen when compared with placebo (157). Long-term use of benzodiazepines has also been tempered by concern over dependence and possible withdrawal seizures. Most recommend avoidance of benzodiazepines in the treatment of fibromyalgia or chronic fatigue syndrome.

## Anti-inflammatory Agents

Anti-inflammatory agents have received modest attention despite the lack of evidence that there is an inflammatory basis for fibromyalgia or chronic fatigue syndrome (132,138–141). No nonsteroidal anti-inflammatory agent has proven to be more beneficial than placebo (151,157–159). Systemic corticosteroid therapy was evaluated in a 2-week, double-blind, placebo-controlled, crossover trial involving 20 patients (160). Patients were assigned to treatment with either 15 mg of prednisone per day or placebo. Mean changes in analogue scores of pain, sleep, fatigue, and dolorimeter score showed no difference between the prednisone and placebo treatment periods (140). Recent data suggesting a dysfunction of the HPA axis in some patients with fibromyalgia syndrome or chronic fatigue syndrome may necessitate a reevaluation of corticosteroids in the disorder. However, today there is no indication for the use of systemic corticosteroids in these disorders.

Acetaminophen and tramadol are useful adjuncts for management of pain symptoms. Caution is advised in the use of tramadol in individuals with a history of substance abuse. The incidence of dependency on this weak opioid agonist in individuals with no history of substance abuse appears to be low. As a general rule, narcotic analgesic use in fibromyalgia should be discouraged.

## Exercise Therapy

At least one controlled trial has demonstrated that cardiovascular fitness training is more effective in reducing global symptoms in patients with fibromyalgia than simple flexibility exercises (161). Unfortunately in clinical practice, relatively few patients are able to comply with a long-term aerobic activity, and some patients will not participate at all because of immediate postexertion exacerbation of symptoms. Nevertheless, for patients who are able to participate in regular long-term aerobic exercise programs, many are able to successfully wean off other medication and become more functional. Those who do not tend to develop a vicious cycle of worsening pain and muscle deconditioning. Although vigorous regular exercise may be the most beneficial, significant benefit is derived from low level aerobic fitness that can be accomplished with simple activities such as a regular walking program.

## Other Approaches

Electromyography feedback has been shown to be of benefit in psychosomatic disorders such as functional diarrhea and tension headache. With this procedure, patients receive auditory feedback of ongoing muscle tension in scalp muscles determined with the use of surface electrodes placed on the forehead. Typically, the feedback is presented in the form of pulse sounds that are proportional to the level of scalp muscle tension. Patients then attempt to control their muscle tension to obtain relief. One controlled study of biofeedback reported a 50% clinical improvement in two thirds of patients at 6 months

(162). Using the MMPI, no correlation was found between depression and "an overt psychosomatic background" and response to biofeedback.

One randomized trial of electroacupuncture has been conducted in patients with fibromyalgia (163). Improvement was observed in seven of eight outcome measures in the active treatment group, whereas none of those that received sham therapy showed improvement. Pain threshold, which was considered the principle outcome measure, improved by 70% in the electroacupuncture group as compared with 4% in the control group. There were several limitations to this study. It is unclear whether electroacupuncture is equivalent to conventional acupuncture because some acupuncturists claim that electroacupuncture provides only short-term analgesic benefit whereas conventional acupuncture may provide longer lasting analgesia. Patients may not have been optimally blinded in this study. There was no measure of functional or psychological status. Finally, the time course of when assessments were performed after treatment was not detailed.

Hypnotherapy has shown to be beneficial in some patients with diseases in which psychological factors may contribute to pathogenesis. These include asthma, peptic ulcer disease, and irritable bowel syndrome. Forty patients with fibromyalgia were randomized to either hypnotherapy or physical therapy for 12 weeks with follow-up at 24 weeks. Patients in the hypnotherapy group experienced significantly greater improvement in pain, fatigue, and global assessment at both 12 and 24 weeks (164). Hypnotherapy therefore may be a useful intervention in some patients with particularly refractory symptoms.

A variety of therapies for fibromyalgia has been advocated based on uncontrolled observations. These include local injection of tender points, low-frequency transcutaneous electrical nerve stimulation, cognitive behavioral treatment, chiropractic manipulation, physical therapy, and myofascial therapy. A variety of "alternative" over-the-counter drugs, nutritional supplements, herbs, vitamins, and various remedies have also been advocated. The role of these therapies and their relative cost-efficacy remain uncertain. Patients should be cautioned to view most of these approaches with a healthy degree of skepticism.

## Role of Patient Education

The optimal management of patients with fibromyalgia should include a discussion of the diagnosis, the natural history of the disorder, aggravating and alleviating factors, and treatment. Knowledge of the condition appears to lessen anxiety and allow better coping strategies. Patients and their families should be instructed to view fibromyalgia as a disorder that is not crippling. In addition, they should learn that although it is generally a chronic condition, effective therapy is available, although there is no specific "cure." When possible, patients should be encouraged to take an active self-help-oriented approach rather than a passive approach to management of their condition.

## Suggested Approach to Management

The management of fibromyalgia should include an assessment of severity of symptoms and particularly their functional impact (Fig. 3). For patients with mild symptoms and minimal functional impact, patient education and low-level aerobic exercise may be sufficient. For most patients, the use of antidepressant therapies form the cornerstone of current treatment approaches. For these patients, initiating therapy with low-dose tricyclic in addition to low-level aerobic exercise is reasonable. The starting dose of amitriptyline generally should be 10 mg given at bedtime. Occasionally, in patients who

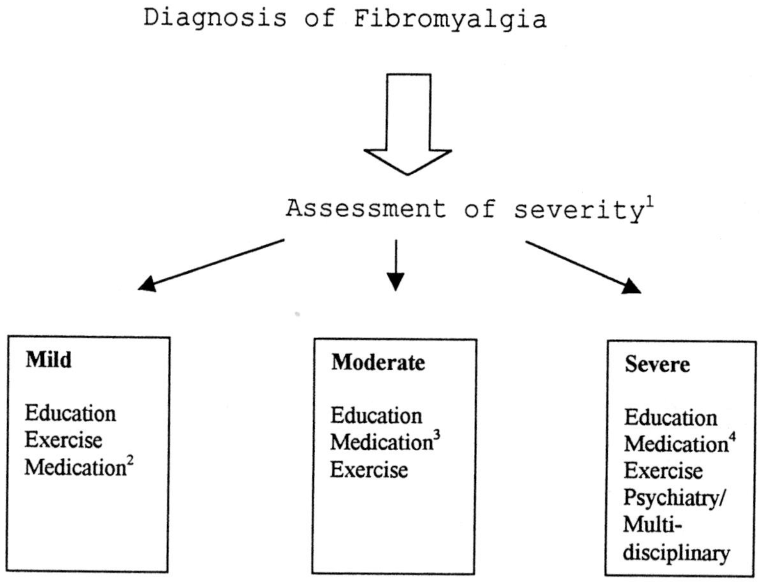

Diagnosis of Fibromyalgia

Assessment of severity[1]

| Mild | Moderate | Severe |
|------|----------|--------|
| Education<br>Exercise<br>Medication[2] | Education<br>Medication[3]<br>Exercise | Education<br>Medication[4]<br>Exercise<br>Psychiatry/<br>Multi-<br>disciplinary |

**FIG. 3.** Management scheme for management of fibromyalgia syndrome. *1.* Assessment of severity includes evaluation of pain, sleep, and fatigue symptoms and functional impairment (e.g., impact of symptoms on employment). *2.* Medication for mild symptoms might include only low-dose tricyclic. *3.* Medication for moderately severe symptoms might include the combination of a selective serotonin reuptake inhibitor with low-dose tricyclic. *4.* Medication regimen for severe symptoms would initially include that recommended for moderate symptoms but may require revision in coordination with a psychiatrist.

are particularly sensitive to side effects, as little as 5 mg/day may be effective. Nortriptyline may be better tolerated than amitriptyline by some patients and should be tried at the same doses as amitriptyline. If there is no response to the initial dose and side effects are tolerable after 1 week, the dose should be increased on a weekly basis thereafter. In general, doses that exceed 50 mg/day confer little additional benefit if there is no response to lower doses. For patients with more severe symptoms and for those with associated depression without agitation or severe anxiety, a selective serotonergic receptor inhibitor combined with low-dose tricyclic appears to be most effective. For patients with more severe or agitated depression, psychiatric input may be required for optimal management. For some very symptomatic patients with or without major depression, pain management or multidisciplinary approaches may be required.

## REFERENCES

1. Layzer RB. Muscle metabolism during fatigue and work. *Baillieres Clin Endocrinol Metab* 1990;4:441–459.
2. Layzer RB. Asthenia and the chronic fatigue syndrome. *Muscle Nerve* 1998;21:1609–1611.
3. Goldenberg DL. Fibromyalgia, chronic fatigue syndrome and myofascial pain syndrome. *Curr Opin Rheumatol* 1997;9:135–143.
4. Wolfe F, Anderson J, Harkness D, et al. A prospective longitudinal multicenter study of service utilization and costs in fibromyalgia [see comments]. *Arthritis Rheum* 1997;40:1560–1570.
5. Simms RW. Fibromyalgia syndrome: current concepts in pathophysiology, clinical features and management. *Arthritis Care Res* 1996;9:315–328.
6. Simms RW. Is there muscle pathology in fibromyalgia syndrome? *Rheum Dis Clin North Am* 1996;22:245–266.
7. Kirmayer LJ, Robbins JM, Kapusta MA. Somatization and depression in fibromyalgia syndrome. *Am J Psychiatry* 1988;145:950–954.

142. Hickie I, Lloyd A, Wakefield D, Park G. The psychiatric status of patients with chronic fatigue syndrome. *Br J Psychiatry* 1990;156:534–540.

143. Hickie I, Hooker AW, Hadzi-Pavlovic D, et al. Fatigue in selected primary care settings: sociodemographic and psychiatric correlates. *Med J Aust* 1996;164:585–588.

144. Buchwald D. Fibromyalgia and chronic fatigue syndrome: similarities and differences. *Rheum Dis Clin North Am* 1996;22:219–243.

145. Moldofsky H. Sleep, neuroimmune and neuroendocrine functions in fibromyalgia and chronic fatigue syndrome. *Adv Neuroimmunol* 1995;5:39–56.

146. Goldenberg DL, Simms RW, Geiger A, Komaroff AL. High frequency of fibromyalgia in patients with chronic fatigue seen in a primary care practice. *Arthritis Rheum* 1990;33:381–387.

147. Lane TJ, Manu P, Matthews DA. Depression and somatization in the chronic fatigue syndrome. *Am J Med* 1991; 91:335–344.

148. Abbey SE, Garfinkel PE. Chronic fatigue syndrome and depression; cause, effect, or corvariate. *Rev Infect Dis* 1991;13[Suppl 1]:S73–S83.

149. Potter W, Rudorfer M, Manjii H. The pharmacologic treatment of depression. *N Engl J Med* 1991;325:633–642.

150. Carette S, McCain GA, Bell DA, Fam AG. Evaluation of amitriptyline in primary fibrositis. A double-blind placebo-controlled study. *Arthritis Rheum* 1986;29:655–659.

151. Goldenberg DL, Felson DT, Dinerman HA. A randomized controlled trial of aamitriptyline and naproxen in the treatment of patients with fibromyalgia. *Arthritis Rheum* 1986;39:1371–1377.

152. Goldenberg D, Mayskiy M, Mossey C, et al. A randomized double-blind crossover trial of fluxetine and amitriptyline in the treatment of fibromyalgia. *Arthritis Rheum* 1996;39:1852–1859.

153. Jaaeschke R, Adachi J, Guyatt G, et al. Clinical usefulness of amitriptyline in fibromyalgia: the results of 23 N-of-1 randomized control trials. *J Rheumatol* 1991;18:447–451.

154. Careette S, Bell MJ, Reynolds WJ, et al. Comparison of amitriptyline, cyclobenzaprine and placebo in the treatment of fibromyalgia. A randomized double-blind clinical trial [see comments]. *Arthritis Rheum* 1994;37: 32–40.

155. Bennett RM, Gatter RA, Campbell SM, et al. A comparison of cyclobenzaprine and placebo in the management of fibrositis. A double-blind controlled study. *Arthritis Rheum* 1988;31:1535–1542.

156. Sussman N, Stahl S. Update on the pharmacology of depression. *Am J Med* 1996;101:26S–36S.

157. Russell IJ, Fletcher EM, Michalek JE, et al. Treatment of primary fibrositis/fibromyalgia syndrome with ibuprofen and alprazolam. A double-blind placebo-controlled study. *Arthritis Rheum* 1991;34:552–560.

158. Yunus MB, Masi AT, Aldag JC. Short term effects of ibuprofen in primary fibromyalgia syndrome: a double-blind placebo-controlled triall. *J Rheumatol* 1989;16:527–532.

159. Quijada-Carreera J, Valenzuela-Castano A, Povedano-Gomez J, et al. Comparison of tenoxicam and bromazepan in the treatment of fibromyalgia: a randomized double-blind placebo-controlled trial. *Pain* 1996;65: 221–225.

160. Clark S, Tindall E, Bennett RM. A double-blind crossover trial of prednisone versus placebo in the treatment of fibrositis. *J Rheumatol* 1985;12:980–983.

161. McCain GA. Role of physical fitness training in the fibrositis/fibromyalgia syndrome. *Am J Med* 1986;81: 73–77.

162. Ferraccioli G, Ghirelli L, Scita F, et al. DMG-biofeedback training in fibromyalgia syndrome. *J Rheumatol* 1987;14;820–825.

163. Deluze C, Bosia L, Zirbs A, et al. Electroacupuncture in fibromyalgia: results of a controlled trial [see comments]. *BMJ* 1992;305:1249–1252.

164. Haanen HC, Hoenderdos HT, van Romunde LK, et al. Controlled trial of hypnotherapy in the treatment of refractory fibromyalgia. *J Rheumatol* 1991;18:72–75.

*Diseases of Skeletal Muscle,*
edited by Robert L. Wortmann.
Lippincott Williams & Wilkins, Philadelphia © 2000

# 13

# Rhabdomyolysis

## Paul Bolin Jr.

*Department of Medicine, Section of Nephrology, East Carolina University*
*School of Medicine, Greenville, North Carolina 27858*

The term rhabdomyolysis represents a perhaps underrecognized syndrome of muscle injury that results in a spectrum of clinical findings ranging from minimally sore muscles to life-threatening electrolyte abnormalities and acute renal failure (Table 1). Physiologically, rhabdomyolysis is best defined as injury to striated muscle that alters the integrity of the cell membrane sufficiently to allow spillage of intracellular contents. Rhabdomyolysis is typically generalized but may be limited to an individual muscle group. The resulting clinical syndrome can be brief and reversible or prolonged and self-sustaining due to secondary injury from extravasated intracellular components.

The first description of rhabdomyolysis was probably written in the book of Numbers describing a plague in the Israelites who had eaten quail that had fed on hemlock seeds (1). Reports of fatal rhabdomyolysis after ingestion of quail continue today, although these are limited to spring ingestions in Mediterranean areas. This unique geographic distribution is due to migration patterns and feeding habits of old world quail. In contrast, new world quail do not ingest hemlock seeds and are nonmigratory. Thus, rhabdomyolysis after quail ingestion has not been reported in North America.

Initial clinical observations of acute renal failure after massive muscle injury in World War II and further studies by Bywaters and Beall (2) stimulated much of our present knowledge of acute renal failure. Since these seminal observations, an expanding list of drugs, chemicals, and infectious agents has been associated with rhabdomyolysis.

## CLINICAL FEATURES

Mild elevations in serum and urine myoglobin not infrequently develop with intense muscular activity and are typically accompanied by minor symptoms of myalgia, weakness, and fatigue (3). These symptoms usually resolve within 24 to 48 hours without sequela. In severe rhabdomyolysis, patients present with profound muscle pain and weakness. It is not unusual to find areas of focal pain and induration when local muscle groups are involved. Serum creatine kinase levels are quite high and generally peak at 12 to 36 hours after onset of the syndrome. Patients with severe consequences of rhabdomyolysis will have serum creatine kinase levels of 100,000 IU/L or higher. Hyperkalemia, hypocalcemia, hyperphosphatemia, and hyperuricemia may also develop.

In a single center study, 16.5% of patients with rhabdomyolysis developed acute renal failure, and the degree of elevation of creatine kinase, potassium, and phosphorus levels allowed prediction of acute renal failure. Fifty-eight percent of patients with acute renal

**TABLE 1.** *Reported causes for rhabdomyolysis*

| | |
|---|---|
| 1. Ischemia | 7. Drugs *(continued)* |
|     Muscle compression |     Amiodarone |
|     Vascular occlusion |     Chloroquine |
|     Sickle cell anemia |     Cocaine |
|     Carbon dioxide arteriography |     Heroin |
|     Reperfusion |     Methadone |
| 2. Direct muscle injury |     Salicylate overdose |
|     Trauma |     Phencyclidine |
|     Crushing injury |     Malignant hypothermia |
|     Burns |     Malignant neuroleptic syndrome |
|     Temperature extremes |     HMG-CoA reductase inhibitors |
|       Electrical injury |       Lovastatin |
|       Lightning strikes |       Dravastatin |
|     Compartment syndromes |       Simvastatin |
| 3. Sustained muscular activity |     Clofibrate |
|     Status asthmaticus |     Gemfibrozil |
|     Seizures |     Quinine derivatives |
|     Delirium tremens |     Corticosteroids |
|     Prolonged labor |     Glycyrrhizinic acid |
| 4. Toxins |     Succinylcholine |
|     Ethanol | 8. Infections |
|     Isopropyl alcohol |     Legionella species |
|     Carbon monoxide |     Francisella tularensis |
|     Ethylene glycol |     Streptococcus species |
|     Toluene |     Staphococcal species |
|     Envenomation |     Vibrio species |
|       Snakes |     Clostridium tetani |
|       Spiders |     Influenza virus |
|       Wasps |     HIV coxsackie virus |
|     Chlorophenoxy herbicides | 9. Genetic disorders |
| 5. Immunologic diseases |     Myophosphorylase deficiency |
|     Dermatomyositis |     Phosphorylase b kinase deficiency |
|     Polymyositis |     Phosphofructokinase deficiency |
| 6. Metabolic disorders |     Phosphoglycerate kinase deficiency |
|     Hypokalemia |     Phosphoglycerate mutase deficiency |
|     Hyponatremia |     Lactate dehydrogenase deficiency |
|     Hypophosphatemia |     Carnitine palmitoyltransferase deficiency |
|     Diabetes mellitus |     Long-, medium-, and short-chain fatty acid |
|     Hypothyroidism |       acyl-CoA dehydrogenase deficiency |
| 7. Drugs |     Mitochondrial myopathies |
|     Amphetamines |     Muscular dystrophy |
|     Amphotericin |     Paroxysmal myoglobinuria |

HMG-CoA, 3-hydroxy-3-methylglutaryl-coenzyme A; HIV, human immunodeficiency virus.

failure had peak creatine kinase levels greater than 16,000 IU/L, whereas only 11% of patients without renal failure had levels greater than 16,000 IU/L (4). It is not uncommon to see a second peak in the serum creatine kinase occurring approximately 48 hours after onset. This is attributed to secondary damage caused by the release of cellular contents. A high index of suspicion for developing a compartment syndrome should be maintained during this period.

Compartment syndromes can both derive from rhabdomyolysis or can be a cause of rhabdomyolysis. A compartment syndrome results when increased interstitial pressure within a closed osseofascial compartment causes vascular (usually microvascular) compromise. This compromise may lead to severe muscle necrosis. Compartment syndromes are caused by increased pressure within the compartment or by substantial external pressure. External pressures can be exerted by a constricting cast or by compression that may occur during an unconscious state or surgery (5). Increased intracompartmental pressure can result from bleeding, edema, or inflammation and has been reported as a complication of anticoagulation (6), drug-induced rhabdomyolysis (5,7), and infection (8).

A compartment syndrome typically causes pain that is more severe than would be expected for the disease or injury. Additional symptoms may include tenderness, weakness, and paresthesia of the involved part. Peripheral pulses, however, almost always remain palpable, despite significant microvascular compromise and intracompartmental pressure elevation.

In the setting of suspected rhabdomyolysis, a urinalysis can be used to screen for myoglobinuria. When myoglobin is present, urine tests positive for hemoglobin but no red cells are seen on microscopic examination. The urine sediment will contain muddy brown casts in the setting of acute renal failure.

Hyperkalemia typically develops rapidly in the course of rhabdomyolysis due to release of potassium from cells. Serum concentrations may reach levels as high as 140 mEq/L. Acute precipitation of calcium in injured muscle can result in profound hypocalcemia. The serum urate level is also elevated in rhabdomyolysis, and the large amount of urate presented to the kidney may contribute to the development of acute renal failure (9). Hyperuricemia results from the increased urate produced by the breakdown of purine nucleotides and nucleosides released from cells and decreased urinary uric acid excretion resulting from acidosis or renal failure. In that setting, one may develop acute uric acid nephropathy, a condition analogous to the tumor lysis syndrome.

Muscle damage results in release of creatine phosphate, which is spontaneously dehydrated to creatinine. Although frequently taught, myoglobinuric acute renal failure is not associated with low blood urea nitrogen to creatinine ratio (10).

## PATHOPHYSIOLOGY

### Mechanism of Muscle Injury

An average 70-kg man has approximately 28 kg of striated muscle, which requires large quantities of ATP to maintain cellular integrity and contractility. Muscle ATP generation accounts for 30% of total body oxygen consumption at rest and 85% during intense muscular activity. Any process that impairs ATP production or the ability of skeletal muscle to maintain adequate ATP levels can cause rhabdomyolysis. Any factor that increases cytosolic calcium can accentuate the activity of phospholipase $A_2$ and enhance cellular injury (11). Cellular injury may be further potentiated by cytokine release triggered by intestinal endotoxins, which may be absorbed under stress conditions associated with rhabdomyolysis.

### Mechanism of Renal Injury

Myoglobin, a monomeric heme protein, is not thought to be directly nephrotoxic. However, casts containing myoglobin can occlude tubules, leading to intrarenal obstruction (12). If arterial volume, blood pressure, and renal perfusion are intact, infusion of muscle extract or myoglobin has no adverse effect on renal function (13). Myoglobin, in contrast to hemoglobin, is less avidly bound to protein and is thus more freely filtered by the glomerulus. Filtered myoglobulin enters proximal tubular cells by pinocytosis, where the intact molecule is taken up by lysosomes. Under conditions of low pH, the heme molecule is split into globulin and ferrihemate. Whereas globulin does not cause nephrotoxicity, ferrihemate is nephrotoxic and is toxic at any urine pH (14). Transportation of ferrihemate out of the proximal tubule requires ATP. The toxicity of ferrihemate is limited if it is removed from the cell. Under the conditions of low ATP stores, ferrihemate builds up, generating toxic superoxide radicals. These superoxide radicals lead to lipid peroxidation, which can cause structural and functional alterations in proximal tubular cells (15). This effect can be potentiated during reperfusion with additional free radical generation, leading to a second wave of injury (16). The importance of reperfusion is highlighted by studies of glycerol-induced rhabdomyolysis where isoflurane was found to be protective by blocking mitochondrial-driven oxidant stress (17).

## DIFFERENTIAL DIAGNOSIS

### Ischemia

Ischemia resulting from a variety of mechanisms can result in ATP depletion to levels sufficiently low to allow rhabdomyolysis. Reperfusion injury is important in the progression of ischemic rhabdomyolysis. Muscle compression associated with prolonged coma, as seen with drug overdose or alcohol intoxication, probably causes rhabdomyolysis by this mechanism. However, similar elevations of intramuscular pressure are seen with no evidence of rhabdomyolysis in healthy adults with drug overdoses, suggesting additional factors may be involved (18). Other ischemic causes of rhabdomyolysis include acute (but not chronic) vascular occlusion, carbon dioxide arteriography (19), and intravascular sludging in sickle cell disease. Rhabdomyolysis occurring after positioning for surgery in patients with end-stage renal failure is probably underrecognized due to preexisting renal failure (20).

### Direct Muscle Injury

Trauma and burns lead to direct muscle injury and secondary rhabdomyolysis. Extremes of temperature and electrical injury directly damage muscle and cause membrane abnormalities, setting into play cytokine cascades that damage muscle.

### Sustained Muscular Activity

Excess sustained muscular activity, such as can occur in status asthmaticus, status ellipticus, delirium tremens, and prolonged labor during pregnancy, are all associated with rhabdomyolysis. This syndrome can develop after anaerobic and aerobic exercise and is more common after excessive eccentric exercise in contrast to concentric exercise (21).

### Toxins

A number of agents that are directly toxic to muscular membranes have been associated with rhabdomyolysis (22). The most widely studied of these is ethanol (23). Ethanol is associated with other risk factors for rhabdomyolysis, including compression, electrolyte disturbances, and withdrawal syndrome. Carbon monoxide is frequently associated with rhabdomyolysis. This most likely develops as a consequence of carbon monoxide displacing oxygen from hemoglobulin.

## Immunologic Diseases

Polymyositis and dermatomyositis can be associated with rhabdomyolysis. In fact, rhabdomyolysis may be the presenting syndrome in rare instances. Whether this can be attributed to vasculopathy causing ischemia or other factors that alter cellular energy metabolism is unclear.

## Metabolic Diseases

Rhabdomyolysis is seen both with hyponatremia and after rapid correction of hyponatremia (24). Asymptomatic rhabdomyolysis has been reported in as many as 28% of patients with hypokalemia (25) and 36% of patients with hypophosphatemia (26). Symptomatic rhabdomyolysis is typically seen in patients with electrolyte disorders and other concurrent risk factors, especially ethanol (27). Diabetic myonecrosis is associated with both small- and large-vessel atherosclerosis, although a clear mechanism is not understood (28).

## Drugs

A variety of medications can cause rhabdomyolysis (22). Mood-altering drugs are associated with rhabdomyolysis either due to prolonged coma such as heroine or by an effect on muscle tone, such as phencyclidine. Cocaine abuse is frequently associated with rhabdomyolysis due to the combined effect of increased muscle activity and ischemia (29).

Rhabdomyolysis has been associated with a variety of cholesterol-lowering agents including nicotinic acid, clofibrate, and the 3-hydroxy-3-methylglutaryl-coenzyme A (HMG-CoA) reductase inhibitors (30). Concurrent use of HMG-CoA reductase inhibitors and drugs that inhibit cytochrome P450, such as erythromycin and fluconazole, can lead to rhabdomyolysis (31). Some newer agents in this class have only been associated with myalgias but without overt rhabdomyolysis. Whether this represents an advance in this class of agents, lag time in reporting events in new agents, or earlier physician recognition of this complication is unclear. Concurrent administration of cyclosporin and an HMG-CoA reductase inhibitor with or without the presence of renal insufficiency increases the risk of developing rhabdomyolysis. Rhabdomyolysis and myopathy have been associated with administration of corticosteroids in severe asthma (32).

## Infections

A number of viral infections are associated with rhabdomyolysis, including influenza, human immunodeficiency virus, coxsackievirus, and a number of the herpes virus family (8,33). Influenza is the most frequently reported viral cause. Legionella is the most frequently reported bacterial cause of rhabdomyolysis. However, reports of necrotizing streptococcal myositis are increasing (34). Diffuse muscle injury seen in many of these cases may be due to immunologic cross-reactivity between streptococcal proteins and myosin (35).

## Genetic Disorders

Several disorders of glycogenolysis, glycolysis, and lipid metabolism have been associated with rhabdomyolysis. Common to all of these disorders is an abnormality of muscle energy metabolism and, under certain conditions, an inability to maintain adequate levels of ATP (see Chapter 9).

## MANAGEMENT

The management of rhabdomyolysis is directed at reversing any known contributing condition, controlling symptoms, and attempting to prevent renal failure. A high index of suspicion with early recognition is pivotal in the successful prevention of acute renal failure in rhabdomyolysis. Maintaining adequate hydration is the single most important intervention. This relieves volume contraction that coexists with massive rhabdomyolysis, increases tubular filtrate flow and urine output, and, by dilution, increases urinary pH, reducing the formation of ferrihematuria. Experience with hydration compared with historical control subjects without hydration has highlighted the importance of giving adequate fluids. Initially, intravenous infusion rates exceeding 500 mL/hour may be required. Hydration at rates that provide good urine flow should continue for several days after the initial intervention as long as volume overload does not develop (36). If oliguria develops or persists after adequate hydration, the use of mannitol 0.5 g/kg body weight as a 20% intravenous solution with or without high-dose intravenous furosemide in doses from 80 to 240 mg should be considered. Although a number of studies have demonstrated the protective effect of mannitol against myoglobinuric renal failure, recent studies have failed to demonstrate a protective effect beyond inducing solute diuresis (37). Mannitol may have a theoretic negative effect by depleting ATP stores.

Although not established clinically, experimental models have demonstrated the efficiency of iron chelators in the prevention of myohemoglobinuric acute renal failure (38). The role of urinary alkalization is controversial, although physiologically an alkaline urine can reduce ferrihematuria. It appears that adequate hydration without alkalization is equally efficacious in preventing myoglobin-induced acute renal failure. However, alkalinization of the urine and allopurinol therapy are important if acute uric acid nephropathy is present or thought to be a factor. In the setting of acute renal failure, a urine uric acid to urine creatinine ratio of greater than 1 is indicative of uric acid nephropathy (39).

Hypocalcemia may develop early in the management of rhabdomyolysis. However, infusions of calcium should be avoided unless the patient develops specific symptoms that can be attributed to hypocalcemia because of the significant risk of developing rebound hypercalcemia in the recovery phase. Hyperkalemia typically develops in the first 24 hours after significant rhabdomyolysis. The hyperkalemia of rhabdomyolysis is less responsive to the medical therapies typically used to treat other causes of hyperkalemia. Nebulized β-antagonists and infusions of calcium, glucose, and insulin work by shifting potassium into cells. The damaged muscle membranes prevent this shift from occurring effectively. Relatively mild hyperkalemia in the presence of hypocalcemia can prove cardiotoxic, highlighting the need for cardiac monitoring.

Patients with accelerating hyperkalemia and oliguria may need urgent dialysis. In this setting, dialysis is better initiated early in the process rather than after prolonged attempts at medical therapy. One should consider continuous vein-to-vein hemodialysis with a biocompatible filter due to enhanced cytokine clearance. Plasma exchange therapy is considered controversial in rhabdomyolysis (40). One must be vigilant for complications of rhabdomyolysis, including infection, disseminated intravascular coagulation, thrombocytopenia, adult respiratory distress syndrome, and multiple organ failure.

When a compartment syndrome is present or suspected, pressures should be measured (41). Normal resting pressures range between 0 and 15 mm Hg. Ischemia develops at a pressure of 50 mm Hg, or higher, and causes necrosis. Surgical decompressive should be considered at a pressure of 30 mm Hg or if the gradient between the compartment and the diastolic pressure is less than 30 mm Hg (18,42).

## REFERENCES

1. Rutecki GW, Ognibene AJ, Geib JD. Rhabdomyolysis in antiquity: from ancient descriptions to scientific explanation. *Pharos* 1998;61:18–22.
2. Bywaters EG, Beall D. Crushed injuries with impairment of renal function. *Br Med J* 1941;1:427–432.
3. Ritter WS, Stone MJ, Willson JT. Reduction in myoglobinuria anemia after physical conditioning. *Arch Intern Med* 1997;139:644–647.
4. Ward MM. Factors predictive of acute renal failure in rhabdomyolysis. *Arch Intern Med* 1988;148:1553–1557.
5. Rutgers PH, Harst F, Koumans RKJ. Surgical implications of drug-induced rhabdomyolysis. *Br J Surg* 1991;78: 490–492.
6. Griffiths D, Jones DH. Spontaneous compartment syndrome in patient on long-term anticoagulations. *J Hand Surg* 1993;18:41–42.
7. Chow LTC, Chow W. Acute compartment syndrome: an unusual presentation of gemfibrozil induced myositis. *Med J Aust* 1993;158:48–49.
8. Paletta CI, Lynch R, Knutsen AP. Rhabdomyolysis and lower extremity compartment syndrome due to influenza B virus. *Ann Plastic Surg* 1993;30:272–273.
9. Knochel JP, Carter NW. The role of muscle in cell injury and pathogenesis of acute renal failure after exercise. *Kidney Int* 1976;10:S54–S58.
10. Gabow PA, Kaehny WD, Kelelher SP. The spectrum of rhabdomyolysis. *Medicine* 1982;61:141–152.
11. Knochel JP. Mechanisms of rhabdomyolysis. *Curr Opin Rheumatol* 1993;5:725–731.
12. Zager RA. Rhabdomyolysis and myohemoglobinuric acute renal failure. *Kidney Int* 1996;49:314–326.
13. Bywaters EGL, Popjakg. Experimental crush injury, peripheral circulatory collapse and other effects of muscle necrosis in the rabbit. *Surg Gynecol Obstet* 1942;75:612–626.
14. Braun SR, Weiss FR, Keller AI. Evaluation of the renal toxicity of heme proteins and their derivatives: a role in the genesis of acute tubular necrosis. *J Exp Med* 1970;131:443–460.
15. Zager RA. Mitochondrial free radical production induces lipid peroxidation during myohemoglobinuria. *Kidney Int* 1996;49:741–751.
16. Odeh M. The role of reperfusion induced injury and the pathogenesis of the crushed syndrome. *N Engl Med* 1991;324:1417–1421.
17. Lochhead, KM, Kharasch ED, Zager RA. Anesthetic effects on the glycerol model of rhabdomyolysis-induced acute renal failure in rats. *J Am Soc Nephrol* 1998;9:305–309.
18. Owen CA, Mubarak SJ, Hargens AR, et al. Intramuscular pressures with limb compression. *N Engl J Med* 1979; 300:1169–1172.
19. Rundback JH, Shah PM, Wong J et al. Livedo reticularis, rhabdomyolysis, massive intestinal infarction and death after carbon dioxide arteriography. *J Vasc Surg* 1997;26:337–340.
20. Ori Y, Korzets A, Gruzman C, et al. Postoperative rhabdomyolysis in patients with end-stage renal failure. *Am J Kidney Dis* 1998;31:539–544.
21. Armstrong R, Warren G, Warren J. Mechanisms of exercising induced muscle fiber injury. *Sport Med* 1991;12: 184–207.
22. Pascuzzi RM. Drugs and toxins associated with myopathies. *Curr Opin Rheumatol* 1998;10:511–520.
23. Ferguson E, Blachley J, Carter N, Knochel J. Derangements of muscle composition, ion transport and oxygen consumption and chronically alcoholic dogs. *Am J Physiol* 1984;Vol.246:F700–F709.
24. Rizzieri DA. Rhabdomyolysis after correction of hyponatremia due to psychogenic polydipsia. *Mayo Clin Proc* 1995;70:473–476.
25. Singhal PC, Venkatesan J, Gibbons N. Prevalence and predictors of rhabdomyolysis in patients with hypokalemia. *N Engl J Med* 1990;323:1488.
26. Singhal PC, Kumar A, Pesroches L, Gibbons N. Prevalence and predictors of rhabdomyolysis in patients with pophosphatemia. *Am J Med* 1992;92:458–464.
27. Knochel JP. Hypophosphatemia and rhabdomyolysis. *Am J Med* 1992;92:455–457.
28. Bjornakov EK, Carry MR, Katz FH, Lefkowitz J, Ringel SP. Diabetic muscle infarction: a new perspective on pathogenesis and management. *Neuromusc Dis* 1995;5:39–45.
29. Pogue VA, Nurse HM. Cocaine-associated acute myoglobinuric renal failure. *Am J Med* 1989;86:183–186.
30. Golman JA, Fishman AB, Lee JE, Johnson RJ. The role of cholesterol-lowering agents in drug-induced rhabdomyolysis and polymyositis. *Arthritis Rheum* 1989;32:358–359.
31. Grunden JW, Fisher KA. Lovastatin-induced rhabdomyolysis possibly associated with clarithromycin and azithromycin. *Ann Pharmacother* 1997;31:859–863.

32. Williams TJ, O'Hehir RE, Czarny D, et. al. Acute myopathy in severe acute asthma treated with intravenously administered corticosteroids. *Am Rev Respir Dis* 1988;137:460–463.

33. Singh V, Scheld WM. Infectious etiologies of rhabdomyolysis: three case reports and review. *Clin Infect Dis* 1996;22:642–649.

34. Hoge CW, Schwartz B, Talkington DF, et al. The group A streptococcal infections and the emergence of streptococcal toxic shock-like syndrome: a retrospective population based study. *JAMA* 1993;269:384–389.

35. Cunningham MW, Quinn A, Immunological cross reactivity between the class I epitope of streptococcal M protein and myosin. *Adv Exp Med Biol* 1997;418:887–892.

36. Better OS. The crush syndrome revisited (1940–1990). *Nephron* 1990;55:97–103.

37. Zager RA, Foerder C, Bredl C. The influence of mannitol an myohemoglobinuric acute renal failure: functional, biochemical, and morphological assessments. *J Am Soc Nephrol* 1991;2:848–855.

38. Zager RA, Burkhart K, Conrad DS, Gmur DJ. Iron, heme oxygenase, and glutathione: effects on myohemoglobinuric proximal tubular injury. *Kidney Int* 1995;48:1624–1634.

39. Kelton J, Kelley WN, Holmes EW. A rapid method for the diagnosis of acute uric acid nephropathy. *Arch Intern Med* 1978;138:612–615.

40. Szpirt WM. Plasmapheresis is not justified in treatment of rhabdomyolysis and acute renal failure. *J Cardiovasc Surg* 1996;37:153–159.

41. Allen MJ. Compartment syndromes of the lower limb. *J R Coll Surg Edinburg* 1990;35:S33–S36.

42. Skejldal S, Stamsoe K, Alho A, et al. Acute compartment syndrome: for how long can muscle tolerate increased tissue pressure? *Eur J Surg* 1992;158:437–438.

# PART III

## Approach to the Patient

*Diseases of Skeletal Muscle,*
edited by Robert L. Wortmann.
Lippincott Williams & Wilkins, Philadelphia © 2000

# 14

# History, Physical Examination, and Laboratory Tests in the Evaluation of Myopathy

Lawrence J. Kagen

*Department of Medicine, Weill Medical College of Cornell University,
New York, New York; Department of Medicine, Division of Rheumatology,
Hospital for Special Surgery, New York, New York 10021*

The muscular system represents one of the largest tissue systems of the body. By some estimates it accounts for 40% to 45% of body weight. Most of what we see and appreciate in ourselves, and in others, can in one way or another relate to the actions of this contractile tissue. Whether it is the ease with which we move, the quality of our voices, or the expression of our skills or performance, the voluntary or skeletal muscles present our image to the world. Yet, in many instances, myopathies or disorders of muscle may go unnoticed for long periods of time. The reasons for this relates to the subtlety or insidious development of certain myopathic disorders and to the difficulty of assigning symptoms to dysfunction of the skeletal muscles even when evident. Furthermore, once a diagnosis of myopathy has been made, it can be difficult to assess changes or progress in the clinical state of the patient with precision.

## HISTORY AND PHYSICAL EXAMINATION

The first techniques used in the evaluation of patients include the history and physical examination. Unfortunately, these can have shortcomings in some instances. The symptoms of a myopathy include fixed weakness; premature fatigue or exercise intolerance; and postexertional ache, cramps, or myalgia.

Insofar as the history is concerned, the vocabulary of both physician and patient may not be sufficiently precise. Weakness, fatigue, tiredness, and lack of energy may be associated with many disorders and may not call to mind the possibility of a myopathy to the patient or to the physician. In some instances deficiencies of performance or weakness may be ascribed to the natural course of aging rather than to a specific diagnosable or treatable disorder. It may indeed be difficult to determine whether the symptoms of exercise intolerance or premature fatigue are due to poor conditioning, inappropriate expectations, or a disease.

Techniques of physical examination also may not be sensitive enough to detect weakness or loss of contractile power in its early stages. All this presents the paradox of a large and evident tissue system whose disorders and changes can remain enigmatic or concealed. Consequently, the history and physical examination must be performed with rigor if they are to prove useful in the detection and quantification of myopathies.

Many categories of illness affect the muscular system. Their classification may be arbitrary to a degree, particularly in the distinctions between hereditary or genetic disorders and those listed as metabolic or acquired. Because it is likely that multifactorial influences affect the expression of myopathy in particular individuals, divisions of this nature can be discretionary to some extent.

## Weakness

Weakness is the cardinal finding in patients with myopathy. Because of its importance, the evaluation of the patient should attempt an assessment of which muscle groups are involved and the degree to which they are affected. Most myopathic states primarily affect proximal muscle groups. With regard to the upper extremity, patients report difficulty in lifting objects, especially overhead. Activities of daily living, including brushing hair, using a hair dryer, hanging up clothing, or putting objects into cabinets or refrigerators, will be difficult. Distal muscles used in fine manipulation, writing or opening jars, often will have preserved function. Involvement of the distal musculature, if it does occur, is seen late in the course or in more progressive or severe forms of myopathy. Inclusion body myositis, myositis in patients with circulating anti-signal recognition particle (anti-SRP) antibodies, and myotonic dystrophy are noteworthy, because they can be characterized by distal weakness early in their courses. In the lower extremity, proximal muscle weakness is characterized by difficulty in arising from a chair or low toilet seat, climbing stairs, going down stairs with a reciprocating gait, getting in and out of an automobile, or lifting the legs to put on shoes and socks. Stepping up onto a sidewalk can also be difficult. Weakness of musculature about the hip may be manifested by the Trendelenburg gait. Weakness of distal foot musculature is demonstrated by a high steppage gait. Tripping on curbs or uneven surfaces is not unusual early in the course of most myopathic disorders.

Gower's sign may be evident in children with pelvic-girdle muscle weakness from muscular dystrophy or myositis. This is assessed by observing the child rise from a supine position from the floor. Normal children will first sit up and then stand by flexing the knees and extending the arms to the side of the body to push up from the floor. Gower's sign is exhibited when instead the child rolls over to a prone position, pushes off the floor with the arms, and brings the legs to a flexed position under the trunk. The legs are then extended with the help of the hands and arms.

Muscles of the trunk may also be affected, although this is somewhat more difficult to recognize. Rising from the supine position in bed can be difficult and accomplished only with a lateral rolling maneuver while swinging the legs downward and pressing against the bed with the arms.

Respiratory muscle involvement if present can be extremely subtle in its manifestation. Shortness of breath is usually not an early feature of most myopathies, perhaps because weakness of other musculature curtails activity. Nevertheless, this sign can occur early in some disorders, such as acid maltase deficiency, carnitine deficiency, or in inflammatory myopathies with associated interstitial lung disease. Weakness of facial musculature is uncommon in most myopathies, with the exception of facioscapulohumeral dystrophy and myotonic dystrophy. Ptosis of the eyelids, with the exception of myasthenia gravis and the Kearn-Sayres type of mitochondrial myopathy, is also unusual. Palatal weakness, with swallowing difficulties and change in phonation, can be early manifestations in patients severely affected with dermatomyositis and polymyositis.

**TABLE 1.** *Muscle strength grading*

| Grade | |
| --- | --- |
| 0 | No detectable contraction |
| 1 (trace) | Contraction palpable—no motion |
| 2 (poor) | Motion—but not against gravity |
| 3 (fair) | Can overcome gravity only |
| 4 (good) | Can overcome moderate resistance |
| 5 (normal) | Can overcome considerable manual resistance |

After obtaining the history and determining which areas of musculature are involved, quantification of functional performance should be approached. How far can the patient walk and up how many stairs? How much can be lifted? Questions of this type provide a framework or base from which to measure progress over time.

Loss of muscle strength or motor function is the most important feature of most myopathies, and the physical examination is essential in documenting the severity of involvement and confirming the nature and degree of dysfunction indicated by the history. In general, myopathic processes cause only a symmetric weakness of proximal muscles. Asymmetric, distal or proximal and distal weakness, or abnormalities of any other portion of the neurologic examination indicate a neuropathic process.

The more objective information the examiner provides at the initial evaluation, the easier it is to chart the course of disease and the effects of therapy. This is an area that requires experience and skill on the part of the examiner and cooperation on the part of the patient. Pain, fatigue, and malaise can interfere with effort and complicate objective assessment of muscle function. Too often treating physicians are frustrated by not being able to accurately determine if strength is improving or worsening. One begins with observation of function. Gait, including toe and heel walking, should be assessed. The ability to rise from a chair, to step onto a footstool or step, and to rise from the supine position should be recorded. The physical examination of the strength of individual muscle groups is generally recorded in a numerical grading system (Table 1). This system is subject to variability because of its dependence on patient effort and observer consistency. In addition, not all grades represented will generally be equally applicable to patients with myopathy. Most patients will score more than 3 and less than 5, which makes discrimination difficult at times. This again emphasizes the importance of characterization of function in clinical assessment. A scheme for assessment of functional performance is shown in Table 2. The time-stands test, or measuring the length of time it takes the pa-

**TABLE 2.** *Muscle function grading*

| | |
| --- | --- |
| 1. Transfer from supine to sitting | _____ |
| 2. Transfer from sitting to standing | _____ |
| 3. Stair climbing | _____ |
| 4. Hair combing, tooth brushing | _____ |
| 5. Donning jacket or shirt | _____ |
| 6. Donning trousers | _____ |
| 7. Lifting objects (e.g., groceries) | _____ |
| 8. Household maintenance | _____ |

Score: 0, cannot do; 1, can do partially or with aid; 2, can do alone. Maximum score, 16.

**TABLE 3.** *Distribution of weakness in musculoskeletal disorders*

Proximal musculature
  Most myopathies, e.g., inflammatory myopathies and muscular dystrophies
Distal musculature
  Inclusion body myositis, myositis with anti-SRP antibodies
  Myotonic dystrophy, distal dystrophies
  Neurogenic disorders
Facial
  Facioscapulohumeral dystrophy
  Myasthenia gravis (e.g., ptosis)
  Myotonic dystrophy
  Mitochondrial myopathy (Kearns-Sayres)
  Disorders of the central nervous system and cranial nerves (e.g., stroke, Bell's palsy)
Palatal and bulbar musculature
  Central nervous system disorders
  Inflammatory myopathies

SRP, signal recognition particle.

tient to rise from a chair ten times without using their hands for assistance, is useful in quantifying lower extremity proximal muscle strength.

The pattern of weakness displayed clinically may be of value in differential diagnosis. Table 3 indicates some general concepts of the distribution of weakness in musculoskeletal disorders.

## Myalgia

Myalgia, or painful muscles, is described by a variety of terms that probably reflect the intensity of the symptoms. These include stiff, sore, ache, pain, spasm, cramp, and charlie horse and result from numerous causes (Table 4). Severe muscle pain and stiffness as isolated or dominant complaints are rare in myopathic disorders. Muscle pain or soreness at rest can be an early feature of inflammatory muscle disorders. This is less common in dermatomyositis and polymyositis than in certain viral myositis syndromes. Polymyalgia rheumatica and fibromyalgia syndromes do present in this way, however. Muscle stiffness can at times be confused with, or coexist with, subjective feelings of pain. Stiffness is an accompaniment of myotonic syndromes and certain connective tissue disorders such as

**TABLE 4.** *Common causes of myalgia*

Inflammatory myopathies (proximal)
Connective tissue disorders (e.g., rheumatoid arthritis, polymyalgia rheumatica)
Infectious myopathies (systemic, localized, bacterial, viral)
Metabolic myopathies, e.g., hypothyroidism, exertional intolerance related to
  disorders of glycogen, or lipid metabolic pathway disorders
Drug-induced myopathies (e.g., due to lipid-lowering agents)
Fibromyalgia
Lower motor neuron disorders
  Myalgia with cramps and/or fasciculations
Claudication syndromes
  Ischemia (arterial insufficiency)
  Neurogenic (e.g., due to spinal stenosis)

rheumatoid arthritis and polymyalgia rheumatica. Cramps, painful sustained and involuntary contractions, usually signify disease of the lower motor neuron, dystonic manifestations, or Brody's disease. Cramplike spasms of several muscle groups, which are provoked by certain repetitive stresses (e.g., writer's or musician's cramps) and generally relieved by avoidance of the provoking activity and stretching exercises, are not usually related to myopathy. Pain on exertion can be associated with ischemia or spinal claudication and usually is noted in the lower extremities of elderly individuals. In younger patients, certain rare metabolic myopathies of glycogen or lipid metabolism and mitochondrial disorders may present with exertional pain. The myopathy associated with the use of lipid-lowering agents also is manifested in this way.

## Movement Abnormalities

Abnormal movements of muscle occurring spontaneously (e.g., twitching or fasciculations), dystonic reactions, or persistent involuntary contractions (myokymia) are usually associated with disorders of the nervous system rather than with myopathic diseases. Lower motor neuron disorders or anterior horn cell diseases are marked by fasciculations, whereas disorders in higher coordinating centers may be associated with dystonic reactions. Abnormally delayed relaxation after contraction, myotonia, can be associated with myopathies. Myotonic muscular dystrophy and hyperkalemic periodic paralysis are examples of disorders affecting adults with myotonic manifestations. Severe hypothyroidism may also be associated with both delayed contraction and relaxation.

## Muscle Volume

In most myopathic disorders, muscle volume is preserved initially, so that weakness appears out of proportion to any loss of volume that may be evident. Later in the course of disease, atrophy can become a prominent feature. In patients with lower motor neuron dysfunction, on the other hand, atrophy and weakness occur early and concomitantly. Whereas atrophy is the usual consequence of chronic myopathy, several processes cause apparent muscle enlargement. Pseudohypertrophy can develop in Duchenne, Becker's, limb-girdle, and oculopharyngeal muscular dystrophies and in spinal muscular atrophy, sarcoidosis, and cystocercosis.

## Family History

The family history can be of great importance in diagnosis. It may be difficult, however, to obtain an accurate family history for several reasons. Lack of knowledge and unwillingness to involve others in medical examinations can limit the amount of information acquired about family members. In addition, phenotypic expression of genetic abnormalities in a number of disorders can be quite varied not only between generations but even between affected siblings. Whereas certain inherited myopathies such as Duchenne muscular dystrophy have a generally recognizable form among all affected individuals, others (e.g., acid maltase deficiency, myotonic dystrophy, facioscapulohumeral dystrophy, and the mitochondrial myopathies) may have markedly varied or incomplete presentations among similarly genetically affected family members. Therefore, it is of importance if the diagnosis is not definitively ascertained to review the family history in detail and if possible to seek to examine relatives in whom a question of a neuromuscular disorder has been raised.

## ANCILLARY TESTS

After the clinical history and examination have indicated the likelihood of a myopathic disorder, several ancillary types of tests may be performed to further explore and define this condition, including laboratory tests of blood serum, electromyography, muscle-imaging techniques, and biopsy. Here we consider the laboratory evaluations generally used (Table 5).

### Serum Enzymes

Assay of certain enzymatic activities in serum is the most commonly used approach for the initial laboratory evaluation of patients suspected of having a myopathy. Unfortunately, none of the enzymes commonly assayed occurs only in skeletal muscle. Creatine kinase elevations can be found not only in disorders of skeletal muscle but in certain cardiac, smooth muscle, and central nervous system diseases as well. Extremely high levels of creatine kinase, however, are generally associated with skeletal muscle disease. Lactate dehydrogenase, aldolase, and the aminotransaminases are present in many tissues, and elevations of these enzymes therefore have less specificity. In skeletal muscle disease, increases in serum activities of these latter enzymes are also frequently less dramatic and less rapid than those of creatine kinase. Only rarely will diseases of skeletal muscle cause an elevation of one of the other enzymes in the presence of a normal creatine kinase level. They are of use, however, in supporting creatine kinase findings, both initially and in follow-up. In interpreting enzyme values, the clinician should keep in mind that most assays reflect enzymatic activity rather than molecular content, so that artifacts induced by specimen handling, dilution, or the presence of inhibitors may affect the final values reported by the laboratory.

### *Creatine Kinase*

In clinical practice, estimation of serum creatine kinase activity has proven to be one of the most useful and practical guides to the presence and severity of myopathies (1). Creatine kinase is present in highest concentrations in excitable tissues (muscle and nervous system). By its action of catalyzing the interconversion of ATP and creatine phosphate,

$$\text{creatine} + \text{ATP} \underset{}{\overset{CK}{\rightleftarrows}} \text{creatine phosphate} + \text{ADP}$$

it controls the flow of energy (in the form of high-energy phosphate) within the cell (see Chapter 2). This enzyme, in its most common form, is a dimer composed of two polypeptide subunits, M and B. There are therefore three forms, MM, MB, and BB. The MM form is predominant in skeletal muscle, accounting for over 90% to 95% of the total creatine kinase. In addition, small amounts of the MB form are present. Cardiac muscle also

---

**TABLE 5.** *Ancillary laboratory tests*

---

Serum enzyme activities: creatine kinase, aldolase, AST, ALT, and lactate dehydrogenase
Serum and urine myoglobin levels
Urinary creatine excretion-elevated in myopathic and atrophic states
Measurements of lactate and ammonia with forearm ischemic exercise

---

AST, aspartate aminotransferase; ALT, alamine aminotransferase.

contains primarily MM and in addition a greater relative concentration of the MB iso-form, 20% to 30%. The BB isoform is the major constituent of smooth muscle and tis-sue of the central nervous system, accounting for 95% to 100% of the total creatine ki-nase in those tissues (2–5).

In diseases of skeletal muscle, creatine kinase leaks or extravasates from the muscle fibers. Increases in serum creatine kinase-MM activity are therefore noted. With injury or inflammation, rapid rises in creatine kinase-MM levels in the circulation occur earlier and in higher concentrations than do those of the other commonly tested enzymes. Cre-atine kinase-MB is present in a higher percentage in embryonal muscles. Accordingly, the content of this isoenzyme changes with age. Creatine kinase-MB values in the range of 20% to 30% have been found in skeletal muscle of children under 1 year of age. Occa-sionally, disproportionate increases in creatine kinase-MB are also seen in adults. This unexpected finding can occur after the release of creatine kinase-MB from skeletal mus-cle cells whose creatine kinase-MB content has increased as the result of chronic dam-age and regeneration. For this reason, serum creatine kinase-MB levels up to 20% to 30% of total creatine kinase have been observed in patients with muscular dystrophy, der-matomyositis, and polymyositis, in the absence of clinical evidence of cardiac disease (6–10). Increases in creatine kinase-MB levels in skeletal muscle have also been found in long distance runners and in other individuals after chronic exertion and exercise (11–14). Because of this, the presence of increased levels of creatine kinase-MB in serum of patients with skeletal muscle disorders should not be assumed to invariably represent cardiac damage.

In addition to these isoforms of creatine kinase, other variants may rarely be seen. Mi-tochondrial creatine kinase, a larger polymeric form of the enzyme, may be present in serum after marked widespread tissue damage. Macroenzyme forms, complexes of crea-tine kinase with other proteins such as IgG, have also been observed in the circulation (15–20).

Posttranslational hydrolytic cleavage of the creatine kinase-M subunit gives rise to iso-forms of both creatine kinase-MM and creatine kinase-MB, which may be distinguished electrophoretically. Quantification of these isoforms has been suggested to be a value in estimating the time of release of creatine kinase-MB in terms of assessment of early acute versus chronic muscle damage (21). Recent studies have indicated the presence of a poly-morphism with at least two members for the creatine kinase-M component. Whether muscle performance in one or another parameter may relate to this genetic influence re-mains to be explored (22).

### *Transaminases*

Aspartate aminotransaminase (AST) catalyzes the reaction shown in the following equation:

$$\begin{array}{ccc} \text{glutamic acid} & & \alpha\text{-ketoglutaric acid} \\ + & \xrightleftharpoons[\text{AST}]{} & + \\ \text{oxaloacetic acid} & & \text{aspartic acid} \end{array}$$

It is found in many tissues of the body, especially heart, liver, skeletal muscle, and kid-ney. Elevations of serum levels of this enzyme also occur in the course of muscle disease but are less striking than those of creatine kinase. Alanine aminotransaminase (ALT) is also found in skeletal muscle but in much smaller amounts. Elevations of ALT are there-fore observed less commonly in myopathies but may be seen with severe muscle damage.

### Lactate Dehydrogenase

Lactate dehydrogenase (LDH) catalyzes the interconversion of lactate and pyruvate and is found throughout the tissues of the body (23).

$$\text{pyruvate} + \text{NADH} \overset{\text{LDH}}{\rightleftharpoons} \text{lactate} + \text{NAD}$$

It is a tetramer composed of two subunits and therefore exists in 5 isoforms (LDH-1, LDH-2, LDH-3, LDH-4, LDH-5). The proportions and type of each isoform vary between muscles and even between myofibers within a muscle. Fast-twitch (type II) fibers are richer in LDH than are the slow-twitch (type I) fibers and contain more of the cathodal forms of the enzyme (LDH-4 and LDH-5). The anodal isoforms (LDH-1 and LDH-2) are relatively increased in type I fibers. Certain muscles such as the gastrocnemius and triceps brachii contain the cathodal forms primarily, whereas the gluteus medius and soleus are richer in the anodal isoforms (24,25). In muscle disease, therefore, serum levels of LDH increase, but the patterns of isoforms found may be variable depending on the muscles involved and the age of the affected individual. Cardiac muscle is richest in LDH-1 (26).

### Aldolase

Aldolase also is widely distributed in body tissues. It catalyzes the splitting of fructose phosphate into two, three-carbon fragments:

$$\text{fructose-1,6-diphosphate} \overset{\text{aldolase}}{\rightarrow} \text{glyceraldehyde-3-phosphate} + \text{dihydroxyacetone phosphate}$$

Type A is the major form in skeletal muscle. Increases in circulating levels of aldolase may be seen, not only in myopathies but in liver, hematologic, and disorders of other tissue (27).

### Myoglobin

This oxygen-carrying respiratory protein is found only in cardiac and skeletal muscle and therefore has greater specificity for muscle tissue than do the enzymes mentioned above. Increases in serum myoglobin levels occur during the course of myopathy, and changes in these levels may be used to reflect and assess changes in the clinical state of patients. Moreover, serum myoglobin values can demonstrate changes in the clinical state of patients earlier than those of the enzymes. Normally, myoglobin is not detectable in the urine. However, in circumstances of massive trauma, burns, or other conditions causing rhabdomyolysis where large amounts of myoglobin are liberated rapidly from the muscle cell into the circulation, myoglobin will be filtered through the glomerulus and appear in the urine. Persistent states of myoglobinuria are associated with a risk of renal failure (28,29). Urinary concentrations of myoglobin do not directly mirror serum myoglobin levels. This is so because of several factors. First, due to renal tubular resorption, a circulation threshold exists below which myoglobin will not appear in the urine. Second, when the threshold is exceeded, water resorption and resulting urine concentration can produce higher concentrations of myoglobin in the urine than are simultaneously present in the serum. Finally, acids and proteolytic factors in urine can denature and destroy myoglobin. This artifactually will lower urine myoglobin values. For greatest accuracy, tests on urine for myoglobin should be made on fresh samples.

## Creatine

Creatine appears in the urine in increased amounts during the course of muscle disorders. It is synthesized in the liver and taken up by the muscle cell to be used to store energy in the form of creatine phosphate. Creatinine is the breakdown product of creatine and is released by the muscle cell into the circulation. The renal threshold for creatinine is low, and therefore its excretion can be seen as a measure of muscle mass. The threshold for creatine, on the other hand, is high so that its daily excretion represents only 5% to 6% of that of creatinine. In myopathic states, creatine excretion is increased. This is due to two factors. First, the uptake of creatine from the plasma by the muscle cell is decreased, and second its retention and storage within the cell is impaired. Both conditions lead to increased creatine loads delivered to the kidney. Atrophy of muscle from any cause may also result in relative increases in creatine excretion compared with that of creatinine for these reasons. In addition, in atrophic states there is less total conversion of creatine to creatinine by the reduced amount of muscle tissue. Creatinuria with increased creatine-to-creatinine ratios can therefore be seen in active muscle disease and in neurologic disorders and other states marked by atrophy of skeletal muscle (30).

## Forearm Ischemic Exercise Testing

The metabolic changes that occur in normal skeletal muscle when it exercises under ischemic conditions result in increased production of lactate and ammonia. Under these conditions, lactate is the end product of glycolysis and ammonia is a byproduct of the purine nucleotide cycle (see Chapter 2). The forearm ischemia exercise test (Table 6) is used to screen for inborn errors of glycogen metabolism or glycolysis and myoadenylate deaminase deficiency. This testing exploits the abnormal biochemistry that results from the particular enzyme deficiency. Patients with glycogen storage disease cannot generate lactate, and those deficient in myoadenylate deaminase deficiency cannot generate ammonia (Table 7).

In normal individuals, venous lactate and ammonia levels will both increase three- to sixfold after forearm ischemic exercise. Those with myophosphorylase deficiency or another

---

**TABLE 6.** *Protocol for forearm ischemic exercise testing*

A sample of venous blood is drawn from the nondominant arm without using a tournequet[a] and analyzed for lactate and ammonia concentrations.

A sphygmomanometer cuff is secured around the upper arm of the dominant side and inflated to and maintained at a pressure at least 20 mm Hg above systolic pressure. The patient then squeezes a tennis ball (or other object) with the dominant hand as vigorously as possible at the rate of one squeeze every 1 to 2 s.

After 2 min of exercise,[b] the cuff is deflated. Venous samples for lactate and ammonia concentrations are obtained from the dominant arm 2 min after the cuff is deflated.[c]

---

[a]Tourniquet use should be minimal, if necessary, because venous stasis use could artifactually raise blood levels of lactate and ammonia.

[b]Two minutes is arbitrary. Some individuals will only be able to exercise for 90 s. Those who can exercise for a full 2 min may not be exerting enough effort. In that case, exercises should be continued until the individual cannot actually make a fist. Insufficient effort may give a false-positive result.

[c]In experimental settings, samples are often drawn at 1, 2, 5, and 10 min postexercise. This is not necessary in the clinical setting.

**TABLE 7.** *Results from forearm ischemic exercise testing*

| Sample time | Normal | | Myophosphorylase deficiency | | Myoadenylate deaminase deficiency | |
|---|---|---|---|---|---|---|
| | Lactate | Ammonia | Lactate | Ammonia | Lactate | Ammonia |
| Baseline | 0.9 | 15 | 0.9 | 18 | 1.0 | 24 |
| 1 min | 5.9 | 110 | 0.9 | 95 | 3.9 | 24 |
| 3 min | 4.3 | 90 | 1.0 | 80 | 2.4 | 27 |
| 5 min | 2.0 | 50 | 0.9 | 40 | 1.6 | 29 |

Lactate in mEq/L; ammonia in μmol/L.
Similar results will be seen in individuals with deficiencies of debrancher enzyme, phosphofructokinase, phosphoglycerate kinase, phosphoglycerate mutase, or lactate dehydrogenase.

glycogen storage disease can generate ammonia under these conditions but cannot generate lactate (31). Myoadenylate deaminase-deficient individuals, in contrast, can generate lactate but not ammonia (32).

The major limitation of this test is that some normal individuals cannot or will not exercise with enough intensity to produce the anaerobic conditions necessary to produce lactate. When that occurs, a false-positive result may be seen (33). Accordingly, any positive test must be followed by a muscle biopsy and enzyme analysis for the putative defect. Adequate exercise will cause an "ischemic pain" and the inability to clench one's fist. This symptom clears instantly when the tourniquet is removed in normal subjects but may result in persistent cramping and transient contracture in a patient with a glycogen storage disease.

## APPROACH TO THE PATIENT WITH UNSUSPECTED ABNORMAL ELEVATION OF SERUM CREATINE KINASE ACTIVITY

A frequent problem confronting clinicians is the patient with an unexplained elevation of serum creatine kinase activity. Typically this occurs when blood chemistries have been ordered for a reason unrelated to suspicion of myopathy. These may have been part of a routine screening or health assessment profile or they may have been the result of investigation into another matter. Nonetheless, the elevated creatine kinase level, usually not specifically requested, is noted and the question arises of how this should be pursued. This is the kind of clinical problem for which an evidence-validated algorithm could be of use. Unfortunately, such an instrument does not exist, and this leaves many physicians in a quandary. However, logic can be applied to this situation (Fig. 1).

First, one attempts to determine any clinical evidence of myopathy. A history of weakness, myalgia, weight loss, fever, rash, or exposure to potentially toxic medications or other environmental factors should be sought. Certain common predisposing conditions such as alcohol or cocaine use, administration of lipid-lowering agents, strenuous exercise, cryptic hypothyroidism, or electrolyte imbalance may become evident in this way. In these cases, elimination or correction of the underlying situation should resolve the problem. In the case of an individual devoted to strenuous exercise, an attempt should be made to measure the creatine kinase after an interval of rest.

After these common factors have been explored and dealt with, a number of individuals still remain with unexplained serum creatine kinase elevation. They can be divided into two groups: those with borderline or mildly elevated levels and those with marked elevations. In the first group are some who for genetic or constitutional reasons have circulating levels of this enzyme higher than that expected in the general population. Men

```
                 CK unexpectedly found elevated
                             ⇓
                           repeat
                             ⇓
                   CK remains elevated
                             ⇓
                 obtain family history
                 medication, drug & toxin history
                 examine for weakness, neurological
                 abnormalities, check thyroid status
                       ⇓                      ⇓
                no evident              diagnosis
                diagnosis               discovered
                 ⇓          ⇓                ⇓
       CK borderline     CK markedly      appropriate
       or mildly elevated  elevated       treatment &
            ⇓                 ⇓            follow up

    continue observation      consider further
    with monitoring of        evaluation
    strength, general health  EMG, biopsy, MRI
    status & CK overtime
              ⇓                    ⇑
            deterioration of
            status or rise in CK
```

**FIG. 1.** Approach to asymptomatic individuals with elevated serum creatine kinase activity.

have higher serum values on average than do women. African-Americans have higher serum values than do whites. Serum creatine kinase of Asians and Hispanics may also be higher than that of whites (34). Family members of individuals affected with muscular dystrophies, glycogen storage diseases, or malignant hyperthermia may also have increased levels of creatine kinase. Most of these individuals will not have an identifiable myopathy. However, they should be observed over time by monitoring their general health status and motor function. Any change in health status or decline in function provides impetus for extensive evaluation. For those with marked elevations, more extensive evaluation may be warranted.

Evaluation for suspected problem cases can be difficult. Electromyography, magnetic resonance imaging, and muscle biopsy of symptomatic areas can be obtained. It should be kept in mind that muscle biopsy done blindly in an area that is not symptomatic may be unrevealing. Moreover, the types of analyses to be applied to the biopsy specimen, such as routine histologic examination or more extensive histochemistry, electron microscopy, or biochemical study, are most effectively used when exploring specific clinical suspicions. In the absence of any clues, biopsy alone may prove to be disappointing.

## REFERENCES

1. Wu AHB, Perryman MB. Clinical applications of muscle enzymes and proteins. *Curr Opin Rheumatol* 1992;4: 815–820.
2. Jockers-Wretou E, Pfleiderer G. Quantitation of creatine kinase isoenzymes in human tissues by an immunological method. *Clin Chim Acta* 1975;58:223–232.
3. Dawson DM, Fine IH. Creatine kinase in human tissues. *Arch Neurol* 1975;16:175–180.
4. Mercer DM. Separation of tissue and serum creatine kinase isoenzymes by ion-exchange column chromatography. *Clin Chem* 1974;20:36–40.
5. Eppenberger HM. A brief summary of the history of the detection of creatine kinase isoenzymes. *Mol Cell Biochem* 1994;133/134:9–11.

6. Edwards YH, Tipler TD, Morgan-Hughes JA, et al. Isozyme patterns and protein profiles in neuromuscular disorders. *J Med Genet* 1982;19:175–183.
7. Goto I, Nagamine M, Katsuki S. Creatine phosphokinase isozymes in muscles. Human fetus and patients. *Arch Neurol* 1969;20:422–429.
8. King DT, Fu PC, Wishon GM. Persistent creatine kinase MB isoenzyme without cardiac disease. *Arch Pathol Lab Med* 1978;102:481–482.
9. Adornato BT, Engel WK. MB-creatine phosphokinase elevation not diagnostic of myocardial infarction. *Arch Intern Med* 1977;137:1089–1090.
10. Larca LJ, Coppola JT, Honig S. Creatine kinase MB isoenzyme in dermatomyositis: a noncardiac source. *Ann Intern Med* 1981;94:341–343.
11. Siegel AJ, Silverman LM, Holman L. Elevated creatine kinase MB isoenzyme levels in marathon runners. Normal myocardial scintograms suggest noncardiac source. *JAMA* 1982;246:2049–2051.
12. Davies B, Daggett A, Watt DAL. Serum creatine kinase and isoenzyme responses of veteran class fell runners. *Eur J Appl Physiol* 1982;48:345–354.
13. Lang H, Wursburg U. Creatine kinase, an enzyme of many forms. *Clin Chem* 1982;28:1439–1447.
14. Miles MP, Schneider CM. Creatine kinase isoenzyme MB may be elevated in healthy young women after submaximal eccentric exercise. *J Lab Clin Med* 1993;122:197–201.
15. James GP, Harrison RL. Creatine kinase isoenzymes of mitochondrial origin in human serum. *Clin Chem* 1979; 25:943–947.
16. Urdal P, Landaas S. Macrocreatine kinase BB in serum and some data on its prevalence. *Clin Chem* 1979;25: 461–465.
17. Laureys M, Sion J-P, Slabbynck H, et al. Macromolecular creatine kinase type 1: a serum marker associated with disease. *Clin Chem* 1991;37:430–434.
18. Lee KN, Csako G, Bernhardt P, Elin RJ. Relevance of macrocreatine kinase type 1 and type 2 isoenzymes to laboratory and clinical data. *Clin Chem* 1994;40:1278–1283.
19. Backer ET, Hafkenscheid JCM, van Wermeskerken RKA. Complexes of creatine kinase and immunoglobulins in serum identified by a nonimmune binding method. *Clin Chem* 1991;37:173–179.
20. Wyss M, Smeitink J, Wevers RA, Wallimann T. Mitochondrial creatine kinase: a key enzyme of aerobic energy metabolism. *Biochim Biophys Acta* 1992;1102:119–166.
21. Panteghini M. Creatine kinase MB isoforms. *J Clin Immunoassay* 1994;17:30–34.
22. Rivera MA, Dionne FT, Simoneau J-A, et al. Muscle specific creatine kinase gene polymorphism and $Vo_2$ max in the HERITAGE family study. *Med Sci Sports Exerc* 1997;29:1311–1317.
23. Markert CL. Lactate dehydrogenase. Biochemistry and function of lactate dehydrogenase. *Cell Biochem Funct* 1984;2:131–134.
24. Gollnick PD, Armstrong RB. Histochemical localization of lactate dehydrogenase isoenzymes in human skeletal muscle fibers. *Life Sci* 1976;18:27–31.
25. Takasu T, Hughes BP. Lactate dehydrogenase isoenzyme patterns in human skeletal muscle. *J Neurol Neurosurg Psychiatry* 1969;32:175–179.
26. Bruns DE, Emerson JC, Intemann S, et al. Lactate dehydrogenase isoenzyme-1. Changes during the first day after acute myocardial infarction. *Clin Chem* 1981;27:1821–1823.
27. Rutter WJ, Rajkumar T, Phenhoet E, Kochmann M. Aldolase variants: structure and physiological significance. *Ann NY Acad Sci* 1968;151:102–117.
28. Kagen LJ. Myoglobin: methods and diagnostic uses. *Crit Rev Clin Lab Sci* 1978;9:273–302.
29. Herrera GA. Myoglobin and the kidney. An overview. *Ultrastruct Pathol* 1994;18:113–117.
30. Vignos PJ Jr, Goldwyn J. Evaluation of laboratory tests in diagnosis and management of polymyositis. *Am J Med Sci* 1972;263:291–308.
31. McArdle B. Myopathy due to a defect in muscle glycogen breakdown. *Clin Sci* 1951;10:13–33.
32. Fishbein WN. Myoadenylate deaminase deficiency: inherited and acquired forms. *Biochem Med* 1985;33: 158–169.
33. Valen PA, Nakayama DA, Veum JA, et al. Myoadenylate deaminase deficiency and forearm ischemic exercise testing. *Arthritis Rheum* 1987;30:661–668.
34. Harris EK, Wong ET, Shaw ST Jr. Statistical criteria for separate reference intervals: race and gender groups in creatine kinase. Clin Chem 1991;37:1580–1582.

*Diseases of Skeletal Muscle,*
edited by Robert L. Wortmann.
Lippincott Williams & Wilkins, Philadelphia © 2000

# 15

# Autoantibodies and Muscle Disease

Ira N. Targoff

*Department of Medicine, Veterans Affairs Medical Center and*
*University of Oklahoma Health Sciences Center, Oklahoma City, Oklahoma 73014*

Autoantibodies are commonly found in some forms of idiopathic inflammatory myopathy, especially polymyositis and dermatomyositis. These autoantibodies can be divided between two general categories: those antinuclear antibodies (ANAs) found in a variety of connective tissue diseases versus those specific for myositis. The latter have been termed myositis-specific autoantibodies (MSAs). In patients with polymyositis and dermatomyositis, the MSAs are directed against fundamental intracellular antigens, antigens found in all cells, rather than to antigens that are specific for muscle or other tissues. These autoantibodies demonstrate the presence of autoimmunity of these diseases. They are important clinically and biologically due to their disease specificity, but their role in the pathogenesis of the idiopathic inflammatory myopathies remains unknown. There is no current evidence that they participate in muscle damage. Most individual MSA specificities are found in only a small proportion of patients but tend to be associated with particular clinical features, thus defining subgroups of patients. Testing for the presence and specificity of serum autoantibodies can be useful in the evaluation of patients with suspected muscle disorders. Often such testing is performed to help with diagnosis of idiopathic inflammatory myopathies and for further information about the likely manifestations to be expected from a patient's illness.

The ANA test, using indirect immunofluorescence on cells, is the most common test used to screen for the autoantibodies found in systemic rheumatic diseases such as systemic lupus erythematosus, scleroderma, and Sjögren's syndrome. As in these other connective tissue diseases, polymyositis and dermatomyositis patients have a high frequency of positive ANA tests (Table 1), often present in high or moderate titers. The frequency is highest among those polymyositis and dermatomyositis patients with overlap syndromes of myositis with other connective tissue disorders. Forms of inflammatory myopathy other than polymyositis and dermatomyositis such as inclusion body myositis or granulomatous myositis have a much lower frequency of positive ANAs, and noninflammatory myopathies (i.e., metabolic, neuropathic) have a normal frequency. Although the presence of a positive ANA can be helpful in pointing to the possibility of polymyositis or dermatomyositis in patients with signs of myopathy, the result is nonspecific, and the possibility of positives in other conditions must be considered. For example, chronic infections can cause clinical presentations with many features of a connective tissue disease and a positive ANA. Furthermore, the ANA is positive in 5% of the normal population, and such incidental positives are more likely in patients with other manifestations of autoimmunity. Generally, those for whom the ANA is a manifestation of their disease

**TABLE 1.** *Autoantibodies in polymyositis and dermatomyositis*

| Name | Antigen | Molecular weight (kDa) | Tests | IIF | Frequency (%) | HLA | Clinical | Comments (Ref.) |
|---|---|---|---|---|---|---|---|---|
| ***Myositis-specific autoantibodies*** | | | | | | | | |
| Antisynthetases | | | | | | | | |
| Jo-1 | Histidyl-tRNA synthetase | 50 | ID, IPP, WB, EIA, AAI | Cyto | 18–20 | DR3, DRw52 DRB1*0501 | Antisynthetase syndrome | PM > DM (2,38) rare in JDMS |
| PL-7 | Threonyl-tRNA synthetase | 80 | ID, IPP, AAI, WB[a] | Cyto | ≤3 | DRw52 | Antisynthetase syndrome | PM ≤ DM (38) |
| PL-12 | Alanyl-tRNA synthetase + tRNA[alac] | 110 | IPP, AAI, WB[a] | Cyto | ≤3 | DRw52 | Antisynthetase syndrome | ILD > Myo[b] (33) |
| EJ | Glycyl-tRNA synthetase | 75 | IPP, WB, AAI, AAI | Cyto | ≤2 | DRw52 | Antisynthetase syndrome | DM > M (85) |
| OJ | Isoleucyl-tRNA synthetase (multienzyme complex)[a] | 150 | IPP, AAI WB[d] | Cyto | ≤1 | DRw52 | Antisynthetase syndrome | ILD = Myo[b] (37) |
| KS | Asparaginyl-tRNA synthetase | 65 | IPP, AAI, ID | Cyto | ≤1 | | Antisynthetase syndrome | ILD > Myo[b] (29) |
| *Nonsynthetase autoantibodies* | | | | | | | | |
| SRP | Signal recognition particle[e] | 54/72 7SL-RNA | IPP, WB, EIA | Cyto | [a]4 | DR5, DRw52 | | Severe, acute, resistant PM (59) |
| Mi-2 | CHD3/CHD4 (HDAC complex)[f] | 206/218[f] | ID, IPP, EIA | Nucl | ≤8 | DR7; DRw53 | | DM; all subgroups (2,64,73) |
| ***Myositis-associated autoantibodies***[a] | | | | | | | | |
| PM-Scl | Unidentified | 100 75[h] | ID, IPP, WB EIA | Nucleo/ Nuclear | ≤8 | DR3 | | PM/SSc/arthritis overlap[i] ("scleromyositis") (74,93,100) |
| U1RNP | U1 small nuclear ribonucleoprotein (U1 snRNP) | A, 70K | ID, IPP, WB, EIA | NucSp | 12 | | | MCTD, other overlap syndromes |
| Non-U1 snRNPs | | | | | | | | |
| U2 snRNP | A', B'' | IPP, WB | NucSp | <1 | | PM/SSc overlap syndrome[j] | | |
| U4/6 snRNP | | IPP | NucSp | <1 | | PM/SSc overlap syndrome | | |
| U5 snRNP | | IPP | NucSp | <2 | | PM or overlap syndrome (82,83) | | |
| U3 snRNP | | IPP | NucSp | <2 | | Scleroderma | | |
| Ku | DNA-binding proteins | 70,80 | ID, IPP, WB | NucSp | <1 | | | Myo/SSc/SLE Overlap (107) |
| Ro/SSA | RNA-protein | 60 | ID, IPP, WB, EIA | Cyto/Nuc | 10 | DR3,DQ1,2 | | Myo often with SS or SLE |
| 56 kD | Ribonucleoprotein particle | 52 | WB,EIA | Nuc | 20 | | | Myo often with anti-Jo-1 |
| | | 56 | WB | Nuc | 87 | | | Myo, all subgroups (118) |

| | Antigen | MW | Method | Frequency | Pattern | HLA | Clinical |
|---|---|---|---|---|---|---|---|
| KJ | Unidentified translation factor | 120 | ID,WB | <1% | Cyto | DRw52 | PM,ILD,RP (124) |
| Fer | Elongation factor 1α | 48 | IPP | <1% | Cyto | | Myo (152) |
| Mas | tRNA[ser]-related antigen | All tRNA | IPP | 1% | Cyto | DR4,DR53 | Myo, alcohol-rhabdomyolysis; chronic hepatitis (2) |
| MJ | Unidentified | 135 | IPP,WB | <10% | Nuc | | Juvenile DM (122) |
| | Nuclear pore | | IIF | <2 | Nuc Pore | | French-Canadian (125) |
| hPMS1 | DNA repair | 110 | IPP | 13% | | | Myo (136) |
| Other | Proteasome | | | | | | |
| | Endothelial cell | | | | | | |
| | Muscle membrane | | | | | | |
| | Muscle-specific proteins | | | | | | |

**Antisynthetase syndrome:** Characteristic syndrome associated with antibodies to aminoacyl-tRNA synthetases, usually including myositis (95%) along with ILD (75%), arthritis (50%), Raynaud's phenomenon (60%), Mechanic's hands (60%), fevers with exacerbations (80%), and response to steroids but recurrence with taper.

[a]WB is inconsistently positive with anti-PL-7 and anti-PL-12

[b]>95% of patients with anti-Jo-1 have evidence of myositis, but only 60% of U.S. anti-PL-12 patients have myositis (lower % in Japan). Anti-KS patients is similar. Anti-OJ may be < anti-Jo-1 but uncertain due to low frequency.

[c]Most sera with anti-PL-12 (anti-AlaRS) have antibodies that react directly with tRNA[ala]. A smaller proportion of sera with other antisynthetases react with the cognate tRNA of the antigenic synthetase.

[d]IleRS is the major antigen for most anti-OJ patients but many sera react with other components of the multi-enzyme synthetase complex (lysyl-, glutamyl-prolyl-, and/or leucyl-tRNA synthetases).

[e]Anti-SRP may react predominantly with 54 kDa or with higher MW components.

[f]Anti-Mi-2 sera react with both Mi-2α (CHD3) and Mi-2β (CHD4), related but different helicase proteins with 75% homology, which are components of histone deacetylase complexes (HDAC).

[g]PM-Scl antigen is a complex of 11 proteins of which the 100 kDa is the largest and major antigen, and 75 kDa another common antigen.

[h]Anti-PM-Scl can be associated with SSc, PM, or DM alone, or myo-SSc overlap ("scleromyositis"). Arthritis is commonly a major feature of the syndrome.

[i]Antibodies to specific proteins of non-U1 snRNPs in the absence of anti-Sm are rare but when present are often associated with overlap syndromes involving myositis.

[j]In Japan, anti-Ku is often precipitin-positive and associated with overlap syndromes of SLE, SSc, and myositis. In the United States, anti-Ku is often precipitin negative and associated with SLE.

**IIF**, indirect immunofluorescent pattern; **HLA**, human leukocyte antigen; **ID**, immunodiffusion; **IPP**, immunoprecipitation; **WB**, Western blot; **EIA**, enzyme immunoassay; **AAI**, aminoacylation inhibition (testing for inhibition of activity of antigenic synthetase enzyme); **Cyto**, cytoplasmic; **nuc**, nuclear; **sp**, speckled; **nucleo**, nucleolar; **Myo**, myositis; **ILD**, interstitial lung disease; **SSc**, systemic sclerosis (scleroderma); **SS**, Sjögren's syndrome; **JDMS**, juvenile DM.

From Ref. 135; with permission.

tend to have a higher titer than those with incidental asymptomatic positive tests. Thus, the ANA should be interpreted cautiously, and a positive or negative result cannot be used by itself to confirm or exclude the presence of polymyositis or dermatomyositis.

The frequency of positive ANAs varies in different clinical subgroups of idiopathic inflammatory myopathies. Among the subgroups of polymyositis and dermatomyositis as defined by Bohan and Peter (1) (see Chapters 4 and 5), ANAs are least common in myositis with malignancy but can occur in that setting (2,3). The frequency of positive ANAs is about the same in children as it is in adults with dermatomyositis (60% to 75%) (4). Some data suggest that in juvenile dermatomyositis, the frequency of positive ANAs is higher in patients with recent onset. In one study, positive ANAs are found in 40% of patients with polymyositis and 62% of dermatomyositis when connective tissue disease-associated patients are excluded (2). There is a higher frequency of ANA in connective tissue disease-overlap syndromes, at least 77%, or higher, depending on the overlapping condition. Features such as arthritis of connective tissue disease or Raynaud's phenomenon without overt overlap syndromes also may be more common in patients with myositis and an ANA, because they are more frequent in patients with certain defined antibodies, discussed below.

The prevalence of ANA positivity is much lower in inclusion body myositis compared with polymyositis or dermatomyositis but is higher than in the normal population (2,5–7). Myositis, myopathy, or weakness that is part of a vasculitis such as polyarteritis nodosa or an antineutrophil cytoplasm antibody-associated vasculitis is generally not associated with positive ANAs on standard substrates. Except for the association with chronic infections noted above, ANA is not a part of infectious myositis.

Among other diseases associated with muscle weakness, ANAs can occur in myasthenia gravis but are lower in frequency. There is a small incidence of overlap with connective tissue diseases, including polymyositis and dermatomyositis (8), and this possibility should be considered when the ANA is positive in myasthenia gravis.

A variety of ANA patterns may be seen in polymyositis and dermatomyositis (9), including nuclear speckled, nuclear homogeneous, nucleolar, cytoplasmic, or mixed patterns (Fig. 1). This reflects the substantial heterogeneity of autoantibody specificity between patients. The pattern can give a clue to the likely underlying specificities and can sometimes help guide specific testing, but the possibility of masking one pattern with another should be kept in mind. An experienced observer can sometimes identify subtleties in the pattern that point to particular autoantibodies (10), but most specific antibodies in polymyositis and dermatomyositis cannot be reliably identified by ANA testing alone.

Several of the known MSAs discussed below react with cytoplasmic antigens, leading to cytoplasmic patterns of cell staining. These are not always reported as positive ANA tests when they are the only changes observed. Specific testing for myositis autoantibodies is usually indicated when the ANA is positive. However, in some cases, particularly anti-Jo-1 or anti-SRP, ANA tests are negative at the screening dilution even for cytoplasmic staining. Thus, testing for some MSAs may be indicated even when the ANA is negative.

The frequency of positive ANAs in polymyositis and dermatomyositis can be affected by other technical factors. The most commonly used substrate is human cultured cells, such as the HEp-2 human epithelial line or other transformed human cell lines. Older studies and procedures using tissue sections from rodent liver or kidney failed to detect many autoantibodies of clinical significance in either disease. In a direct comparison with the same reader, microscope, and technique, positive ANAs in sera from patients with polymyositis and dermatomyositis rose from 33% to 78% when changing from mouse kidney sections to HEp-2 cells (9). In addition to higher frequency, human cells may also give higher titers. The factors responsible include ease of interpretation with larger cells and nuclei, fresher cells at the time of fixation, greater expression of some antigens in actively growing cells, and the preferential reaction of some autoantibodies with the human form of the antigen. ELISA methods using cell extracts or pooled purified antigens have been introduced. ELISA techniques have practical advantages but also have a potential to lose sensitivity due to loss of antigens.

## MYOSITIS-SPECIFIC AUTOANTIBODIES

Several MSAs have been identified in the serum of patients with polymyositis or dermatomyositis. These are found almost exclusively in patients with myositis or myositis syndromes. Although the MSAs are specific, they are far from sensitive for myositis. Even the most common, anti-Jo-1, is present in at most 20% of patients with idiopathic inflammatory myopathy. Taken together, MSAs are present in less than half of patients. Thus, although their presence can provide powerful support for a diagnosis of polymyositis or dermatomyositis, their absence does not provide significant evidence against the diagnosis.

With extremely rare exception, each patient will have only one MSA (11). In addition, they are invariably present from the earliest samples taken from patients with overt disease. It is highly likely that the MSAs serve as markers, each defining a small subgroup of patients with characteristic clinical associations.

### Anti-Aminoacyl-tRNA Synthetases ("Anti-synthetases")

Each cell has 20 different aminoacyl-tRNA synthetase activities, with a separate enzyme for each amino acid (12) (although the synthetases for glutamic acid and proline are fused into a single 170-kDa protein [13]). For the cell to maintain fidelity of translation and produce a polypeptide with the correct amino acid sequence, it is crucial for the tRNAs to be charged with the correct amino acid. For this purpose, each synthetase must properly recognize its specific amino acid and the specific tRNAs for that amino acid (14). The tRNA synthetase activities have been divided into two classes. Certain features are shared among members of the same class and differ from the other class, including the overall structure and organization of the molecules, certain amino acid sequence motifs, the site of first attachment of the amino acid to the tRNA, and others (15). This may reflect separate evolutionary origin of the class I and class II enzymes (16). They retain signature sequences defining their amino acid specificity and significant sequence homology for a given amino acid between species (17). Synthetases for nine amino acids (glu-pro, ile, leu, met, lys, gln, arg, asp), most of which are class I, are incorporated into a large multienzyme complex along with at least three nonsynthetase proteins. Other synthetases are independent, usually free in the cytoplasm.

Anti-synthetase antibodies react with the enzyme protein, and most do not immunoprecipitate the cognate tRNAs if the protein is removed. This implies that the tRNAs are immunoprecipitated indirectly through their affinity for the protein. The tRNA synthetases have relatively high affinity for their tRNA substrates, and tRNA may at some points exist in a complex with the enzyme. It is possible that the anti-synthetase helps to stabilize this complex, accounting for the immunoprecipitation of the specific tRNA.

Anti-Jo-1 was originally defined as a precipitating antibody in Ouchterlony immunodiffusion against calf thymus extract, using prototype serum from patient "Jo"[1] (18,19).

---

[1]The original "Jo-2" is lost, but other sera occasionally have associated, unidentified precipitins.

The highly specific double immunodiffusion is still often used to test for anti-Jo-1 and is sensitive enough to detect this antibody in most patients. The Jo-1 antigen is histidyl-tRNA synthetase, an enzyme that binds histidine to its cognate transfer RNA (tRNA[his]) to form histidyl-tRNA (histidine aminoacylation) for the amino acid to be incorporated into the growing polypeptide chain during protein synthesis (20,21). Anti-Jo-1 antibodies inhibit histidine aminoacylation in vitro, and this inhibition is specific because aminoacylation with other amino acids is not inhibited (20). Inhibition of the antigen's function is a characteristic feature of many autoantibodies and suggests reaction with functional sites (22).

Histidyl-tRNA synthetase is required in all cells for protein synthesis and is present predominantly in the cytoplasm (23). Anti-Jo-1 often gives a finely speckled or homogeneous cytoplasmic pattern by indirect immunofluorescence (10). The fluorescence tends to be weak and is often absent at the screening dilution (9), so that some sera with anti-Jo-1 have a negative ANA test. Although anti-Jo-1 can also bind to the nucleus (24), the nuclear or nucleolar patterns that are not infrequently encountered clinically with anti-Jo-1 sera probably represent coexistent autoantibodies.

Autoantibodies to other aminoacyl-tRNA synthetases have been described (Table 1). Each anti-synthetase is specific for the individual aminoacyl-tRNA synthetase without cross-reaction with others. Non-Jo-1 anti-synthetases were found when anti-PL-7 and anti-PL-12, named for "precipitin lines" defined by prototype sera, also immunoprecipitated specific sets of tRNAs, which could be distinguished by electrophoresis from the Jo-1 tRNA and from each other (Fig. 2) (25). Anti-PL-7 specifically inhibited threonyl-

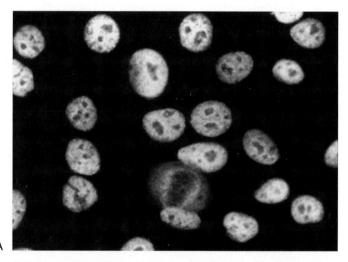

A

**FIG. 1.** ANA patterns in myositis. Indirect immunofluorescence on HEp-2 cells for antinuclear antibody testing using sera from patients with various myositis-specific antibodies. **A:** Anti-Mi-2 serum showing pure nuclear staining (without cytoplasmic staining) that spares nucleoli. **B:** Anti-PM-Scl serum showing bright nucleolar staining and nuclear staining of moderate intensity. Both patterns are typical of anti-PM-Scl. **C:** Anti-synthetase serum showing a granular type of cytoplasmic staining. Anti-OJ (anti-isoleucyl-tRNA synthetase) was used. Some anti-synthetase sera show nuclear staining, probably representing a coexistent antibody. **D:** Anti-SRP showing typical cytoplasmic staining, usually without nuclear staining.

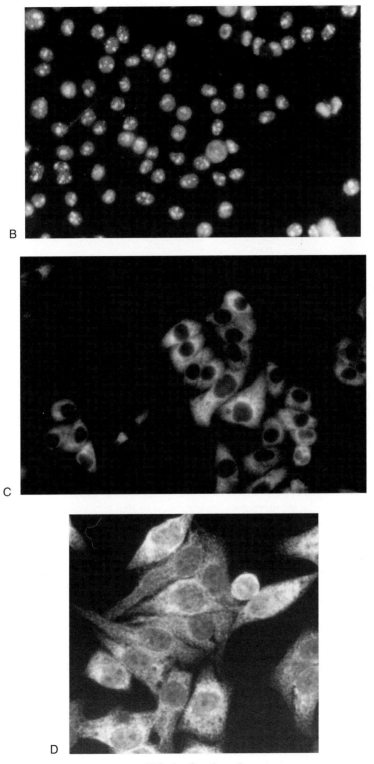

**FIG. 1.** *Continued.*

*DISEASES OF SKELETAL MUSCLE*

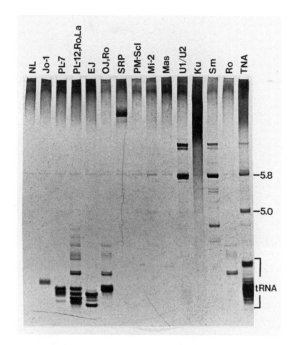

**FIG. 2.** Tender point counts in the general population. (From Ref. 22, with permission.)

tRNA synthetase and anti-PL-12 specifically inhibited alanyl-tRNA synthetase (Table 1) (26,27). Using similar methods, demonstrating immunoprecipitation of a distinctive set of tRNAs and specific inhibition of the antigen's functional enzymatic activity, anti-EJ antibodies were shown to react with glycyl-tRNA synthetase, anti-OJ antibodies with isoleucyl-tRNA synthetase (Fig. 3) (28), and anti-KS antibodies with asparaginyl-tRNA synthetase (29). As with anti-Jo-1, several of these have been confirmed by demonstration of reaction with recombinant forms of the enzymes (30–32).

Almost all anti-PL-12–positive sera have antibodies that react directly with tRNA$^{ala}$ in addition to the antibodies to alanyl-tRNA synthetase (27,33). The antibodies react specifically with certain forms of tRNA$^{ala}$ at a binding site that includes the anticodon (34). It is now clear that some sera with other anti-synthetases also have antibodies that react directly with the cognate tRNA, although it is less frequent than with anti-PL-12. This difference between anti-PL-12 and other anti-synthetases remains unexplained.

### Clinical Associations

The clinical associations of the anti-synthetases are generally similar to each other. The "anti-synthetase syndrome" includes a myositis (either polymyositis or dermatomyositis) (Fig. 4) and several extramuscle features (Table 2) (2,35). Patients with any of the anti-synthetases may have the full expression of this syndrome but may also present with incomplete forms of the syndrome in which any of the features, including myositis, may be absent.

Myositis occurs at some point in the course of almost all anti-Jo-1–positive patients. Most patients have some evidence of myositis when they are first evaluated. Overt polymyositis or dermatomyositis is most common, but patients who present with other

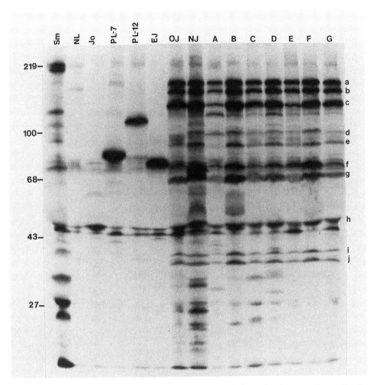

**FIG. 3.** Immunoprecipitation from HeLa cells with anti-OJ and other anti-synthetase autoantibodies. Polyacrylamide gel electrophoresis showing the proteins immunoprecipitated by autoantibodies reacting with aminoacyl-tRNA synthetases. Most anti-synthetases react with and immunoprecipitate a single synthetase enzyme protein (lanes Jo, PL-7, PL-12, and EJ). Anti-OJ autoantibodies precipitate the multienzyme synthetase complex, consisting of isoleucyl-tRNA synthetase (*band b*), which is usually the major antigen, along with at least nine other proteins and containing synthetase activity for nine amino acids (Glu, Pro, Ile, Leu, Met, Lys, Gln, Arg, Asp). (From Ref. 37, with permission.)

manifestations, such as arthritis or interstitial lung disease, may have an elevated creatine kinase level representing asymptomatic myositis or may develop myositis later in their course. Rarely, patients with other anti-Jo-1 manifestations have been followed for long periods without developing myositis (36).

Certain anti-synthetases are more likely than anti-Jo-1 to have a course that is free of any sign of myositis (36). Only 60% of patients with anti-PL-12 and 80% with anti-OJ antibodies have myositis (33,37). Anti-KS was discovered among patients with interstitial lung disease and no myositis (29). Some anti-KS patients with myositis have been found, but it is the least common anti-synthetase in myositis. Like anti-Jo-1, myositis is more common among anti-PL-7 and anti-EJ patients. There may also be differences between ethnic groups as to which features develop, because myositis was entirely absent among Japanese patients with anti-PL-12 (38) or anti-KS (29). However, a study from the United Kingdom did not show a difference in the frequency of myositis between anti-PL-12 patients (83%) and anti-Jo-1 patients (84%) (35).

The abnormalities present usually fulfill the Bohan and Peter criteria for the diagnosis of polymyositis or dermatomyositis. Polymyositis is more common than dermatomyositis in patients with anti-Jo-1 antibodies in some, but not all, studies (2,39,40). Dermato-

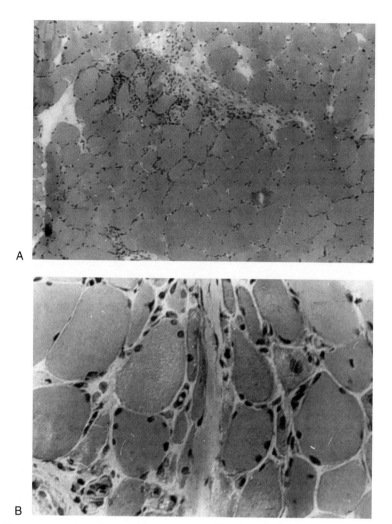

**FIG. 4.** Histology of muscle in myositis patients with myositis-specific autoantibodies. **A:** Muscle biopsy from a patient with anti-Jo-1–positive polymyositis showing endomysial infiltration with mononuclear cells, a finding typical of polymyositis patients. **B:** Muscle biopsy from a patient with anti-Mi-2–positive dermatomyositis showing perifascicular atrophy, a finding typical of dermatomyositis.

myositis appears to be more common than polymyositis among the small number of non-Jo-1 anti-synthetase patients thus far studied (33,41). Anti-synthetases are distinctly less common among children (4), but they can occur (42,43). Similarly, only very rarely have anti-synthetases been seen in malignancy-associated dermatomyositis (2,3). Despite a recent report (7), there are no convincing descriptions of anti-synthetases in inclusion body myositis. Anti-Jo-1 has very rarely been reported in polymyositis that was apparently induced by D-penicillamine (44). Anti-synthetase–associated myositis usually responds to treatment with prednisone, but it is more likely to recur when treatment is reduced than is myositis without MSAs (2,45). One study found that the onset of myositis in patients with anti-Jo-1 (but not anti-Jo-1–negative myositis) was more likely to occur in the spring than at other times of the year (46).

**TABLE 2.** *Clinical features of the antisynthetase syndromes*

Myositis
Polymyositis or dermatomyositis
Interstitial lung disease
Arthritis
Raynaud's
Fever
Mechanic's hands

The presence of anti-synthetase antibodies is associated with an increased frequency of extramuscle features. Most striking and clinically important is the frequent association with interstitial lung disease. This condition may vary in severity but can lead to significant morbidity and mortality (47). It can be the presenting feature, with myositis discovered incidentally. It can also be acute and rapidly progressive with an adult respiratory distress syndrome picture (48) or bronchiolitis obliterans organizing pneumonia (49). The myositis that may be suppressed by treatment for the interstitial lung disease sometimes appears as immunosuppressive therapy is tapered or may be unrecognized due to the severity interstitial lung involvement. Most patients with anti-synthetases who do not have myositis have had interstitial lung disease (36).

Additional features encountered in patients with anti-synthetases include arthritis, Raynaud's phenomenon, fevers, and "mechanic's hands" (Table 2). The arthritis is present in 50% to 90% of cases and is usually nonerosive but can be significant and deforming, with swan-neck and other changes as seen in rheumatoid arthritis (50). The fingers (proximal interphalangeal and metacarpophalangeal joints) and knees are most commonly involved. Severe arthritis is sometimes associated with calcinosis (51). Fever typically appears in association with exacerbations of the disease. The term mechanic's hands applies to hyperkeratosis typically on the edges of the fingers (see Fig. 3, Chapter 4). This change has been associated with overlap syndromes and is histologically similar to dermatomyositis (52).

The list of features associated with the anti-synthetase syndrome is similar to that of the mixed (or undifferentiated) connective tissue disease associated with anti-U1nRNP antibodies. The anti-synthetase syndrome is sometimes thought of as an "overlap" syndrome (53). The features of some patients with anti-Jo-1, especially early in the course, can be similar to those seen in mixed connective tissue disease. However, typical anti-synthetase syndrome is quite different from typical mixed connective tissue disease. Anti-synthetase patients tend to have more severe myositis, typically require more intense treatment for the myositis, have more recurrences of myositis as treatment is withdrawn, and are more likely to have myositis alone without overlap features. In addition, interstitial lung disease is more common and tends to be more severe among anti-synthetase patients. In contrast, features typically associated with systemic lupus erythematosus, sclerodactyly, and esophageal dysfunction are seen more commonly in patients with anti-U1RNP antibodies. Anti-PM-Scl antibodies can also be associated with a syndrome that includes features of scleroderma and myositis (10). This syndrome, sometimes termed scleromyositis, can be clinically similar to the anti-synthetase syndrome but is usually associated with milder myositis.

Anti-Jo-1 patients have anti-Ro/SSA60 autoantibodies more commonly than MSA-negative myositis patients. This difference is significant (2,40) and possibly may relate to immunogenetic associations of the antibodies. Anti-La/SSB antibodies may also occur. A higher frequency of Sjögren's syndrome, often associated with anti-Ro/SSA antibodies, has been reported in the anti-synthetase syndrome (35). Patients with anti-Jo-1 antibodies have an increased frequency of anti-Ro52 (58%) (54,55)

## Anti-SRP

The signal recognition particle (SRP) is a ribonucleoprotein found in the cytoplasm of all cells that is involved in translocation, a process by which proteins are transferred from the cytoplasm into the endoplasmic reticulum. This highly conserved particle is composed of six proteins and a small RNA, labeled 7SL. Proteins that are destined for secretion, membrane incorporation, or certain organelles include signal sequences near their amino-terminal ends. These are recognized by the SRP during the synthesis of the protein at the ribosome. SRP binds to the docking protein on the endoplasmic reticulum, resulting in the opening of pores for translocation of the proteins to occur (56).

As expected from the location of the antigen, anti-SRP sera usually give a cytoplasmic ANA pattern but can be negative. Anti-SRP antibodies show a characteristic picture by immunoprecipitation, which typically includes the six proteins and the 7SL RNA (57,58). Consequently, this method is highly specific for detection of this autoantibody. The antibody reacts with proteins of the SRP and does not appear to react with deproteinized 7SL RNA. Immunoprecipitation is by far the best test for clinical detection of anti-SRP antibodies (57–59). A small percentage of patients have anti-Ro/SSA antibodies, but few other non-MSA autoantibodies have been found in patients with anti-SRP.

### *Clinical Associations*

Anti-SRP is uncommon, present in less than 5% of myositis patients overall. Males and females and adults and children have been reported (43,57). All patients described to date have had myositis. Almost all have had polymyositis. Muscle histology may show a paucity of inflammation despite clear evidence of myopathy with prominent necrosis.

Typically, the myositis is severe with markedly elevated serum creatine kinase levels. Several features that are common among anti-SRP patients are relatively atypical in polymyositis. First, many anti-SRP patients have an acute or rapid onset of severe myositis (2,57). Second, cardiac involvement, characterized by rhythm disturbances or cardiomyopathy, seems to be more common. The distribution of muscles involved may also be atypical with more frequent distal weakness (2). Third, this syndrome is relatively resistant to treatment. Complete remission is rarely attained despite the use of immunosuppressive agents (45). Once initiated, treatment can rarely be completely withdrawn without exacerbation (2).

Despite this poor prognosis, treatment should be attempted. Most patients have partial response to prednisone and may benefit significantly from other treatments. Comparatively, patients with anti-SRP antibodies are more likely to benefit from treatment than those with inclusion body myositis. Patients with anti-SRP antibodies have a greater incidence of disability and mortality than patients without MSA or with other MSAs. The 5-year survival in one study of a small number of patients with anti-SRP antibodies was approximately 25% (2).

These patients do not have an increased frequency of the features typical of the anti-synthetase syndrome. Lung involvement, arthritis, Raynaud's phenomenon, and connective tissue disease overlap are uncommon. For example, interstitial lung disease was found in 1 of 10 anti-SRP patients, compared with two thirds of patients with anti-Jo-1 antibodies, and 1 of 30 MSA-negative patients with polymyositis or dermatomyositis (57).

The onset of myositis in anti-SRP patients, in contrast to the common onset in spring (peak in April) of anti-Jo-1 patients, more commonly occurred later in the year, peaking in November (46). No seasonal predominance was found for those without MSAs. Individual patients may diverge from this trend. These findings suggest that an environmental factor may be involved in the development of the polymyositis, further defining the uniqueness of this subgroup.

### Anti-Mi-2 (anti-CHD3/4)

Anti-Mi autoantibodies were first identified with a complement fixation test using prototype Mi serum (60). The structure of the Mi-2 antigen has been well characterized in several recent studies using immunoprecipitation and molecular cloning (Fig. 5) (61–66). Mi-2 antigen is composed of a series of proteins of 34, 50, 63, 65, 75, 150, 200, and 240 kDa, of which the 240 kDa is the strongest (63). The 240-kDa protein has been shown to be the major antigen (63–65). Cloning of the 240-kDa protein also revealed at least two different but closely related forms, originally labeled Mi-2α and Mi-2β (66). They are approximately 75% identical to each other in amino acid sequence, with certain functional regions showing much higher identity (64,65,67).

Both forms of Mi-2 are apparent helicases, because they contain all seven of the amino acid sequence motifs common to a group of helicases defined by the "DEAD/H" sequence (asp-glu-ala-[asp or his]). These unwinding enzymes are involved in numerous

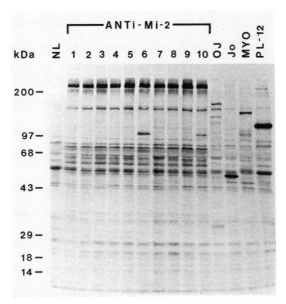

**FIG. 5.** Immunoprecipitation from HeLa cells with anti-Mi-2 autoantibodies. Polyacrylamide gel electrophoresis showing the proteins immunoprecipitated by autoantibodies to Mi-2 antigen. Lanes 1 to 10 show immunoprecipitation with different anti-Mi-2–positive sera; other lanes show immunoprecipitation with normal serum (*NL*), serum from a myositis patient (*MYO*), or serum with anti-OJ, anti-Jo, or anti-PL-12. The main antigenic protein is the strong band at 230 to 240 kd (Mi-2α [CHD3] and Mi-2β [CHD4] are not separable on this gel). The 150-kDa protein is approximately the size of isoleucyl-tRNA synthetase (compare lane OJ to band b in Fig. 3). Other components of Mi-2 antigen (apparent components of NuRD complex) are at 70, 65, 63, 50, and 34 kDa (the latter band is weak and just above a weak artifact line).

fundamental processes in the cell, one of which is transcriptional regulation. Of these proteins, Mi-2 most resembles in molecular sequence the human SNF2 protein involved in global activation of transcription by modifying ("remodeling") the chromatin structure, presumably opening it to allow access (65). Supporting this impression, Mi-2 proteins were found to be part of the newly recognized family labeled "CHD" because they contain "chromo" domains (*chr*omatin *o*rganization *mo*difier), *h*elicase domains, and *D*NA-binding domains. Mi-2α and Mi-2β have been designated CHD3 and CHD4, respectively (68). CHD proteins generally are believed to be involved in chromatin-mediated regulation of gene expression. Mi-2 also contains PHD finger structures which have been associated with this function (68). Recently, Mi-2 has been found to be part of a complex that contains histone deacetylase enzymes that alter chromatin structure by affecting histone acetylation (69,70).

### Clinical Associations

Almost all patients with anti-Mi-2 antibodies have dermatomyositis (2,40,62,65,71). Anti-Mi-2 patients without myositis are extremely rare, and patients without the rash of dermatomyositis are uncommon. The myositis sometimes presents acutely and can be severe. The presence of this autoantibody confers the best prognosis for survival among subsets of idiopathic inflammatory myopathy (2). Rarely, rash without myositis may be seen, but "amyopathic dermatomyositis" appears to be less common among anti-Mi-2 patients than among dermatomyositis patients overall. Patients may initially have severe myositis without cutaneous features but may develop typical Gottron's papules years later while still on treatment. The rashes seen are usually those typical in dermatomyositis: the "V" sign (involvement of the base of the neck tapering to the chest) or the "shawl" sign (involvement of upper back and shoulders) (2). Anti-Mi2 is almost as common in children with dermatomyositis as in adults and is the most common MSA in children (43). Anti-Mi-2 has been seen in occasional patients with overlap syndromes and occasionally coexists with anti-Ro or anti-U1RNP. It is not associated with an increased rate of interstitial lung disease or Raynaud's phenomenon. A small number have had a malignancy (62) but at a prevalence less than the 10% to 20% rate reported for all malignancy in dermatomyositis.

In the United States, anti-Mi-2 occurs in 15% to 20% of patients with dermatomyositis (62). Anti-Mi-2 has been found in all populations studied but was distinctly more frequent in a population from Guatemala (43). Preliminary data suggest that it is more frequent in Mexican patients as well. Some increase was also found in Asian Indian patients. It was not increased in Polish patients (72). This difference in frequency between populations may relate to genetic or environmental factors. However, genetic factors clearly influence production of anti-Mi-2, because a strong association with human leukocyte antigen (HLA) DR7 exists (71).

## MYOSITIS-ASSOCIATED AUTOANTIBODIES

Some antibodies to intracellular cytoplasmic and nuclear antigens are associated with inflammatory myopathies but are also commonly found in other conditions. These have been termed myositis-associated autoantibodies (MAAs). Although less specific than the MSAs, their presence is more predictive than only finding a positive ANA. They are not all mutually exclusive. Like the MSAs, they tend to be present from the earliest samples and persist despite treatment.

## Connective Tissue Disease Overlap Autoantibodies

### *Anti-snRNPs*

Anti-U1RNP was described in the early 1970s as an autoantibody associated with systemic lupus erythematosus and a lupus-related overlap syndrome termed mixed connective tissue disease, of which myositis was a feature (73,74). The antigen was known to have RNA and protein components and to have a relationship to the antigen Sm. Once the biochemical nature of the antigen was defined, these antibodies greatly facilitated our understanding of RNA processing (75,76). Anti-U1RNP is directed at the U1 small nuclear ribonucleoprotein, which is the most abundant snRNP involved in mRNA splicing. It contains the U1 RNA along with 11 proteins, including 3 specific for the U1snRNP (70K, A, C) and 8 that comprise the Sm group of proteins also shared by other spliceosomal snRNPs (those containing the U2, U4, U5, or U6 RNAs and the less abundant U7, U11, or U12 RNAs). Sera with anti-U1RNP antibodies react with one or more of the three U1-specific proteins and may also react with the U1 RNA directly (77,78). Sera with anti-Sm react with one or more of the shared Sm proteins, usually B/B' and D. Most anti-Sm sera also show reactivity with U1RNP, but many sera react with U1RNP without anti-Sm reactivity. Rarely, sera have been described that react specifically with individual spliceosomal snRNPs other than U1RNP, including anti-U2RNP (79), anti-U4/6RNP, anti-U5RNP (80), and others. These react with one or more of the proteins specific for the antigenic snRNP. Anti-U2RNP are commonly associated with anti-U1RNP and are typically recognized by immunoprecipitation of U1 and U2 RNAs without U4,5,6. Anti-U5RNP has been described in association with anti-U1RNP and anti-Sm, but it occasionally occurs without anti-U1RNP (81).

### *Clinical Association*

Anti-U1RNP antibodies are essential for the diagnosis of mixed connective tissue disease. Anti-U1RNP antibodies are typically present in high titer and anti-Sm antibodies are not present. Patients with mixed connective tissue disease have features of systemic lupus erythematosus, scleroderma, and polymyositis. Patients with anti-U1RNP can have any one of these conditions alone or any combination. This disease may begin as "mixed" or undifferentiated and evolve into a single disease. Inflammatory myositis arising in the context of systemic lupus erythematosus is not unusual, and anti-U1RNP is common in such patients. Anti-Sm is closely associated with systemic lupus erythematosus, but myositis can occur in such patients. One study found anti-Sm in 7% of their 224 myositis patients, compared with 16% with anti-U1RNP (45). Myositis is often milder and more responsive to treatment in connective tissue disease overlap syndromes. This tends to be true of anti-U1RNP–associated myositis. Nevertheless, very significant myositis can occur (82).

Patients with anti-U1RNP antibodies can also have autoantibodies with other MAAs or MSAs, including anti-synthetases (33), although the combination is rare. Anti-U1RNP is usually present from the onset of illness and persists, but occasional exceptions have occurred in which it appears during follow-up (83). In general, correlation of anti-U1RNP titer with disease activity has not been consistent (84), and the antibody usually persists despite remission (85).

Specific anti-U2RNP is uncommon, but many of the reported cases have had myositis or scleroderma-polymyositis overlap (79). Anti-U4/U6 is very rare (80), but one such patient has had dermatomyositis. Anti-U5RNP is also very rare, but all reported cases have had myositis or scleroderma with myositis (80,81).

### *Anti-PM-Scl*

Wolfe et al. (86) first reported anti-PM-1 antibodies in a high proportion of patients with myositis, often with an overlap syndrome. Subsequent studies defined a unique specificity, anti-PM-Scl, that turned out to be directed at the same antigen as anti-PM-1 (87). Anti-PM-Scl was named for the frequent association with an overlap syndrome of myositis and scleroderma. Anti-PM-Scl antibodies show a mixed pattern of immunofluorescent staining the nucleoli strongly and the nuclei significantly (88).

The PM-Scl antigen includes a series of at least 11 proteins (89–91). This includes one protein of 100 kDa (92) that is the major antigen, reacting with at least 90% of anti-PM-Scl sera. A second protein that is also a frequent antigen aberrantly migrates as a 70- to 75-kDa protein by polyacrylamide gel electrophoresis but has a calculated molecular weight of 40 kDa based on its cDNA sequence (93). Other PM-Scl proteins migrate between 20 and 40 kDa (94). No clinical implications of these differences in component reactivity have yet been found.

The function of the PM-Scl antigen is not completely understood, but there are important clues from recent studies. A yeast homologue to the 100-kDa protein has been identified, which appears to function in small ribosomal RNA processing (95). It may also play a role in regulation of transcription of certain proteins because it interacts with the E12 and E47 transcription factors important in regulating growth and differentiation, and its expression is regulated by growth factors (96).

### *Clinical Associations*

Most patients with anti-PM-Scl have an overlap syndrome with features of myositis and scleroderma (91). Most patients who do not have the overlap syndrome have myositis or scleroderma alone (91,97–100). The myositis may be either quite mild and readily responsive to prednisone treatment (10,72) or more severe. About half of those with myositis have typical cutaneous features of dermatomyositis such as Gottron's papules. At least 80% of those with scleroderma have limited cutaneous involvement distal to the elbows (91). Raynaud's phenomenon is quite a common, and interstitial lung disease, calcinosis, and mechanic's hands can occur (41). Arthritis is present in almost all patients in some series (98,99). Sometimes prominent and deforming arthritis can be the presenting feature. This overlap syndrome with features of mild myositis, mild scleroderma, and arthritis has been called "scleromyositis" (10). As noted, this constellation of features can resemble that of the anti-synthetase syndrome, but the typical patient with anti-PM-Scl antibodies has a milder and more treatment-responsive muscle disease.

Positive ANAs are very common in this syndrome, and defined autoantibodies are more common than in polymyositis or dermatomyositis overall. The autoantibodies to the UsnRNPs can also be associated with scleroderma-myositis overlap, but anti-PM-Scl antibodies are not usually associated with systemic lupus erythematosus.

Anti-PM-Scl antibodies are mutually exclusive with MSAs and also with scleroderma-specific antibodies. Therefore, they identify a distinct subgroup. Genetic factors also strongly influence production of anti-PM-Scl antibodies. They are found predominantly in whites and are very rare in Japanese. A strong association is found between anti-PM-Scl antibodies and HLA-DR3 (91,97,98), DQw2, and DQB1*0201 (91).

## *Anti-Ku*

The Ku antigen has two proteins of 70 and 80 kDa and binds nonspecifically to free ends of double-stranded DNA (101,102). Anti-Ku is associated with a large protein of 350 kDa, DNA-dependent protein kinase, in a complex referred to as DNA-pk, that is involved in DNA repair. The 350-kDa protein can also be an antigen.

Anti-Ku was originally described in Japanese patients with an overlap syndrome of polymyositis, scleroderma, and systemic lupus erythematosus (103). The anti-Ku precipitin is found in a lower proportion of patients with polymyositis-scleroderma overlap in the United States than in Japan (104,105). It can be seen in patients with scleroderma or systemic lupus erythematosus without myositis (106). Anti-Ku also occurs in other conditions such as primary pulmonary hypertension (107). This decreases its utility as a diagnostic tool, but it can still be helpful for confirmation in patients with a typical picture. Anti-Ku antibodies are commonly associated with other autoantibodies commonly encountered in systemic lupus erythematosus or scleroderma but are not usually found in patients with an MSA.

## Other Antibodies Associated with Overlap Syndromes

Antibodies to Ro/SSA occur in about 10% to 20% of patients with myositis and a higher proportion of those with anti-synthetase antibodies (40). Both anti-60kd Ro and anti-52kD Ro (54) may be seen together, but there is an unusually high frequency of anti-52kD Ro without anti-60kd Ro. Anti-Ro is most often seen in systemic lupus erythematosus, Sjögren's syndrome, and overlap syndromes. When anti-Ro is seen in myositis, an overlap with Sjögren's syndrome should be excluded. Sjögren's syndrome can be associated with a myositis mediated by vasculitis (108). Myositis patients with anti-Ro may also have anti-La in about one fourth of cases.

Anti-centromere antibodies or anti-U3RNP (anti-fibrillarin) antibodies can be found in patients with scleroderma and myositis (40,109). Autoantibodies associated with thyroid disease are occasionally seen, and rheumatoid factor is present in a small number (2). There have been numerous case reports of polymyositis or an inflammatory myopathy in association with primary biliary cirrhosis (110). In some cases, the biliary cirrhosis has been asymptomatic (111,112). These patients usually have anti-mitochondrial antibodies. An association of mitochondrial myopathy and primary biliary cirrhosis has been reported (113).

## Other Myositis-associated Autoantibodies

An autoantibody to a 56-kDa component of large nuclear ribonucleoproteins has been described (114,115) and is very common, occurring in up to 86% of adults with polymyositis or dermatomyositis, 92% of children with dermatomyositis, and 75% of patients with cancer-associated myositis (116). It was also found in a small proportion of patients with systemic lupus erythematosus or other connective tissue diseases. The exact nature of the antigen has not been further characterized. The titer appears to vary with disease activity in the few adults studied and in ANA-positive children. In some cases, the ANA was negative, despite the nuclear localization of the antigen.

Anti-MJ is an autoantibody described in adults with dermatomyositis and more commonly in the juvenile form (117). In a juvenile dermatomyositis cohort from Argentina, anti-MJ was present at twice the frequency of anti-PM-Scl or anti-Mi-2 (118). It does not identify patients with particular clinical features. Disease can be mild or severe and associated with vasculitis. Although a few patients have had an overlap syndrome, thus far it has not been described in patients without myositis. Anti-MJ antibodies react with an unidentified 130-kDa cellular protein (117).

Anti-Mas autoantibodies were reported in two patients with myositis occurring in association with an alcohol-related myopathy. The two patients had similar HLA types (2). A similar antibody has been found in association with liver disease (119) and in other myositis patients without an alcohol-related myopathy. The antigen that has been identified as a serine-tRNA, but it is not directed at a synthetase enzyme.

Anti-Fer (120) is directed at elongation factor $1\alpha$ and was first described in a patient with myositis. Anti-tRNA$^{MET}$ antibodies have also been reported in myositis (121). Those are extremely rare, and therefore their true clinical associations are unknown.

Anti-KJ antibody was originally reported in two patients with myositis, interstitial lung disease, and Raynaud's phenomenon, a syndrome similar to the anti-synthetase syndrome (122). However, instead of being directed at a synthetase enzyme, it was directed at a different protein associated with the process of translation, possibly an unidentified translation factor. This led to the hypothesis that the MSAs may be directed at this process in general, because the synthetases are crucial for translation to occur. However, anti-ribosomal antibodies are specific for systemic lupus erythematosus and rare in idiopathic inflammatory myopathies, whereas other autoantibodies to tRNA-related antigens have commonly not been associated with myositis.

Antinuclear pore antibody was found in a small proportion of French Canadian patients with myositis (123). This antibody is directed at pore structures on the nuclear membrane. An antibody to a component of the proteasome has been found in some myositis patients but is not specific for myositis (124).

Antibodies to the muscle cell membrane protein are found in many patients with myositis (71% with polymyositis, 15% with dermatomyositis) but are also found in some patients with other connective tissue diseases but not in normal subjects (125). These antibodies did not react with other cell lines. Due to the accessibility of their antigens, such autoantibodies have the potential for pathogenic significance and are therefore interesting, but their lack of disease specificity makes them less useful for diagnosis.

## Significance of the "Myositis Autoantibodies"

The nature of the relationship between MSAs and MAAs to polymyositis and dermatomyositis remains uncertain. It is not known whether these autoantibodies are involved in the pathogenesis of these diseases, contribute to any of their manifestations, or are reflections of inciting events or other factors. In favor of a pathogenic role is the very strong association with the disease and with particular subgroups and evidence that dermatomyositis is mediated by a humoral attack on muscle microvasculature, with consistent deposition of membrane attack complete of complement in small blood vessels of muscle and skin (126–130). Against a pathogenetic role is that analyses of inflammatory infiltrates indicate a T-cell–mediated attack on muscle fibers in polymyositis (131,132) where no signs of immunoglobulin or complement deposition are found. Also, these autoantibodies are heterogeneous in specificity and low in frequency, with some myositis patients having no identified autoantibody.

Their origin is also unknown. Hypotheses proposed for the generation of autoantibodies in other connective tissue disease such as molecular mimicry (133) or presentation of fragments during apoptosis (134) have also been suggested for the autoantibodies of myositis (135,136). Studies of the epitopes recognized by MSAs and MAAs have generally shown the presence of multiple epitopes but often with a common predominant epitope (22,95,135,137–139). These and other studies suggest that the immune responses are driven by the recognized autoantigens. These findings are compatible with several hypotheses for autoantibodies generation. Genetic factors clearly also play a role in their production as demonstrated by the many HLA associations that have been recognized (2,43,93,140,141) (Table 1).

Testing for autoantibodies in patients with myositis may be helpful clinically for diagnosis and classification due to their disease and subgroup specificity (142). Tests should be used that maximize specificity, such as immunodiffusion or immunoprecipitation. Alternately, a screening test followed by a confirmatory test can be used (e.g., ELISA followed by immunoblot). Although some studies have suggested a general correlation of antibody titer and disease activity (143), in most patients they persist in significant titer after treatment and disease suppression. Thus, the value of titers of most MSAs or MAAs is uncertain, and titers are seldom used for assessing disease activity. When reliable tests for MSAs are positive in patients with a compatible clinical picture, it has been suggested that this could establish the diagnosis without the need for muscle biopsy (142). Their presence appears to be at least as specific as other criteria of Bohan and Peter (1), and they might serve as a sixth criterion for diagnosing polymyositis or dermatomyositis. The effects on the sensitivity and specificity of adding this to the criteria have not been formally tested.

## AUTOANTIBODIES IN OTHER NEUROMUSCULAR CONDITIONS

In evaluating patients for muscle weakness, other neuromuscular conditions must often be considered. Certain forms of autoimmune-mediated neuropathies are also associated with characteristic autoantibodies, including myasthenia gravis, Lambert-Eaton myasthenia syndrome, and other paraneoplastic syndromes. Unlike the cellular antigens studied in inflammatory myopathies, these are typically directed at organ-specific antigens. In addition to disease specificity and diagnostic utility, there is more evidence for pathogenicity of these autoantibodies.

### Acetylcholine Receptor Antibodies

These autoantibodies are directed at the nicotinic acetylcholine receptor (AChR) of the motor endplate. They react predominately with the α-subunits of the receptor, recognizing a "major immunogenic region." Anti-AChR antibodies are relatively specific for myasthenia gravis, and there is good evidence that they are responsible for the disease manifestation (144). The usual clinical radioimmunoassay for anti-AChR, which uses an α-bungarotoxin-labeled human receptor, detects these antibodies in 85% of patients (144,145). Even some of the radioimmunoassay-negative patients have evidence of anti-AChR antibodies when other methods are used. Those test for blocking or "modulating" effects on the receptor. Antibody binds the receptor in vivo, with complement activation (146,147). This result in damage to the endplate, as shown by simplification (loss of the complex folds) of the postsynaptic membrane. Anti-AChR antibodies causes a reduction in the number of AChRs by cross-linking them, thus inducing accelerated loss (144,148). The pathogenicity of anti-AChR antibodies is shown by induction of a myasthenia gravis-like disease in animals using anti-AChR antibodies from patients with myasthenia, improvement of disease after removal of the antibodies by plasmapheresis, and the phenomenon of neonatal myasthenia gravis associated with transplacental transfer of anti-AChR antibodies.

Patients with myasthenia gravis commonly have involvement of extraocular muscles, which is not usually seen in inflammatory myopathies other than orbital myositis. Negative anti-AChR antibody tests are more common in myasthenia gravis when involvement is limited to ocular muscles, but such patients are less likely to be confused with those with polymyositis. A negative test does not exclude myasthenia. False-positive tests can occasionally be seen in Lambert-Eaton syndrome and systemic lupus erythematosus.

Other autoantibodies may circulate in patients with myasthenia gravis, including anti-striational antibodies, which react with various muscle proteins such as the ryanodine receptor (sarcoplasmic reticulum calcium release channel protein) (149). The frequency of these antibodies increase with age. They are also present in 80% to 90% of patients with a thymoma. Some antistriational specificities, especially those directed at ryanodine or titin, are more closely associated with this tumor and can be useful in predicting its presence clinically.

### Antibodies to the Calcium Channels

The Lambert-Eaton myasthenic syndrome has been associated with autoantibodies to the voltage-gated calcium channels in the presynaptic region, otherwise termed the nerve terminal (150,151) These antibodies cause a reduction of release of acetylcholine.

### Autoantibodies in Neuropathies

Certain neuropathies that can be confused with myopathies or myositis can be associated with autoantibodies. Several autoantibodies have been associated with neuropathies, including those associated with paraneoplastic neuropathies such as anti-Hu and those seen in inflammatory polyneuropathies. Such autoantibodies may have a pathogenic role in the neuropathy.

### REFERENCES

1. Bohan A, Peter JB. Polymyositis and dermatomyositis. Parts 1 and 2. *N Engl J Med* 1975;292:344–347, 403–407.
2. Love LA, Leff RL, Fraser DD, et al. A new approach to the classification of idiopathic inflammatory myopathy: myositis-specific autoantibodies define useful homogeneous patient groups. *Medicine (Baltimore)* 1991;70:360–374.
3. Nishikai M, Sato A. Low incidence of antinuclear antibodies in dermatomyositis with malignancy. *Ann Rheum Dis* 1990;49:422.
4. Feldman BM, Reichlin M, Laxer RM, Targoff IN, Stein LD, Silverman ED. Clinical significance of specific autoantibodies in juvenile dermatomyositis. *J Rheumatol* 1996;23:1794–1797.
5. Gutmann L, Govindan S, Riggs JE, Schochet SS. Inclusion body myositis and Sjögren's syndrome. *Arch Neurol* 1985;42:1021–1022.
6. Yood RA, Smith TW. Inclusion body myositis and systemic lupus erythematosus. *J Rheumatol* 1985;12:568–570.
7. Koffman BM, Rugiero M, Dalakas MC. Immune-mediated conditions and antibodies associated with sporadic inclusion body myositis. *Muscle Nerve* 1998;21:115–117.
8. Kobayashi T, Asakawa H, Komoike Y, et al. A patient with Graves' disease, myasthenia gravis, and polymyositis. *Thyroid* 1997;7:631–632.
9. Reichlin M, Arnett FC. Multiplicity of antibodies in myositis sera. *Arthritis Rheum* 1984;27:1150–1156.
10. Jablonska S, Chorzelski TP, Blaszczyk M, et al. Scleroderma/polymyositis overlap syndromes and their immunologic markers. *Clin Dermatol* 1993;10:457–472.
11. Gelpi C, Kanterewicz E, Gratacos J, Targoff IN, Rodriguez-Sanchez JL. Coexistence of two anti-synthetases in a patient with the antisynthetase syndrome. *Arthritis Rheum* 1996;39:692–697.

12. Mirande M. Aminoacyl-tRNA synthetase family from prokaryotes and eukaryotes: structural domains and their implications. *Prog Nucleic Acid Res Mol Biol* 1991;40:95–142.

13. Cerini C, Kerjan P, Astier M, et al. A component of the multi-synthetase complex is a multifunctional aminoacyl-tRNA synthetase. *EMBO J* 1991;10:4267–4277.

14. Carter CW. Cognition, mechanism, and evolutionary relationships in aminoacyl-tRNA synthetases. *Annu Rev Biochem* 1993;62:715–748.

15. Eriani G, Delarue M, Poch O, et al. Partition of tRNA synthetases into two classes based on mutually exclusive sets of sequence motifs. *Nature* 1990;347:203–206.

16. Cusack S, Hartlein M, Leberman R. Sequence, structural and evolutionary relationships between class 2 aminoacyl-tRNA synthetases. *Nucleic Acids Res* 1991;19:3489–3498.

17. Raben N, Borriello F, Amin J, et al. Human histidyl-tRNA synthetase: recognition of amino acid signature regions in class 2a aminoacyl-tRNA synthetases. *Nucleic Acids Res* 1992;20:1075–1081.

18. Nishikai M, Reichlin M. Heterogeneity of precipitating antibodies in polymyositis and dermatomyositis: characterization of the Jo-1 antibody system. *Arthritis Rheum* 1980;23:881–888.

19. Wasicek CA, Reichlin M, Montes M, Raghu G. Polymyositis and interstitial lung disease in a patient with anti-Jo-1 prototype. *Am J Med* 1984;76:538–544.

20. Mathews MB, Bernstein RM. Myositis autoantibody inhibits histidyl-tRNA synthetase: a model for autoimmunity. *Nature* 1983;304:177–179.

21. Rosa MD, Hendrick JP Jr, Lerner MR, et al. A mammalian tRNA$^{his}$-containing antigen is recognized by the polymyositis-specific antibody anti-Jo-1. *Nucleic Acids Res* 1983;11:853–870.

22. Raben N, Nichols RC, Dohlman J, et al. A motif in human histidyl-tRNA synthetase which is shared among several aminoacyl-tRNA synthetases is a coiled-coil that is essential for enzymatic activity and contains the major autoantigenic epitope. *J Biol Chem* 1994;269:24277–24283.

23. Dang CV, LaDuca FM, Bell WR. Histidyl-tRNA synthetase, the myositis Jo-1 antigen, is cytoplasmic and unassociated with the cytoskeletal framework. *Exp Cell Res* 1986;164:261–266.

24. Vazquez-Abad D, Carson JH, Rothfield N. Localization of histidyl-tRNA synthetase (Jo-1) in human laryngeal epithelial carcinoma cell line (HEp-2 cells). *Cell Tissue Res* 1996;286:487–491.

25. Bernstein RM, Bunn CC, Hughes GRV, et al. Cellular protein and RNA antigens in autoimmune disease. *Mol Biol Med* 1984;2:105–120.

26. Mathews MB, Reichlin M, Hughes GRV, Bernstein RM. Anti-threonyl-tRNA synthetase, a second myositis-related autoantibody. *J Exp Med* 1984;160:420–434.

27. Bunn CC, Bernstein RM, Mathews MB. Autoantibodies against alanyl-tRNA synthetase and tRNA$^{ala}$ coexist and are associated with myositis. *J Exp Med* 1986;163:1281–1291.

28. Targoff IN. Autoantibodies to aminoacyl-transfer RNA synthetases for isoleucine and glycine: two additional synthetases are antigenic in myositis. *J Immunol* 1990;144:1737–1743.

29. Hirakata M, Suwa A, Nagai S, et al. Anti-KS: identification of autoantibodies to asparaginyl-transfer RNA synthetase associated with interstitial lung disease. *J Immunol* 1999;162:2315–2320.

30. Ge Q, Trieu EP, Targoff IN. Primary structure and functional expression of human glycyl-tRNA synthetase, an autoantigen in myositis. *J Biol Chem* 1994;269:28790–28797.

31. Nichols RC, Raben N, Boerkoel CF, Plotz PH. Human isoleucyl-tRNA synthetase: sequence of the cDNA, alternative mRNA splicing, and the characteristics of an unusually long C-terminal extension. *Gene* 1995;155:299–304.

32. Beaulande M, Tarbouriech N, Hartlein M. Human cytosolic asparaginyl-tRNA synthetase: cDNA sequence, functional expression in *Escherichia coli* and characterization as human autoantigen. *Nucleic Acids Res* 1998;26:521–524.

33. Targoff IN, Arnett FC. Clinical manifestations in patients with antibody to PL-12 antigen (alanyl-tRNA synthetase). *Am J Med* 1990;88:241–251.

34. Bunn CC, Mathews MB. Autoreactive epitope defined as the anticodon region of alanine transfer RNA. *Science* 1987;238:1116–1119.

35. Marguerie C, Bunn CC, Beynon HLC, et al. Polymyositis, pulmonary fibrosis and autoantibodies to aminoacyl-tRNA synthetase enzymes. *Q J Med* 1990;77:1019–1038.

36. Friedman AW, Targoff IN, Arnett FC. Interstitial lung disease with autoantibodies against aminoacyl-tRNA synthetases in the antibodies of clinically apparent myositis. *Semin Arthritis Rheum* 1996;26:459–467.

37. Targoff IN, Trieu EP, Miller FW. Reaction of anti-OJ autoantibodies with components of the multi-enzyme complex of aminoacyl-tRNA synthetases in addition to isoleucyl-tRNA synthetase. *J Clin Invest* 1993;91:2556–2564.

38. Hirakata M, Nakamura K, Okano Y, et al. Anti-alanyl-tRNA synthetase (PL-12) antibodies are associated with interstitial lung disease in Japanese patients. *Arthritis Rheum* 1995;38:S321(abst).

39. Arnett FC, Hirsch TJ, Bias WB, Nishikai M, Reichlin M. The Jo-1 antibody system in myositis: relationships to clinical features and HLA. *J Rheumatol* 1981;8:925–930.

40. Arnett FC, Targoff IN, Mimori T, et al. Interrelationship of major histocompatibility complex class II alleles and autoantibodies in four ethnic groups with various forms of myositis. *Arthritis Rheum* 1996;39:1507–1518.

41. Targoff IN, Trieu EP, Plotz PH, Miller FW. Antibodies to glycyl-tRNA synthetase are associated with polymyositis with interstitial lung disease. *Arthritis Rheum* 1990;33:S72(abst).

42. Chmiel JF, Wessel HU, Targoff IN, Pachman LM. Pulmonary fibrosis and myositis in a child with anti-Jo-1 antibody. *J Rheumatol* 1995;22:762–765.
43. Rider LG, Miller FW, Targoff IN, et al. A broadened spectrum of juvenile myositis: myositis-specific autoantibodies in children. *Arthritis Rheum* 1994;37:1534–1538.
44. Jenkins EA, Hull RG, Thomas AL. D-Penicillamine and polymyositis: The significance of the anti-Jo-1 antibody. *Br J Rheumatol* 1993;32:1109–1110.
45. Joffe MM, Love LA, Leff RL, et al. Drug therapy of the idiopathic inflammatory myopathies: predictors of response to prednisone, azathioprine, and methotrexate and a comparison of their efficacy. *Am J Med* 1993;94:379–387.
46. Leff RL, Burgess SH, Miller FW, et al. Distinct seasonal patterns in the onset of adult idiopathic inflammatory myopathy in patients with anti-Jo-1 and anti-signal recognition particle autoantibodies. *Arthritis Rheum* 1991; 34:1391–1396.
47. Targoff IN. Inflammatory muscle disease. In: Cannon GW, Zimmerman GA, eds. *The lung in rheumatic diseases.* New York: Marcel Dekker, 1990:303–328.
48. Clawson K, Oddis CV. Adult respiratory distress syndrome (ARDS) in myositis patients with anti-Jo-1 antibody. *Arthritis Rheum* 1993;36:S256(abst).
49. Kalenian M, Zweiman B. Inflammatory myopathy, bronchiolitis obliterans/organizing pneumonia, and anti-Jo-1 antibodies—an interesting association. *Clin Diagn Lab Immunol* 1997;4:236–240.
50. Oddis CV, Medsger TA Jr, Cooperstein LA. A subluxing arthropathy associated with the anti-Jo-1 antibody in polymyositis/dermatomyositis. *Arthritis Rheum* 1990;33:1640–1645.
51. Cohen MG, Ho KK, Webb J. Finger joint calcinosis followed by osteolysis in a patient with multisystem connective tissue disease and anti-Jo-1 antibody. *J Rheumatol* 1987;14:605–608.
52. Mitra D, Lovell CL, Macleod TI, Tan RS, Maddison PJ. Clinical and histological features of "mechanic's hands" in a patient with antibodies to Jo-1—a case report. *Clin Exp Dermatol* 1994;19:146–148.
53. Venables PJ. Polymyositis-associated overlap syndromes. *Br J Rheumatol* 1996;35:305–306.
54. Rutjes SA, Vree Egberts WT, Jongen P, et al. Anti-Ro52 antibodies frequently co-occur with anti-Jo-1 antibodies in sera from patients with idiopathic inflammatory myopathy. *Clin Exp Immunol* 1997;109:32–40.
55. Venables PJ. Antibodies to Jo-1 and Ro-52: why do they go together? *Clin Exp Immunol* 1997;109:403–405.
56. Walter P, Lingappa VR. Mechanism of protein translocation across the endoplasmic reticulum membrane. *Annu Rev Cell Biol* 1986;2:499–516.
57. Targoff IN, Johnson AE, Miller FW. Antibody to signal recognition particle in polymyositis. *Arthritis Rheum* 1990;33:1361–1370.
58. Okada N, Minori T, Mukai R, et al. Characterization of human autoantibodies that selectively precipitate the 7SL RNA component of the signal recognition particle. *J Immunol* 1987;138:3219–3223.
59. Reeves WH, Nigam SK, Blobel G. Human autoantibodies reactive with the signal-recognition particle. *Proc Natl Acad Sci USA* 1986;83:9507–9511.
60. Reichlin M, Mattioli M. Description of a serological reaction characteristic of polymyositis. *Clin Immunol Immunopathol* 1976;5:12–20.
61. Nishikai M, Reichlin M. Purification and characterization of a nuclear non-histone basic protein (Mi-1) which reacts with anti-immunoglobulin sera and the sera of patients with dermatomyositis. *Mol Immunol* 1980;17: 1129–1141.
62. Targoff IN, Reichlin M. The association between Mi-2 antibodies and dermatomyositis. *Arthritis Rheum* 1985; 28:796–803.
63. Nilasena DS, Trieu EP, Targoff IN. Analysis of the Mi-2 autoantigen of dermatomyositis. *Arthritis Rheum* 1995; 38:123–128.
64. Ge Q, Nilasena DS, O'Brien CA, Frank MB, Targoff IN. Molecular analysis of a major antigenic region of the 240-kD protein of Mi-2 autoantigen. *J Clin Invest* 1995;96:1730–1737.
65. Seelig HP, Moosbrugger I, Ehrfeld H, et al. The major dermatomyositis-specific Mi-2 autoantigen is a presumed helicase involved in transcriptional activation. *Arthritis Rheum* 1995;38:1389–1399.
66. Seelig HP, Renz M, Targoff IN, et al. Two forms of the major antigenic protein of the dermatomyositis-specific Mi-2 autoantigen. *Arthritis Rheum* 1996;39:1769–1771.
67. Aasland R, Gibson TJ, Stewart AF. The PHD finger: implications for chromatin-mediated transcriptional regulation. *Trends Biochem Sci* 1995;20:56–59.
68. Woodage T, Basrai MA, Baxevanis AD, et al. Characterization of the CHD family of proteins. *Proc Natl Acad Sci USA* 1997;94:11472–11477.
69. Wade PA, Jones PL, Vermaak D, Wolffe AP. A multiple subunit Mi-2 histone deacetylase from *Xenopus laevis* cofractionates with an associated Snf2 superfamily ATPase. *Curr Biol* 1998;8:843–846.
70. Zhang Y, LeRoy G, Seelig HP, Lane WS, Reinberg D. The dermatomyositis-specific autoantigen Mi-2 is a component of a complex containing histone deacetylase and nucleosome remodeling activities. *Cell* 1998;95:279–289.
71. Mierau R, Dick T, Bartz-Bazzanella P, et al. Strong association of dermatomyositis-specific Mi-2 autoantibodies with a tryptophan at position 9 of the HLA-DR beta chain. *Arthritis Rheum* 1996;39:868–876.
72. Hausmanowa-Petrusewicz I, Kowalska-Oledzka E, Miller FW, et al. Clinical, serologic, and immunogenetic features in Polish patients with idiopathic inflammatory myopathies. *Arthritis Rheum* 1997;40:1257–1266.
73. Craft J. Antibodies to snRNPs in systemic lupus erythematosus. *Rheum Dis Clin North Am* 1993;18:311–335.

74. Sharp GC, Irvin WS, Tan EM, et al. Mixed connective tissue disease—an apparently distinct rheumatic disease syndrome associated with a specific antigen (ENA). *Am J Med* 1972;52:148–159.

75. Lerner MR, Steitz JA. Antibodies to small nuclear RNAs complexed with proteins are produced by patients with systemic lupus erythematosus. *Proc Natl Acad Sci USA* 1979;76:5495–5499.

76. Hardin JA, Rahn DR, Shen C, et al. Antibodies from patients with connective tissue disease bind specific subsets of cellular RNA-protein particles. *J Clin Invest* 1982;70:141–147.

77. van Venrooij WJ, Hoet R, Castrop J, et al. Anti-(U1) small nuclear RNA antibodies in anti-small nuclear ribonucleoprotein sera from patients with connective tissue diseases. *J Clin Invest* 1990;86:2154–2160.

78. Hoet RM, Kastner B, Luhrmann R, van Venrooij WJ. Purification and characterization of human autoantibodies directed to specific regions on U1RNA; recognition of native U1RNP complexes. *Nucleic Acids Res* 1993; 21:5130–5136.

79. Craft J, Mimori T, Olsen TL, Hardin JA. The U2 small nuclear ribonucleoprotein particle as an autoantigen. Analysis with sera from patients with overlap syndromes. *J Clin Invest* 1988;81:1716–1724.

80. Okano Y, Targoff IN, Oddis CV, et al. Anti-U5 small nuclear ribonucleoprotein (snRNP) antibodies: a rare anti-U snRNP specificity. *Clin Immunol Immunopathol* 1996;81:41–47.

81. Rider LG, Targoff IN, Leff RL, et al. Association of autoantibodies to the U5-ribonucleoprotein (U5-RNP) with idiopathic inflammatory myopathy (IIM). *Arthritis Rheum* 1994;37:S242(abst).

82. Garton MJ, Isenberg DA. Clinical features of lupus myositis versus idiopathic myositis: a review of 30 cases. *Br J Rheumatol* 1997;36:1067–1074.

83. Targoff IN, Trieu EP, Plotz PH, Miller FW. Antibodies to glycyl-transfer RNA synthetase in patients with myositis and interstitial lung disease. *Arthritis Rheum* 1992;35:821–830.

84. Ter Borg EJ, Horst G, Limburg PC, et al. Changes in levels of antibodies against the 70 kDa and a polypeptides of the U1RNP complex in relation to exacerbations of systemic lupus erythematosus. *J Rheumatol* 1991;18: 363–367.

85. Hoet RM, Koornneef I, de Rooij DJ, et al. Changes in anti-U1 RNA antibody levels correlate with disease activity in patients with systemic lupus erythematosus overlap syndrome. *Arthritis Rheum* 1992;35:1202–1210.

86. Wolfe JF, Adelstein E, Sharp GC. Antinuclear antibody with distinct specificity for polymyositis. *J Clin Invest* 1977;59:176–178.

87. Reichlin M, Maddison PJ, Targoff IN, et al. Antibodies to a nuclear/nucleolar antigen in patients with polymyositis-overlap syndrome. *J Clin Immunol* 1984;4:40–44.

88. Targoff IN, Reichlin M. Nucleolar localization of the polymyositis-Scl antigen. *Arthritis Rheum* 1985;28: 226–230.

89. Reimer G, Scheer U, Peters J-M, Tan EM. Immunolocalization and partial characterization of a nucleolar autoantigen (PM-Scl) associated with polymyositis/scleroderma overlap syndromes. *J Immunol* 1986;137: 3802–3808.

90. Gelpi C, Alguero A, Angeles Martinez M, et al. Identification of protein components reactive with anti-PM/Scl autoantibodies. *Clin Exp Immunol* 1990;81:59–64.

91. Oddis CV, Okano Y, Rudert WA, et al. Serum autoantibody to the nucleolar antigen PM-Scl: clinical and immunogenetic associations. *Arthritis Rheum* 1992;35:1211–1217.

92. Ge Q, Frank MB, O'Brien CA, Targoff IN. Cloning of a complementary DNA coding for the 100-kD antigenic protein of the PM-Scl autoantigen. *J Clin Invest* 1992;90:559–570.

93. Alderuccio F, Chan EKL, Tan EM. Molecular characterization of an autoantigen of PM-Scl in the polymyositis/scleroderma overlap syndrome: a unique and complete human cDNA encoding an apparent 75-kD acidic protein of the nucleolar complex. *J Exp Med* 1991;173:941–952.

94. Ge Q, Wu Y, Trieu EP, Targoff IN. Analysis of fine specificity of anti-PM-Scl autoantibodies. *Arthritis Rheum* 1994;37:1445–1452.

95. Briggs MW, Burkard KT, Butler JS. Rrp6p, the yeast homologue of the human PM-Scl 100-kDa autoantigen, is essential for efficient 5.8 S rRNA 3' end formation. *J Biol Chem* 1998;273:13255–13263.

96. Kho CJ, Huggins GS, Endege WO, et al. The polymyositis-scleroderma autoantigen interacts with the helix-loop-helix proteins E12 and E47. *J Biol Chem* 1997;272:13426–13431.

97. Genth E, Mierau R, Genetzky P, et al. Immunogenetic associations of scleroderma-related antinuclear antibodies. *Arthritis Rheum* 1990;33:657–665.

98. Marguerie C, Bunn CC, Copier J, et al. The clinical and immunogenetic features of patients with autoantibodies to the nucleolar antigen PM-Scl. *Medicine (Baltimore)* 1992;71:327–336.

99. Blaszczyk M, Jablonska S, Szymanska-Jagiello W, et al. Childhood scleromyositis: An overlap syndrome associated with PM-Scl antibody. *Pediatr Dermatol* 1991;8:1–8.

100. Schnitz W, Taylor-Albert E, Targoff IN, et al. Anti-PM/Scl autoantibodies in patients without clinical polymyositis or scleroderma. *J Rheumatol* 1996;23:1729–1733.

101. Mimori T, Hardin JA, Steitz JA. Characterization of the DNA-binding protein antigen Ku recognized by autoantibodies from patients with rheumatic disorders. *J Biol Chem* 1986;261:2274–2278.

102. Mimori T, Hardin JA. Mechanism of interaction between Ku protein and DNA. *J Biol Chem* 1986; 261:10375–10379.

103. Mimori T, Akizuki M, Yamagata H, et al. Characterization of a high molecular weight acidic nuclear protein recognized by autoantibodies in sera from patients with polymyositis-scleroderma overlap. *J Clin Invest* 1981; 68:611–620.

104. Hirakata M, Mimori T, Akizuki M, et al. Autoantibodies to small nuclear and cytoplasmic ribonucleoproteins in Japanese patients with inflammatory muscle disease. *Arthritis Rheum* 1992;35:449–456.
105. Mimori T. Structures targeted by the immune system in myositis. *Curr Opin Rheumatol* 1996;8:521–527.
106. Yaneva M, Arnett FC. Antibodies against Ku protein in sera from patients with autoimmune diseases. *Clin Exp Immunol* 1989;76:366–372.
107. Isern RA, Yaneva M, Weiner E, et al. Autoantibodies in patients with primary pulmonary hypertension: association with anti-Ku. *Am J Med* 1992;93:307–312.
108. Ringel SP, Forstot JZ, Tan EM, et al. Sjögren's syndrome and polymyositis or dermatomyositis. *Arch Neurol* 1982;39:157–163.
109. Okano Y, Steen VD, Medsger TA Jr. Autoantibody to U3 Nucleolar ribonucleoprotein (fibrillarin) in patients with systemic sclerosis. *Arthritis Rheum* 1992;35:95–100.
110. Hughes P, McGavin CR. Sarcoidosis and primary biliary cirrhosis with co-existing myositis. *Thorax* 1997;52:201–202.
111. Bondeson J, Veress B, Lindroth Y, Lindgren S. Polymyositis associated with asymptomatic primary biliary cirrhosis. *Clin Exp Rheumatol* 1998;16:172–174.
112. Yasuda Y, Nakano S, Akiguchi I, et al. Polymyositis associated with asymptomatic primary biliary cirrhosis. *Eur Neurol* 1993;33:51–53.
113. Varga J, Heiman-Patterson T, Munoz S, Love LA. Myopathy with mitochondrial alterations in patients with primary biliary cirrhosis and antimitochondrial antibodies. *Arthritis Rheum* 1993;36:1468–1475.
114. Arad-Dann H, Isenberg DA, Shoenfeld Y, et al. Autoantibodies against a specific nuclear RNP protein in sera of patients with autoimmune rheumatic disease associated with myositis. *J Immunol* 1987;138:2463–2468.
115. Arad-Dann H, Isenberg D, Ovadia E, et al. Autoantibodies against a nuclear 56-kDa protein: a marker for inflammatory muscle disease. *J Autoimmun* 1989;2:877–888.
116. Cambridge G, Ovadia E, Isenberg DA, et al. Juvenile dermatomyositis: serial studies of circulating autoantibodies to a 56kD nuclear protein. *Clin Exp Rheumatol* 1994;12:451–457.
117. Oddis CV, Fertig N, Goel A, et al. Clinical and serological characterization of the anti-MJ antibody in childhood myositis. *Arthritis Rheum* 1997;40:S139(abst).
118. Espada G, Confalone Gregorian M, Ortiz Z, et al. Serum autoantibodies in juvenile idiopathic inflammatory myopathies (IIM) in a cohort of Argentine patients. *Arthritis Rheum* 1998;40:S140(abst).
119. Gelpi C, Sontheimer EJ, Rodriguez-Sanchez JL. Autoantibodies against a serine tRNA-protein complex implicated in cotranslational selenocysteine insertion. *Proc Natl Acad Sci USA* 1992;89:9739–9743.
120. Targoff IN, Hanas J. The polymyositis-associated Fer antigen is elongation factor 1a. *Arthritis Rheum* 1989;32: S81(abst).
121. Wilusz J, Keene JD. Autoantibodies specific for U1 RNA and initiator methionine tRNA. *J Biol Chem* 1986; 261:5467–5472.
122. Targoff IN, Arnett FC, Berman L, et al. Anti-KJ: a new antibody associated with the myositis/lung syndrome that reacts with a translation-related protein. *J Clin Invest* 1989;84:162–172.
123. Uthman I, Vazquez-Abad D, Senecal JL. Distinctive features of idiopathic inflammatory myopathies in French Canadians. *Semin Arthritis Rheum* 1996;26:447–458.
124. Feist E, Dorner T, Kuckelkorn U, et al. Proteasome alpha-type subunit C9 is a primary target of autoantibodies in sera of patients with myositis and systemic lupus erythematosus. *J Exp Med* 1996;184:1313–1318.
125. Stuhlmuller B, Jerez R, Hausdorf G, et al. Novel autoantibodies against muscle-cell membrane proteins in patients with myositis. *Arthritis Rheum* 1996;39:1860–1868.
126. Emslie-Smith AM, Engel AG. Microvascular changes in early and advanced dermatomyositis: a quantitative study. *Ann Neurol* 1990;27:343–356.
127. Kissel JT, Mendell KW, Rammohan KW. Microvascular deposition of complement membrane attack in dermatomyositis. *N Engl J Med* 1986;314:329–334.
128. Kissel JT, Halterman RK, Rammohan KW, Mendel JR. The relationship of complement-mediated microvasculopathy to the histologic features and clinical duration of disease in dermatomyositis. *Arch Neurol* 1991;48: 26–30.
129. Crowson AN, Magro CM. The role of microvascular injury in the pathogenesis of cutaneous lesions of dermatomyositis. *Hum Pathol* 1996;27:15–19.
130. Mascaro JM Jr, Hausmann G, Herrero C, et al. Membrane attack complex deposits in cutaneous lesions of dermatomyositis. *Arch Dermatol* 1995;131:1386–1392.
131. Engel AG, Arahata K. Mitochondrial antibody analysis of mononuclear cells in myopathies. II. Phenotypes of autoinvasive cells in polymyositis and inclusion body myositis. *Ann Neurol* 1984;16:209–215.
132. Dalakas MC. Polymyositis, dermatomyositis, and inclusion-body myositis. *N Engl J Med* 1991;325:1487–1498.
133. James JA, Gross T, Scofield RH, Harley JB. Immunoglobulin epitope spreading and autoimmune disease after peptide immunization: Sm B/B-derived PPPGMRPP and PPPGIRGP induce spliceosome autoimmunity. *J Exp Med* 1995;181:453–461.
134. Casiola-Rosen L, Rosen A. Ultraviolet light-induced keratinocyte apoptosis: a potential mechanism for the induction of skin lesions and autoantibody production in LE. *Lupus* 1997;6:175–180.
135. Targoff IN. Immune manifestations of inflammatory muscle disease. *Rheum Dis Clin North Am* 1994;20: 857–880.

136. Casiola-Rosen L, Pluta A, Plotz PH, et al. HPMS1 is a novel, frequently targeted myositis autoantigen which is cleaved by granzyme B but not by caspases during apoptosis. *Arthritis Rheum* 1998;41:S127(abst).
137. Martin A, Schulman MJ, Tsui FWL. Epitope studies indicate that histidyl-tRNA synthetase is a stimulating antigen in idiopathic myositis. *FASEB J* 1995;9:1226–1233.
138. Ge Q, Wu Y, James JA, Targoff IN. Epitope analysis of the major reactive region of the 100-kd protein of PM-Scl autoantigen. *Arthritis Rheum* 1996;39:1588–1595.
139. Ge Q, Wu Y, Targoff IN. Analysis of epitope reactivity of autoantibodies to glycyl-tRNA synthetase. *Arthritis Rheum* 1994;37:S351(abst).
140. Garlepp MJ. Immunogenetics of inflammatory myopathies. *Bailliere's Clin Neurol* 1993;2:579–597.
141. Garlepp MJ. Genetics of the idiopathic inflammatory myopathies. *Curr Opin Rheumatol* 1996;8:514–520.
142. Targoff IN, Miller FW, Medsger TA Jr, Oddis CV. Classification criteria for the idiopathic inflammatory myopathies. *Curr Opin Rheumatol* 19997;9:527–535.
143. Miller FW, Twitty SA, Biswas T, Plotz PH. Origin and regulation of a disease-specific autoantibody response: antigenic epitopes, spectrotype stability, and isotype restriction of anti-Jo-1 antibodies. *J Clin Invest* 1990;85: 468–475.
144. Drachman DB. Myasthenia gravis. *N Engl J Med* 1994;330:1797–1810.
145. Lewis RA, Selwa JF, Lisak RP. Myasthenia gravis: immunological mechanisms and immunotherapy. *Ann Neurol* 1995;37[Suppl 1]:S51–S62.
146. Shashi K, Engel AG, Lambert EH, Howard FM. Ultrastructural localization of the terminal and lytic ninth complement component (C9) at the motor end-plate in myasthenia gravis. *J Neuropathol Exp Neurol* 1980;39: 160–172.
147. Engel AG, Lambert EH, Howard FM. Immune complexes (IgG and C3) at the motor end-plate in myasthenia gravis: ultrastructural and light microscopic localization and electrophysiologic correlations. *Mayo Clin Proc* 1977;52:267–280.
148. Fambrough DM, Drachman DB, Satyamurti S. Neuromuscular junction in myasthenia gravis: decreased acetylcholine receptors. *Science* 1973;182:293–295.
149. Reyes H. Striational autoantibodies. In: Peter JB, Schoenfeld Y, eds. *Autoantibodies*. Amsterdam: Elsevier Science, BV, 1996:805–809.
150. Sanders DB. Lambert-Eaton myasthenic syndrome: clinical diagnosis, immune-mediated mechanisms, and update on therapies. *Ann Neurol* 1995;37[Suppl 1]:S63–S73.
151. Maselli RA. Pathophysiology of myasthenia gravis and Lambert-Eaton syndrome. *Neurol Clin* 1994;12: 285–303.
152. Targoff IN. Autoantibodies in polymyositis. *Rheum Dis Clin North Am* 1992;18:455–482.

*Diseases of Skeletal Muscle,*
edited by Robert L. Wortmann.
Lippincott Williams & Wilkins, Philadelphia © 2000

# 16

# Skeletal Muscle Imaging for the Evaluation of Myopathies

Jane H. Park and Nancy J. Olsen

*Department of Molecular Physiology and Biophysics and Department of Medicine,*
*Vanderbilt University, Nashville, Tennessee 37232*

Skeletal muscle imaging plays an increasingly important role in the clinical evaluation and understanding of muscle disorders. The three major modalities, computed tomography (CT), ultrasound, and magnetic resonance imaging (MRI), significantly enhance diagnostic approaches to many myopathies. During the last decade, MRI has emerged as the method of choice for the examination of soft tissue muscle abnormalities (1). Although MRI provides the most accurate images for diagnosis and longitudinal management, it may not be the method of choice under all circumstances. The alternative modalities, CT and ultrasonography, are indispensable for evaluation and treatment of some diseases.

Most imaging techniques are noninvasive and thus have distinct advantages over invasive or painful diagnostic procedures such as muscle biopsy and electromyography. Occasionally, intravenous contrast agents are useful. However, in most cases, neither CT nor MRI requires such enhancement to provide optimal information (2). Noninvasive procedures are also easily repeatable and valuable for longitudinal evaluations.

A second advantage of imaging is its ability to examine relatively large volumes of muscle. Muscle biopsies, even those obtained via an open surgical approach, represent a very limited sample of tissue. Disorders such as dermatomyositis (3), polymyositis (4), pyomyositis (5), and sarcoidosis (6) often involve focal areas of muscle. Adjoining tissues may be normal on histologic examination, and there are usually no clinical clues to guide the choice of biopsy site. Thus, the relatively small biopsy sample taken may not reflect the true scope of disease involvement. Imaging also may be useful as an adjunct to guide biopsy location, thus increasing the probability of a positive result (7). MRI is not, however, a replacement for biopsy in decisions such as distinguishing between polymyositis and inclusion body myositis.

A third advantage of most of the currently used imaging procedures is that they can be applied to all types of patients, some of whom may be difficult to study using other techniques. For example, important diagnostic information can be obtained even from very weak patients or very young children for whom functional muscle testing, electromyography, or biopsy may be difficult.

MRI, the most costly imaging technique, has been subjected to a cost-effectiveness analysis (7). Investigators followed 25 patients with inflammatory muscle disease over a period of 2 years. Approximately half of the patients had an MRI evaluation that was then used to determine the best site for biopsy. The remaining patients did not have MRI, and biopsies were done based on clinical impressions alone. Of the patients with preoperative MRI, only 7% had a false-negative biopsy. For the remaining patients without preoperative scanning, 45% had false-negative biopsies. The difference between the two groups was statistically significant. Furthermore, four of the five patients with negative results proceeded to a second biopsy. The costs of the repeat biopsies, longer periods of hospitalization, and increased numbers of laboratory tests drove the total expenses for the non-MRI group of patients to 40% more than the average cost for the MRI group (8).

Needle biopsies are often less costly than open surgical biopsies, and the use of MRI to localize the needle placement site may enhance the utility of this procedure (7,9). Depending on the institution, needle or surgical biopsy with related costs for pathology services may be considerably more expensive than the MRI itself.

A further consideration is whether muscle biopsy could be avoided in some cases by using MRI for diagnostic purposes (10). In the setting of other variables that are consistent with a diagnosis of inflammatory muscle disease, for example, a compatible MRI might provide sufficient evidence to support treatment. The MRI can be repeated to follow responses to therapy if questions arise during the course of treatment. In considering the expenses of muscle biopsy processing, including significant fees for histologic preparation and analysis, the use of MRI is most likely a cost-effective approach in at least some patients.

Each imaging modality has unique advantages and disadvantages depending on factors such as instrument availability, patient variability, specific clinical disease, requirements for rapid image acquisition, and cost (Table 1). Routine radiographs of soft tissues provide only limited information about muscle pathology. Soft tissue calcifications may be detected in patients with inflammatory muscle disorders such as juvenile dermatomyositis and some types of scleroderma (11). Even earlier stages of ectopic mineral deposition may be observed using radionuclide bone scans. Infectious processes can be identified by findings on plain films. Calcified cysticerci due to infection with *Taenia* or gas layers in deep tissues may be seen (12). Gallium ($^{67}$Ga) scanning is considered useful for detection and localization of infection (13). Granulomatous muscle changes in patients with the nodular or myopathic forms of sarcoidosis may be seen as increased uptake of gallium (6).

CT is the modality of choice for abnormalities of cortical bone, calcifications in soft tissues, and abscesses. CT is also the most used technology for percutaneous needle-

**TABLE 1.** *Advantages and disadvantages of muscle imaging techniques*

| Technique | Advantages | Disadvantages |
|---|---|---|
| Plain radiographs | General availability, detects calcification | Radiation exposure, insensitive to soft tissue changes |
| Computed tomography (CT) | General availability, large field of view, soft tissue calcifications, abscesses, gas | Radiation exposure, insensitive to soft tissue changes |
| Ultrasound (US) | General availability, no radiation, portable, images vascularization and blood flow (color Doppler), quantitative | Small field of view, no cross-sections for deep muscles, images operator dependent |
| Magnetic resonance imaging (MRI) | Best images for muscle, bone, and tendons; detects inflammation; large field of view, quantitative | Less available than CT or US, patient discomfort (claustrophobia), exclusion of some patients with indwelling metals, high cost |

guided biopsy. Cross-sectional CT images allow evaluation of deep muscles that are not generally accessible using ultrasound.

Sonography is the primary alternative to MRI for detection of soft tissue abnormalities (12). Ultrasound provides a safe, noninvasive, and relatively inexpensive approach for the evaluation of muscle abnormalities. Virtually all imaging abnormalities of muscle detectable by other imaging techniques can be visualized by ultrasonography, including edematous and fatty changes, calcification, alterations in muscle size, and localization of pathologic changes in selected muscle groups. In addition, abnormal vascularization and rates of blood flow can be effectively monitored with color Doppler.

Areas of muscle that can be included in each sonography examination are necessarily limited, and deep-seated muscles cannot be visualized in cross-section. Furthermore, image analyses may be somewhat subjective and dependent on the experience of the examiner (14). Ultrasound is very useful as an adjunct to other diagnostic investigations, such as in guiding the choice of site for biopsy.

MRI is the method of choice for imaging a wide range of soft tissue muscle disorders because it provides the most accurate images for diagnosis and tissue characterization. MRI offers distinct advantages in the study of muscle because of its high spatial resolution, exquisite sensitivity to anatomic differences in tissues, the options to accentuate or modulate tissue contrast, manipulation of images in different planes, and visualization of major blood vessels without contrast. The disadvantages for some patients include claustrophobia, indwelling metals, positioning difficulties, and cost.

The muscles to be imaged with MRI may be positioned within the body coil (main bore of the magnet) or in a specialized coil, which provides closer proximity to the muscles (Fig. 1). For example, in imaging the thigh muscles, use of the body coil has the advantage of allowing bilateral evaluations. Placement of the thigh within a relatively small extremity (knee) coil provides enhanced anatomic detail due to coil proximity (3,10).

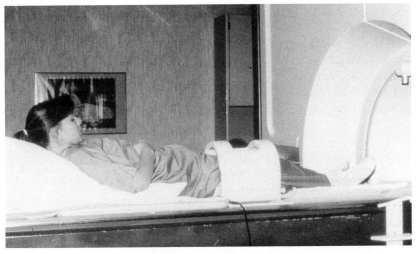

**FIG. 1.** Patient in position for MRI examination of the thigh muscles. The thigh of the patient is centered in an extremity coil, which is actually designed for the knee. The close proximity of the coil to the thigh muscles affords a detailed image of the muscle groups. Alternatively, both legs could be imaged simultaneously using the large main bore of the magnet, the so-called body coil. The patient and bed are then moved into the bore of the magnet for imaging.

Muscles of the shoulder, back, neck, and other regions are visualized with appropriately designed coils. Both axial and coronal images may be useful (15). Coronal images may give a more accurate assessment of the total extent of abnormal muscle involvement, whereas axial images usually provide a greater level of detail. Screening of patients for MRI examinations must include questioning with regard to the possibility of indwelling ferromagnetic metals (Table 2).

Early studies using T1-weighted images alone demonstrated the presence of fat replacement in patients with polymyositis (16). However, inflammatory changes could not be detected. Subsequently, T2-weighted images were used to show muscle inflammation and edema (2,3,17). Both the T1- and T2-weighted images can be obtained during a single session within the magnet lasting approximately 30 minutes or less. Intravenous contrast with gadolinium chelate generally does not enhance the detection of muscle abnormalities and is not routinely recommended (18,19). The T1-weighted image provides an excellent morphologic picture with clear definition of various muscle groups. Normal muscle tissue appears as a homogeneously dark area corresponding to a low signal intensity. In contrast, fat appears bright, corresponding to high signal intensity (Fig. 2). The T2-weighted image shows normal muscle as even darker and inflammation detected as focally distributed bright areas. Fat appears bright in the T2- and T1-weighted images. Thus, coinciding regions of muscle with high signal intensity (brightness) on both images most likely correspond to infiltrating fat.

Fat and inflammation may be closely juxtaposed within muscle tissues, and the high signal intensity (brightness) of fat on the T2-weighted images may obscure coexisting inflammatory changes. One approach to solving this problem is to calculate relaxation times, the T1 and T2 values, within defined regions of interest. These calculations yield very different T1 and T2 values for fat and inflammation (3). The second approach is to use a fat-suppression sequence (short TI inversion [STIR]), which substantially improves visualization of muscle inflammation by increasing the signal intensity (brightness) of inflammation and decreasing the fat signal (Fig. 3) (4,20). STIR sequences have been used extensively for detection and quantitation of inflammation and edema (4).

Conversion of the visual analysis of the images to quantitative values is of great utility for two reasons. First, vague or minimal abnormalities can be confirmed. Second, changes in clinical status or responses to treatment can be characterized more precisely in longitudinal studies of individual patients. The usual approach to quantitation is by measuring relaxation times that relate to molecular motion (3,10,21). Calculated T1 and T2 values are not included as part of routine clinical studies but have been widely used in research investigations (3,10,22).

**TABLE 2.** Considerations for metal screening in magnetic resonance imaging

| Contraindicated | Generally allowed |
| --- | --- |
| Internal cardiac pacemaker, defibrillator, insulin pumps, cochlear implants, etc. | Most orthopedic implants and devices |
| Magnetically activated implants (i.e., ocular implants, magnetic sphincters) | Pellets and bullets, depending on composition and bodily location (as determined by plain film radiography) |
| Aneurysm clips | Dental devices and materials |
| Occupational exposure to metal fragments (sheet metal workers with eye injury) | Intravascular stents and filters (analyzed as nonferromagnetic) |

A detailed discussion of the evaluation criteria for metallic implants, materials, and foreign bodies is presented in Stark DD, Bradley WG. *Magnetic resonance imaging,* 3rd ed. Vol. 1. Mosby, St. Louis 1999: 296–300.

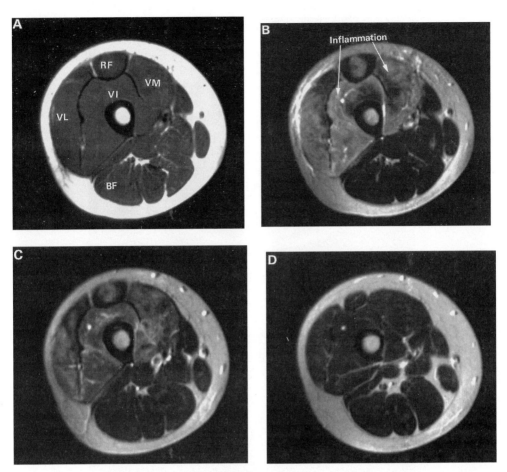

**FIG. 2.** T1- and T2-weighted images of the thigh muscles of a juvenile dermatomyositis patient acquired on three successive visits. **A:** Before treatment, the T1-weighted image appeared normal and showed homogeneous signal intensity (moderately dark) for all muscle groups. *VL*, vastus lateralis; *VM*, vastus medialis; *VI*, vastus intermedius; *RF*, rectus femoris; *BF*, biceps femoris. **B:** The initial T2-weighted image showed increased signal intensity (brightness) in the quadricep muscles, indicative of inflammation. The hamstring muscles were homogeneously dark due to absence of inflammation. **C:** After 3 weeks of prednisone treatment, the T2-weighted image showed considerably less inflammation in the quadriceps. **D:** After 5 months of treatment, the entire T2-weighted image had homogeneously low signal (dark), demonstrating the disappearance of inflammation.

Table 3 shows the application of these calculations in longitudinal evaluations of a patient with juvenile dermatomyositis. This 14-year-old subject was studied four times over a period of 7 months (21). During that time the serum creatine kinase level decreased from 4,962 to 63 IU/mL (normal range, 30 to 210 IU/mL) and his maximum voluntary contraction of quadricep muscles increased from 15 to 40 pounds. Initially elevated T1 and T2 values decreased to normal levels at month 5 and remained within the normal range at month 7. Clinically, this child showed a complete recovery.

The fat-suppressed (STIR) images can also be quantitatively evaluated on the basis of the increased signal intensities (4). For 25 patients with idiopathic inflammatory myopathies, linear regression analyses of signal intensity ratio scores of STIR images showed

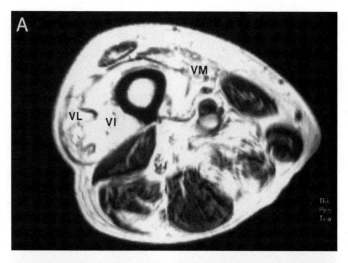

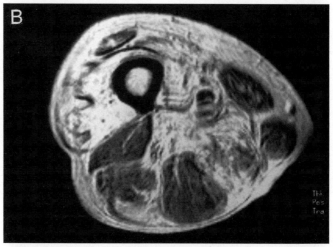

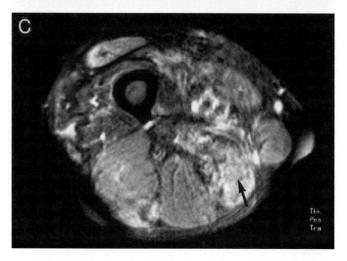

**TABLE 3.** *Calculated T1 and T2 values show improvement in patient with JDM*

| Subject | Month | T1 (ms) | T2 (ms) | CPK (IU) |
|---|---|---|---|---|
| JDM patient | 1 | 1890[a] | 65[a] | 4962 |
| | 1.5 | 1698[a] | 53[a] | 1025 |
| | 5 | 1232 | 39 | 77 |
| | 7 | 1265 | 37 | 63 |
| Control subjects ($n = 8$) | Muscle | 1380 | 38 | 30–210 |
| Control subjects ($n = 8$) | Superficial fat[b] | 350 | 56 | |

[a]$p < 0.001$ vs. control subjects: The high T1 and T2 values for the patient indicate inflammation.
[b]T1 and T2 values for superficial fat were the same in control subjects and patient.
JDM, juvenile dermatomyositis; CPK, creatine phosphokinase.
From Ref. 21, with permission.

a highly significant correlation with disease activity scores. In three patients followed longitudinally, the increased STIR signal intensity ratios paralleled changes in disease activity. Thus, MRI has proved to be a useful asset for assessing clinical status and guiding therapeutic decisions.

## INFLAMMATORY DISEASES

Normal muscle density as detected by CT is close to that of water (23), and active muscle inflammation does not change that density to any significant extent. Therefore, CT is not often used for the evaluation of inflammatory myopathies. However, changes in muscle mass, such as atrophy and fat replacement, are readily detected as areas of decreased muscle density. Infiltrating fat may give the involved muscle a patchwork or "moth-eaten" appearance (8). Calcifications in soft tissues, which are characteristically associated with juvenile dermatomyositis, are very well visualized using CT (14,24).

Ultrasound may be used effectively in some patients with myositis. Soft tissue calcifications are easily visualized on ultrasound as bright intensely reflective echoes (25). Inflammatory changes in muscle tissue can also be detected on ultrasound examination as areas of decreased echogenicity. Muscle atrophy in patients with chronic long-standing polymyositis appear, as areas of increased echo intensity (8). An ultrasound study of muscle in a series of 70 patients with polymyositis, dermatomyositis, inclusion body myositis, and granulomatous myositis showed that two thirds had significantly abnormal echo patterns, either above or below the normal range of values (26). For 12 additional patients, visual analysis of the ultrasound images showed abnormalities, such as atrophy. Overall, 83% of the patients showed pathologic findings on quantitative and visual analyses.

**FIG. 3.** Comparison of T1- and T2-weighted images with a STIR image for detection of inflammation in the thigh muscles of a polymyositis patient. **A and B:** The T1- and T2-weighted images appear almost identical, and detection of inflammation is difficult because of the extensive fat infiltration, especially in the vastus muscles. *VL*, vastus lateralis; *VM*, vastus medialis; *VI*, vastus intermedius. Preservation of muscle tissue is seen in the rectus femoris, biceps femoris, semitendinosus, sartorius, and gracilis. **C:** In the fat-suppressed STIR image, the fat appears dark (note superficial fat and bone marrow), whereas very bright areas of inflammation are readily visible, particularly in the semimembranosus and adductor muscles (*arrow*).

Patients with long-standing myositis generally had higher echointensities than patients with acute muscle syndromes (26). This finding is consistent with the presence of atrophy and lipomatosis in chronic long-standing disorders, whereas patients with acute syndromes are more likely to show inflammatory changes manifested as edema with lower echogenicity in muscles. Lipomatosis was more readily visualized than fibrosis. Patients with dermatomyositis showed, on average, lower echointensities than those with polymyositis, and this finding was independent of disease duration. Muscle atrophy was quantitatively measured as most severe in inclusion body myositis. Polymyositis showed more atrophy than either dermatomyositis or granulomatous myositis. The sonographic changes in this study did not correlate with either elevated serum muscle enzyme levels or with electromyographic abnormalities and thus provided unique information.

MRI is very useful in the evaluation of patients with dermatomyositis and its variants (3,4,21,22,27,28). T1-weighted images are often normal, indicating anatomic integrity and lack of significant fat infiltration or muscle atrophy. However, inflammation within the diseased muscle is observed as areas of brightness or increased signal intensity on T2-weighted and STIR images but not on T1-weighted images (Fig. 4) (3,4). In the thigh, anterior muscles of the quadriceps are more commonly involved than are posterior muscles. Abnormalities may be confined to one muscle of a group, most commonly the vastus lateralis, whereas adjacent muscles can appear normal. MRI has been especially useful in establishing the diagnosis of dermatomyositis in patients with normal serum levels of muscle enzymes (21). Increased signal intensity on T2-weighted or STIR images correlates strongly with disease activity and functional disability (4). Longitudinal studies have documented the utility of MRI in assessing responses to therapeutic interventions (21).

Although inflammation can resolve with therapy, metabolic abnormalities may still be detected in the muscles of adults using $^{31}$P-magnetic resonance spectroscopy (Fig. 5). $^{31}$P-spectroscopy measures the levels of high-energy phosphate compounds, ATP and creatine phosphate, which are required for muscle contraction. The initially low concentrations of ATP and creatine phosphate are increased during treatment but do not return to normal control levels. This may account for the presence of persistent fatigue without apparent inflammation (21). In some cases, however, therapy results in disappearance of inflammation and normalization of ATP levels.

Patients with the juvenile variant of dermatomyositis show MRI changes that are similar to those seen in adults except that calcification is more common in children. Statistically, significant correlations exist between muscle strength and MRI abnormalities in this age group (17,20). As in adults, MRI findings in children do not always correlate with serum levels of muscle enzymes, and therefore the scans provide useful and unique diagnostic information (27,29).

The amyopathic variant of dermatomyositis (dermatomyositis sine myositis) is characterized by normal T1- and T2-weighted images, consistent with other normal laboratory

---

**FIG. 4.** T1- and T2-weighted images of an adult dermatomyositis patient on two successive visits. **A:** T1-weighted images of the thigh were normal on both visits. **B:** On the first visit, T2-weighted images clearly showed that inflammation was present, as indicated by the high signal intensity (brightness) in the quadricep muscles. **C:** After 4 months of prednisone treatment, inflammation was resolved as demonstrated on the T2 images by the homogeneously dark signal in all muscle groups. Resolution of the inflammation was verified by calculation of the T1 and T2 relaxation times.

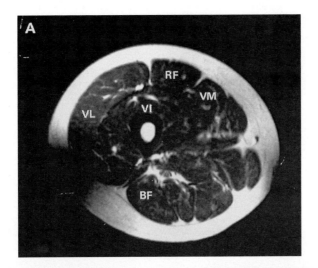

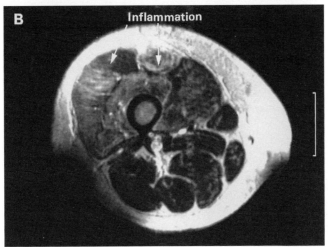

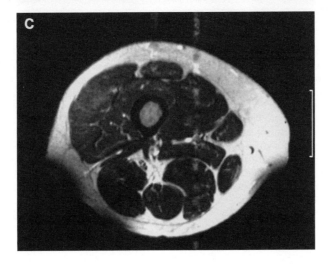

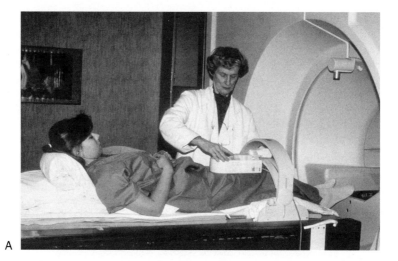

A

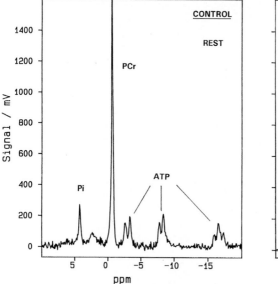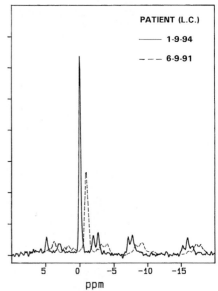

B

**FIG. 5. A:** Patient being prepared for a magnetic resonance spectroscopy ($^{31}P$) examination. The same MRI equipment is used for determination of $^{31}P$ metabolites, ATP and creatine phosphate, with the exception of a different specialized coil, which is placed over the thigh and secured with velcro straps. The patient is able to exercise inside the magnet by contracting the quadricep muscles and thereby raising the foot with an attached weight. Exercise can often accentuate metabolic abnormalities. **B:** $^{31}P$-MR spectra of the quadricep muscles of a normal control subject and the dermatomyositis patient shown in Fig. 4. The spectrum of the patient's diseased muscle shows reduced levels of ATP and creatine phosphate, the two high-energy phosphate compounds required for muscle contraction. After 4 months of treatment, the levels of these compounds were still 40% below normal, despite the resolution of inflammation (– – –). Substantial improvements in ATP and creatine phosphate concentrations were seen after 30 months of therapy (——).

PCr, creatine phosphate; Pi, inorganic phosphorus; ATP, adenosine triphosphate.

and histologic findings in this disorder (22). Abnormalities in energy metabolism in the muscle of these patients consistent with fatigue can be detected during heavy exercise with $^{31}$P-magnetic resonance spectroscopy in some patients (22).

Patterns of muscle abnormalities in polymyositis are usually different from those seen in dermatomyositis. T1-weighted images often show distortion of the normal anatomy with extensive fat infiltration and muscle atrophy (Fig. 3) (4,14). T2-weighted images may show areas of inflammation but not as distinctly as in dermatomyositis muscles (Fig. 3B). Thus, STIR sequences are best for detection of inflammation (Fig. 3C). The abnormalities seen in the thigh muscles of patients with polymyositis are not limited to anterior muscle groups but may involve posterior muscles such as the abductors as well (Fig. 3). Differences in muscle involvement in polymyositis and dermatomyositis are probably a reflection of underlying pathogenetic differences in these two distinct syndromes.

Marked distortions of muscle anatomy are commonly observed on T1-weighted images from patients with inclusion body myositis (Fig. 6) (4,19,30). In one study of upper extremity muscles, MRI abnormalities in the flexor digitorum profundus were detected in 20 of 21 patients, and these changes did not correlate with duration of disease (30). Therefore, scanning of this muscle may be useful in detecting inclusion body myositis relatively early. MRI changes seen in upper and lower extremities of patients with long-standing inclusion body myositis are consistent with extensive fat infiltration and muscle atrophy and are concordant with the extreme weakness usually observed in these patients. $^{31}$P-spectroscopy shows lower levels of ATP and creatine phosphate in inclusion body myositis as compared with polymyositis or dermatomyositis.

Muscle weakness and fatigue are very common complaints in patients with scleroderma (31). The most common muscle disorder in scleroderma is noninflammatory and

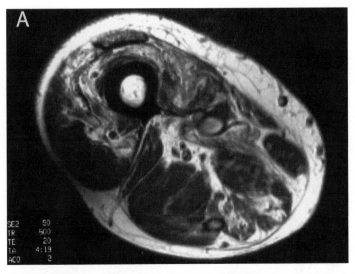

**FIG. 6.** T1- and T2-weighted images of the thigh muscles of a patient with inclusion body myositis. **A:** On the T1-weighted image, high signal intensity (brightness) throughout the quadriceps indicates extensive fat replacement, which will increase with time. There is partial sparing of muscle in the vastus lateralis, as well as both heads of the biceps femoris and gracilis muscles. The pattern of atrophy is variable in this disease. *(Continued on next page.)*

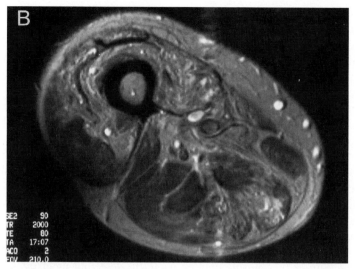

**FIG. 6.** *Continued.* **B:** In the T2-weighted image, the increased signal intensity in the vastus lateralis and biceps muscles indicates the presence of inflammation, as verified by calculation of the T1 and T2 relaxation times.

has been termed a simple myopathy (32). Levels of serum muscle enzymes and electromyography are usually normal. In concordance with these observations, MR images in patients with simple myopathy generally do not show muscle inflammation. Fascial thickening may be observed (33). However, findings consistent with an inflammatory myositis, including inflammatory changes on the T2-weighted images, may be seen in a small percentage of patients (Fig. 7) (31).

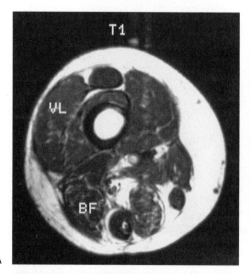
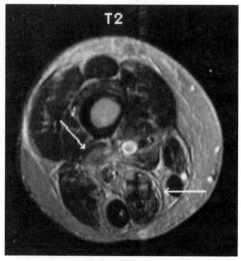

A                                                                                          B

**FIG. 7.** T1- and T2-weighted images of a patient with diffuse scleroderma. **A:** The cross-sectional area of the T1-weighted image of the thigh was decreased, suggesting atrophy. **B:** The T2-weighted images showed increased signal intensity in the short head of the biceps, indicative of inflammation (*upper left arrow*). Thickening of the fascia was observed throughout the thigh.

## INFECTIONS OF MUSCLE

Infections in muscle can occur as spontaneous events, secondary to penetrating wounds, extensions from a contiguous source of infection such as osteomyelitis, or in immunocompromised patients. Identification, localization, and estimation of the extent of infection can be readily ascertained with imaging techniques (34,35).

In pyomyositis, areas of low attenuation surrounded by an enhancing rim and increased muscle volume are observed with CT. Iodinated contrast infusion may be helpful in detecting pyomyositis in some patients (5,36). CT and MRI of the suspicious areas can be used to rule out an abscess and may obviate the need for exploratory surgery (37). CT is also an excellent screening modality for patients with human immunodeficiency virus who are at risk for unusual infections that may occur in unpredictable patterns (38).

Ultrasound is useful for exploring muscles for suspected infections. This technology can be used rapidly and may provide information that indicates the need for more expensive studies such as CT, MRI, or biopsy (25,39). Soft tissue abnormalities detected by ultrasound include thickening of subcutaneous tissue, fluid collections, abscess, and sinus tract formation (40). The findings of muscle swelling and a hypoechoic fluid collection found in pyomyositis may simulate soft tissue sarcoma, muscle neoplasia, or hematoma. Therefore, correlation with the clinical findings and possibly biopsy are required (12). The diagnosis of cellulitis is made clinically, but an associated underlying infectious process such as abscess, osteomyelitis, or septic arthritis can be detected with ultrasound (40).

At present, MRI is the preferred technique for determining the extent of an infection because of its excellent soft tissue contrast, spatial resolution, and multiplanar capabilities. Acute infections are usually observed as bright, irregularly marginated rims surrounding edematous areas with inhomogeneous low signal on T1-weighted images. Abscesses usually show sharp margins and homogeneous internal regions similar to infections. Lesions are much more clearly visualized as areas of high signal intensity (brightness) on T2-weighted or STIR images (36,41).

Chronic infections such as tuberculosis, fungal disease, or actinomycosis may have a different appearance. These lesions may be difficult to distinguish from injury or other masses within the muscles. Distinction between infected and noninfected fluid cannot be made with MRI, even with the use of contrast agents. MRI can help differentiate between cellulitis and more serious necrotizing fasciitis (5). MRI can demonstrate muscle edema associated with bacterial myositis in the early stages using T2-weighted or particularly STIR images (42). MRI is extremely helpful initially in indicating a possible site for aspiration or biopsy and subsequently in monitoring the responses to therapy.

## SARCOIDOSIS

Both nodular and diffuse forms of sarcoid myopathy have been characterized using imaging modalities. MRI is more accurate than CT or ultrasound in detecting and localizing granulomatous abnormalities in muscles, particularly in the diffuse myopathy.

Granulomatous nodules can be detected with CT by revealing well-defined regions of low attenuation (decreased intensity) that can be enhanced with contrast agents (6). However, this is not a particularly sensitive technique for evaluating the nodular form of disease (43). Fatty infiltration, detected as areas of decreased attenuation, and atrophy can be observed in cases of diffuse chronic myopathy (43–45).

Nodular sarcoidosis can also be identified with ultrasound using a 7.5-MHz linear probe (6). In the axial view, a nodule has increased echogenicity in the center and decreased echogenicity at the periphery. Ultrasound is less effective in identifying diffuse myopathic sarcoidosis but can identify areas of atrophy, fatty infiltration, and pseudohypertrophy (43,44).

Sarcoid nodules are readily detected with MRI as areas with star-shaped centers of decreased signal intensity on both T1- and T2-weighted images with outer rims of high signal intensity, particularly on T2-weighted images. The peripheral areas become enhanced with the use of gadolinium. The central portion of the lesion consists of dense connective tissue and hyaline material with low cellularity, accounting for the decreased signal. The periphery has high cellularity and possibly inflammatory granulomas, causing the bright outer rim (6). In chronic diffuse sarcoidosis, the fat infiltration and replacement appear as increased signal intensity on T1- and T2-weighted images of the lower extremities (19). Acute sarcoid myositis shows a mesh pattern with intermediate intensity on the T1 and T2 images (45). The MR images may be normal when the granulomas are small and widely distributed (6). In these cases, gallium scanning will still show increased uptake in the diseased muscles.

## METABOLIC MYOPATHIES

The metabolic myopathies show various patterns of abnormalities on imaging that represent the morphologic consequences of the respective inborn errors (46). CT findings in acid maltase deficiency include significant infiltration of fat with preserved muscle architecture (47,48). Fat infiltration was frequently present in the psoas and erector spinae of adult patients with acid maltase deficiency but absent in the psoas of phosphorylase-deficient patients. This particular distribution is interesting from the perspective of pathophysiology but is not specific for diagnostic purposes. MRI of the thighs in adults with acid maltase deficiency shows severe fatty degeneration that may be asymmetric in distribution. Even with extensive fat replacement, the configuration of the muscle is not distorted and the intermuscular fascia remain intact (46).

Debrancher disease is associated with a diffuse increase in signal intensity on T2-weighted images. The high signal intensity is due to excess glycogen deposition rather than increased water content (49). Fatty replacement is not a major feature of this deficiency.

In myophosphorylase deficiency, the muscles often appear normal with only minimal fat replacement and focal areas of edema or necrosis (46,50). By contrast, MRI in phosphofructokinase deficiency shows focal regions of fat with minimal fatty edema (46).

Only a few imaging studies of muscle have been performed in patients with mitochondrial myopathies (51,52). Both CT and MRI demonstrate muscle deterioration with atrophy and fatty replacement. In some patients, particularly those with ophthalmoplegia, there was selective deterioration of the sartorius and gracilis muscles (52).

[31]P-magnetic resonance spectroscopy has been used extensively to study the biochemical defects of most metabolic muscle diseases. Abnormalities in the generation and utilization of the high-energy compounds, ATP and creatine phosphate, have been detected during rest, exercise, and recovery (see Chapter 9) (53).

## CONGENITAL MYOPATHIES

Congenital myopathies include nemaline myopathy, central core disease, congenital fiber type disproportion, multicore (minicore) disease, and myotubular (centronuclear)

**TABLE 4.** *Selective muscle involvement in congenital myopathies, muscular dystrophy, and mitochondrial disease*

| Disease | Affected muscles | Spared muscles |
|---|---|---|
| Nemaline myopathy | Dorsiflexors and plantar flexors of the feet, tibialis (ant.) gastrocnemius | Quadriceps, rectus femoris, soleus, gracilis, tibialis (post.) |
| Central core disease | Sartorius, gracilis, soleus | Dorsiflexors, rectus femoris |
| Fiber type disproportion | Soleus, tibialis (ant. and post.) | Gastrocnemius |
| Muscular dystrophy | Gastrocnemius, quadriceps, biceps femoris | Sartorius, gracilis, tibialis (post.) |
| Mitochondrial myopathy | Sartorius, gracilis | |

The degree of involvement of the various muscles depends on the length and stage of the disease. The table demonstrates preferential distribution of muscle involvement in the early stages of the myopathies.

myopathy. These rare diseases are characterized by hypotonia, weakness from birth, and muscle fiber abnormalities as detected in biopsies. Imaging with CT, ultrasound, and MRI has clearly demonstrated the different selectivity for affected muscle groups in congenital myopathies and also the sparing of specific groups even with increasing severity (Table 4) (54–57). This disease distribution of muscle abnormalities in congenital myopathies (as well as muscular dystrophies and mitochondrial myopathies) can be clinically useful and interesting, but the mechanism of preservation of muscle groups is not understood.

## MUSCULAR DYSTROPHIES

The muscular dystrophies are a group of inherited disorders that include Duchenne muscular dystrophy, Becker's muscular dystrophy, limb-girdle dystrophy, Emery-Dreifuss dystrophy, facioscapulohumeral dystrophy, distal muscular dystrophy, and oculopharyngeal dystrophy. All these disorders, with the exception of oculopharyngeal dystrophy, have been examined with CT, ultrasound, and MRI.

Ultrasound does not detect abnormalities in the early stages of Duchenne muscular dystrophy. As the disease progresses, two changes are observed. Echointensities are increased, indicating fat infiltration and atrophy (58). Nonuniform involvement of the muscles can be demonstrated and quantitated with ultrasound measurements (58–60).

CTs have been performed in the preclinical or early stages of Duchenne muscular dystrophy. Only slight decreases in intramuscular density and muscle size are observed up to 3 years of age (61). CT can be used quantitatively to monitor the progression of muscle involvement in terms of fat replacement and muscle fiber loss (62). Initially, the gluteus maximus and medius, tensor fasciae latae, biceps femoris, hip adductors, quadriceps, peroneals, and gastrocnemius muscles become infiltrated with fat as indicated by decreased attenuation with CT. Subsequently, the iliopsoas, quadratus lumborum, paravertebral, semimembranosus, semitendinosus, anterior tibialis, and soleus muscles become involved. A significant correlation between CT-detected abnormalities and muscle strength has been observed. The gracilis, sartorius, and posterior tibialis are preserved and may even become hypertrophic. Reasons for selectivity have not been ascertained.

In the early stages of disease, MRI reveals increased T1 relaxation times in the gluteus maximus and quadriceps muscles, possibly indicating interstitial edema. As the disease progresses, the T1 values rapidly decrease due to fat replacement in the muscles (63). Although the distribution of fat in the various muscle groups is similar to that seen with CT, MRI provides an extraordinarily detailed image of fat infiltration that can be evaluated quantitatively (64). In fact, a statistically significant correlation can be found between the MR grade and disease duration, age, and clinical function (65).

There have been discussions as to whether imaging with CT or MRI might improve the accuracy of genetic counseling. Although several investigators have demonstrated muscle abnormalities in Duchenne muscular dystrophy carriers, others have been unable to detect pathologic changes, suggesting a lack of reliability of using the techniques to identify carriers.

The sonographic, CT, and MR images for patients with Becker's muscular dystrophy are similar to those of Duchenne muscular dystrophy but, in accord with the clinical manifestations, are less severe. There is selective involvement of most muscles with relative preservation of the sartorius, gracilis, adductor longus, semitendinosus, and semimembranosus muscles (55,60,61,66). Muscle imaging provides the most accurate information concerning the status of degeneration of both compound and deep-seated muscles in Duchenne and Becker's muscular dystrophy. This knowledge may be important for the planning of rehabilitative care and evaluation of therapeutic measures.

## MYOTONIC DISORDERS

Three types of myotonia can be distinguished clinically: congenital, childhood, and juvenile or adult onset. The congenital and childhood types have only been studied with ultrasound, which showed hyperechogenicity indicative of fat in the muscles (67). A comparative study of ultrasound, CT, and MRI was performed on 57 patients with juvenile-type myotonia (68). Ultrasonography demonstrated that myotonia characteristically showed decreased thickness of the muscles and increased thickness of the subcutaneous fat layers. Echogenicity increases due to fat infiltration in most muscles and correlates well with muscle weakness. CT proves an excellent technology for tracking muscle changes longitudinally. In the early stages, true hypertrophy is observed, but over the course of time fat replacement and atrophy become apparent in the muscles of the spine, neck, shoulder girdle, abdomen, legs, and forearms (68,69). MRI was the most sensitive for tracking alterations longitudinally, as illustrated by long-term atrophy of the anterior tibialis and triceps brachii and more recent fat replacement in the vastus intermedius, sartorius, and soleus. Imaging appears to be more sensitive than the determination of serum creatine kinase levels in detecting myopathy (68).

The intellectual impairment associated with myotonia has prompted numerous CT and MRI studies of brain lesions. A comprehensive MRI investigation of 40 patients demonstrated diffuse atrophy in two thirds, white matter lesions in two thirds, and thickening of the skull in one third (70). The extent of atrophy and white matter disease correlated with mental retardation, disease duration, and the length of the unstable CTG repeat sequence on the affected protein kinase gene. In this study, muscle abnormalities on MR images correlated with dysfunction and less strongly with the CTG repeat length in the defective gene.

## NEUROPATHIC DISORDERS THAT CAUSE MUSCLE WEAKNESS

Most neuropathies, including inflammatory, hereditary, demyelinating, and degenerative disorders, have been studied with imaging modalities. Because the radiologic findings are not often specific, a definitive diagnosis for a patient usually cannot be made on the basis of imaging data. However, CT, ultrasound, and MR images of muscle and nerves can provide useful supplementary data and may afford a reasonable alternative to invasive electromyography and biopsy procedures.

Using CT, denervation can be initially detected as fat and connective tissue deposition that gives the muscles a moth-eaten appearance. With disease progression, atrophy can be visualized along with further decreased density of the muscle, indicating additional fat infiltration. Ultrasonography is especially advantageous in examining small children for screening purposes. It can be applied without sedation, radiation, or motion artifacts. In addition, only ultrasound can detect fasciculations in the deep muscles. MRI remains the modality of choice for providing detailed pictures of hypertrophy, pseudohypertrophy, atrophy, nerve compression, inflammation, and localization of specific changes in an extremity or an individual muscle.

Muscle imaging of the neuropathic patient can be advantageous in a number of circumstances. Early signs of denervation can be ascertained as edema or fasciculations. The distribution of affected muscles can indicate if the denervation is focal, generalized, asymmetric, or symmetric. Characterization of the extent of hypertrophy, pseudohypertrophy, atrophy, and possibly regeneration of muscles may be helpful in selection of biopsy sites, determination of progress after relief of nerve compression, and planning of procedures such as arthrodesis. Longitudinal imaging over time can determine the progression of disease and efficacy of therapeutic procedures.

## FIBROMYALGIA

Patients with fibromyalgia frequently complain of fatigue and muscle weakness. The pathogenesis of these symptoms is not well understood, but muscle abnormalities have been suggested in histologic studies (71). MRI investigations of these individuals have not shown anatomic derangements or inflammatory changes (72). In fact, MRI studies found that the cross-sectional areas of the quadriceps and tibialis anterior muscles of patients were not different from those of normal control subjects (73,74). However, impaired muscle function in fibromyalgia patients was demonstrated by their significantly reduced strength per cross-sectional area of muscle. $^{31}$P MR spectroscopy has demonstrated diminished levels of ATP and creatine phosphate and decreased oxidative metabolism in some patients (71).

## RHABDOMYOLYSIS

Rhabdomyolysis is characterized by destruction of muscle and can result from a wide variety of etiologic factors, including direct trauma, ischemia, excessive activity, myositis, drugs, and metabolic disorders. Thus, the distribution and magnitude of the abnormalities may vary considerably. Accurate identification and localization of the injured muscles may be useful in evaluation and subsequent treatment in compartment syndromes or if fasciotomy is contemplated. In a comparative study of imaging technologies in patients with rhabdomyolysis, MRI showed abnormalities in all patients, CT detected changes in 62%, and ultrasound was abnormal in 42% (75). Muscle biopsy or fasciotomy confirmed that the increased MRI signal (brightness) was due to necrosis or edema. MRI has been used to follow the course of sports-related injuries, such as compartment syndromes (76,77). Decreases in the pathologic MRI parameters correlated with clinical improvement, decreases in serum creatine kinase levels, and return of the limb to more normal diameter. MRI is the preferred imaging technique for detecting the distribution and extent of rhabdomyolysis.

## REFERENCES

1. Hodler J, Yu JS, Steinert HC, Resnick D. MR imaging versus alternative imaging techniques. *Magn Reson Imaging Clin North Am* 1995;3:591–608.

2. Stiglbauer R, Graninger W, Prayer L, et al. Polymyositis: MRI-appearance at 1.5 T and correlation to clinical findings. *Clin Radiol* 1993;48:244–248.
3. Park JH, Vansant JP, Kumar NG, et al. Dermatomyositis: correlative MR imaging and P-31 MR spectroscopy for quantitative characterization of inflammatory disease. *Radiology* 1990;177:473–479.
4. Fraser DD, Frank JA, Dalakas M, et al. Magnetic resonance imaging in the idiopathic inflammatory myopathies. *J Rheumatol* 1991;18:1693–1699.
5. Ma LD, Frassica FJ, Bluemke DA, Fishman EK. CT and MRI evaluation of musculoskeletal infection. *Crit Rev Diagn Imaging* 1997;38:535–568.
6. Otake S. Sarcoidosis involving skeletal muscle: imaging findings and relative value of imaging procedures. *AJR Am J Roentgenol* 1994;162:369–375.
7. Schweitzer ME, Fort J. Cost-effectiveness of MR imaging in evaluating polymyositis. *Am J Radiol* 1995;165:1469–1471.
8. Fleckenstein JL, Reimers CD. Inflammatory myopathies: radiologic evaluation. *Radiol Clin North Am* 1996;34:427–439.
9. Haddad MG, West RL, Treadwell EL, Fraser DD. Diagnosis of inflammatory myopathy by percutaneous needle biopsy with demonstration of the focal nature of myositis. *Am J Clin Pathol* 1994;101:661–664.
10. Olsen NJ, Park JH. Inflammatory myopathies: issues in diagnosis and management. *Arthritis Care Res* 1997;10:200–207.
11. Feldman F. Soft tissue mineralization: roentgen analysis. *Curr Probl Diagn Radiol* 1986;15:161–240.
12. Boutin RD, Brossmann J, Sartoris DJ, et al. Update on imaging of orthopedic infections. *Orthop Clin North Am* 1998;29:41–66.
13. Chiu NT, Yao WJ, Jou IM, Wu CC. The value of $^{67}$Ga-citrate scanning in psoas abscess. *Nucl Med Commun* 1997;18:1189–1193.
14. Reimers CD, Finkenstaedt M. Muscle imaging in inflammatory myopathies. *Curr Opin Rheumatol* 1997;9:475–485.
15. Fujitake J, Ishikawa Y, Fujii H, et al. Magnetic resonance imaging of skeletal muscles in the polymyositis. *Muscle Nerve* 1997;20:1463–1466.
16. Kaufman LD, Gruber BL, Gerstman DP, Kaell AT. Preliminary observations on the role of magnetic resonance imaging for polymyositis and dermatomyositis. *Ann Rheum Dis* 1987;46:569–572.
17. Hernandez RJ, Keim DR, Sullivan DB, et al. Magnetic resonance imaging appearance of the muscles in childhood dermatomyositis. *J Pediatr* 1990;117:546–550.
18. Schedel H, Reimers CD, Vogl T, Witt TN. Muscle edema in MR imaging of neuromuscular diseases. *Acta Radiol* 1995;36:228–232.
19. Reimers CD, Schedel H, Fleckenstein JL, et al. Magnetic resonance imaging of skeletal muscles in idiopathic inflammatory myopathies of adults. *J Neurol* 1994;241:306–314.
20. Hernandez RJ, Keim DR, Chenevert TL, et al. Fat-suppressed MR imaging of myositis. *Radiology* 1992;182:217–219.
21. Park JH, Vital T, Ryder N, et al. MR imaging and P-31 MR spectroscopy provide unique quantitative data for longitudinal management of patients with dermatomyositis. *Arthritis Rheum* 1994;37:736–746.
22. Park JH, Olsen NJ, King LE, et al. MRI and P-31 magnetic resonance spectroscopy detect and quantify muscle dysfunction in the amyopathic and myopathic variants of dermatomyositis. *Arthritis Rheum* 1995;38:68–77.
23. Hawley RJJ, Schellinger D, O'Doherty DS. Computed tomographic patterns of muscles in neuromuscular diseases. *Arch Neurol* 1984;41:383–387.
24. Jouve JL, Cottalorda J, Bollini G, et al. Myositis ossificans: report of seven cases in children. *J Pediatr Orthop B* 1997;6:33–41.
25. Jacobson JA, van HM. Musculoskeletal ultrasonography. *Orthop Clin North Am* 1998;29:135–167.
26. Reimers CD, Fleckenstein JL, Witt TN, et al. Muscular ultrasound in idiopathic inflammatory myopathies of adults. *J Neurol Sci* 1993;116:82–92.
27. Hernandez RJ, Sullivan DB, Chenevert TL, Keim DR. MR imaging in children with dermatomyositis: musculoskeletal findings and correlation with clinical and laboratory findings. *AJR Am J Roentgenol* 1993;161:359–366.
28. Adams EM, Chow CK, Premkumar A, Plotz PH. The idiopathic inflammatory myopathies: spectrum of MR imaging findings. *Radiographics* 1995;15:563–574.
29. Ryder N, Park J, Lawton A, et al. Magnetic resonance imaging and P-31 MR spectroscopy for evaluation of juvenile dermatomyositis. *Arthritis Rheum* 1994;37:S243(abst).
30. Sekul EA, Chow C, Dalakas MC. Magnetic resonance imaging of the forearm as a diagnostic aid in patients with sporadic inclusion body myositis. *Neurology* 1997;48:863–866.
31. Olsen NJ, King LEJ, Park JH. Muscle abnormalities in scleroderma. *Rheum Dis Clin North Am* 1996;22:783–796.
32. Clements PJ, Furst DE, Campion DS, et al. Muscle disease in progressive systemic sclerosis. *Arthritis Rheum* 1978;21:62–71.
33. King LE, Olsen NJ, Puett D, et al. Quantitative evaluation of muscle weakness in scleroderma patients using magnetic resonance imaging and spectroscopy. *Arch Dermatol* 1993;129:246–247.
34. Beltran J. MR imaging of soft-tissue infection. *Magn Reson Imaging Clin N Am* 1995;3:743–751.
35. Magid D. Computed tomographic imaging of the musculoskeletal system. *Radiol Clin North Am* 1994;32:255–274.

36. Gordon BA, Martinez S, Collins AJ. Pyomyositis: characteristics at CT and MR imaging. *Radiology* 1995;71: 279–286.
37. Kinahan AM, Douglas MJ. Piriformis pyomyositis mimicking epidural abscess in a parturient. *Can J Anaesth* 1995;42:240–245.
38. Steinbach LS, Tehranzadeh J, Fleckenstein JL, Vanarthos WJ, Pais MJ. Human immunodeficiency virus infection: musculoskeletal manifestations. *Radiology* 1993;186:833–838.
39. Chem RK, Kaplan PA, Dussault RG. Ultrasound of the musculoskeletal system. *Radiol Clin North Am* 1994: 32: 275–289.
40. Chern CH, Hu SC, Kao WF, et al. Psoas abscess: making an early diagnosis in the ED. *Am J Emerg Med* 1997;15: 83–88.
41. Hernandez RJ, Keim DR, Chenevert TL, et al. Fat-suppressed MRI of myositis. *Radiology* 1992;182:217–219.
42. Wysoki MG, Angeid-Backman E, Izes BA. Iliopsoas myositis mimicking appendicitis: MRI diagnosis. *Skeletal Radiol* 1997;26:316–318.
43. Kurashima K, Shimizu H, Ogawa H, et al. MR and CT in the evaluation of sarcoid myopathy. *J Comput Assist Tomogr* 1991;15:1004–1007.
44. Levine CD, Miller JJ, Stanislaus G, et al. Sarcoid myopathy: imaging findings. *J Clin Ultrasound* 1997;25: 515–517.
45. Shinazoki T, Watanabi H, Aoki J, et al. Imaging features of subcutaneous sarcoidosis. *Skeletal Radiol* 1998; 27:359–364.
46. Fleckenstein JL, Peshock RM, Lewis SF, Haller RG. Magnetic resonance imaging of muscle injury and atrophy in glycolytic myopathies. *Muscle Nerve* 1989;12:849–855.
47. Cinnamon J, Slonim AE, Black KS, et al. Evaluation of the lumbar spine in patients with glycogen storage disease: CT demonstration of patterns of paraspinal muscle atrophy. *Am J Neuroradiol* 1991;12:1099–1103.
48. de Jager AE, van der Vliet TM, van der Ree TC, et al. Muscle computed tomography in adult-onset acid maltase deficiency. *Muscle Nerve* 1998;21:398–400.
49. Marbini A, Gemignani F, Saccardi F, Rimoldi M. Debrancher deficiency neuromuscular disorder with pseudo-hypertrophy in two brothers. *J Neurol* 1989;236:418–420.
50. Fleckenstein JL, Haller RG, Lewis SF, et al. Absence of exercise-induced MRI enhancement of skeletal muscle in McArdle's disease. *J Appl Physiol* 1991;71:961–969.
51. Wysoki MG, Santora TA, Shah RM, Friedman AC. Necrotizing fasciitis: CT characteristics. *Radiology* 1997;203:859–863.
52. Fleckenstein JL, Haller RG, Girson MS, Peshock RM. Focal muscle lesions in mitochondrial myopathy: MR imaging and evaluation. *J Magn Reson Imaging* 1992;2[Suppl]:121.
53. Kent-Braun JA, Miller RG, Weiner MW. Magnetic resonance spectroscopy studies of human muscle. *Radiol Clin North Am* 1994;32:313–335.
54. Wallgren-Pettersson C, Kivi L, Jaaskelainen J, et al. Ultrasonography, CT and MRI of muscles in congenital nemaline myopathy. *Pediatr Neurol* 1990;6:20–28.
55. Lamminen AE. Magnetic resonance imaging of primary skeletal muscle disease: patterns of distribution and severity of involvement. *Br J Radiol* 1990;63:946–950.
56. Termote J-L, Baert A, Crolla D, et al. Computed tomography of the normal and pathological muscular system. *Radiology* 1980;137:439–444.
57. Lamminen A, Jaaskelainen J, Rapola J, Suramo I. High-frequency ultrasonography of skeletal muscle in children with neuromuscular disease. *J Ultrasound Med* 1988;7:505–509.
58. Fischer AQ, Carpenter DW, Hartlage PL, et al. Muscle imaging in neuromuscular disease using computerized real-time sonography. *Muscle Nerve* 1988;11:270–275.
59. Heckmatt J, Rodillo E, Doherty M, et al. Quantitative sonography of muscle. *J Child Neurol* 1989;4:S101–S106.
60. Reimers CD, Schlotter B, Eicke BM, Witt TN. Calf enlargement in neuromuscular diseases: a quantitative ultrasound study in 350 patients and review of the literature. *J Neurol Sci* 1996;143:46–56.
61. Arai Y, Osawa M, Fukuyama Y. Muscle CT scans in preclinical cases of Duchenne and Becker muscular dystrophy. *Brain Dev* 1995;17:95–103.
62. Liu M, Chino N, Ishihara T. Muscle damage progression in Duchenne muscular dystrophy evaluated by a new quantitative computed tomography method. *Arch Phys Med Rehabil* 1993;73:507–514.
63. Matsumura K, Nakano I, Fukuda N, et al. Proton spin-lattice relaxation time of Duchenne muscular dystrophy by magnetic resonance imaging. *Muscle Nerve* 1988;11:97–102.
64. Leroy-Willig A, Willig TN, Henry-Feugeas MC, et al. Body composition determined with MR in patients with Duchenne muscular dystrophy, spinal muscular atrophy, and normal subjects. *Magn Reson Imaging* 1997; 15:737–744.
65. Liu G-C, Jong Y-J, Chaing C-H, Jaw T-S. Duchenne muscular dystrophy: MR grading system with functional correlation. *Radiology* 1993;186:475–480.
66. Kuryama M, Hayakawa K, Konishi Y, et al. MR imaging of myopathy. *Comp Med Imaging Graph* 1989;13:329–333.
67. Ito T, Tanikawa M, Miura H, Treshima N, et al. The movements of fetuses with congenital myotonic dystrophy in utero. *J Perinat Med* 1996;24:277–282.
68. Schedel H, Reimers CD, Nagele M, et al. Imaging techniques in myotonic dystrophy. A comparative study of ultrasound, computed tomography and magnetic resonance imaging of skeletal muscles. *Eur J Radiol* 1992; 15:230–238.

69. Nordal HJ, Dietrichson P, Eldevik P. Fat infiltration, atrophy, and hypertrophy of skeletal muscles demonstrated by X-ray computed tomography in neurological patients. *Acta Neurol Scand* 1988;7:115–122.
70. Bachmann G, Damin MS, Koch M, et al. The clinical and genetic correlates of MRI findings in myotonic dystropy. *Neuroradiology* 1996;38;629–635.
71. Olsen NJ, Park JH. Skeletal muscle abnormalities in patients with fibromyalgia. *Am J Med Sci* 1998;315: 315–358.
72. Kravis MMM, Munk PO, McCain GA, et al. MR imaging of muscle and tender points in fibromyalgia. *JMRI* 1993;3:669–690.
73. Norregaard J, Bulow PM, Vestergaard-Poulsen P, et al. Muscle strength, voluntary activation and cross-sectional muscle area in patients with fibromyalgia. *Br J Rheumatol* 1995;34:925–931.
74. Vestergaard-Poulsen P, Thomsen C, Norregaard J, et al. P-31 spectroscopy and electromyography during exercise and recovery in patients with fibromyalgia. *J Rheumatol* 1995;22:1544–1551.
75. Lamminen AE, Hekali PR, Tinula I, et al. Acute rhabdomyolysis: evaluation with magnetic resonance imaging compared with computed tomography and ultrasound. *Br J Radiol* 1989;62:326–331.
76. Orava S, Laakko E, Mattila K, et al. Chronic compartment syndrome of the quadriceps femoris muscle in athletes. Diagnosis, imaging and treatment with fasciotomy. *Ann Chir Gynaecol* 1998;87:53–58.
77. Fleckenstein JL, Weatherall PT. Parkey RW, et al. Sports-related muscle injuries: evaluation with MRI. *Radiology* 1989;172:793–798.

*Diseases of Skeletal Muscle,*
edited by Robert L. Wortmann.
Lippincott Williams & Wilkins, Philadelphia © 2000

# 17

# Electrophysiologic Evaluation of Muscle Disease

Maren L. Mahowald and *William S. David

*Department of Medicine, University of Minnesota Medical School and Veterans Affairs Medical Center, Minneapolis, Minnesota 55417; and *Department of Neurology, University of Minnesota Medical School and Hennepin County Medical Center, Minneapolis, Minnesota 55415*

Weakness is a common complaint. Physicians evaluating such patients face a formidable diagnostic challenge because the clinical possibilities are vast. True neuromuscular weakness may result from pathologic processes affecting any level of the neuraxis, including muscle (myopathies), neuromuscular junction (neuromuscular transmission disorders such as myasthenia gravis), nerve (neuropathies), anterior horn cells (motor neuron diseases such as amyotrophic lateral sclerosis), spinal cord (myelopathies), or more central processes. Neuromuscular diseases may occur in isolation, in association with an underlying systemic disorder (e.g., rheumatoid arthritis, lupus, vasculitis) or as a consequence of medical treatments (e.g., corticosteroids, gold). As such, weakness may portend a benign or life-threatening disorder. Effective treatments may exist and will vary depending on the relevant disease process. Accurate diagnosis is therefore essential.

Myopathies represent a diverse group of disorders in which the primary disease process affects muscle. Myopathies may be quite protean in their presentation. The "classic" pattern is one of symmetric proximally predominant weakness and atrophy affecting limb and girdle muscles, with preservation of sensation and reflexes. However, many variations in the presentation exist. Patients with myopathies may present with distally predominant or diffuse (proximal equal to distal) weakness. Some experience asymmetric or episodic weakness. In others there is no weakness but rather myalgias or exercise-induced cramping. Still others may present with recurrent myoglobinuria. In infants, myopathies may present as hypotonia only. Therefore, electrodiagnostic studies are very useful in the diagnosis of myopathic diseases because they may be difficult to recognize clinically.

Because the differential diagnosis of patients presenting with weakness in general, and myopathies in particular, is so extensive, physicians have traditionally relied on ancillary laboratory investigations to supplement their clinical examination. Of these, electrodiagnostic studies and biopsy of muscle and nerves have proved the most useful. A detailed review of electrodiagnostic studies is clearly beyond the scope of this chapter, and the interested reader is referred to the several excellent textbooks that exist (1,2).

**TABLE 1.** *Information from electrodiagnostic studies*

1. Differentiate true weakness from limited effort due to psychogenic factors, pain, or upper motor neuron or central nervous system deficits.
2. Localize site of pathology along the neuraxis to muscle, neuromuscular junction, nerve, or anterior horn cell.
3. Characterize the pattern of electrical abnormalities that suggest a differential diagnosis.
5. May elucidate underlying pathologic process such as axonal or demyelinating neuropathy.
6. Assess severity and prognosis.
7. Identify unsuspected subclinical systemic disease.
8. Help select sites for biopsy.

## ELECTRODIAGNOSIS

Buchthal and Clemmenson (3) and Kugelberg (4) were among the first to propose that electrophysiologic findings could be used to differentiate myopathic from neurogenic disorders, with Kugelberg defining the basic electrical abnormalities observed in muscle disease. Since that time, electrophysiologic techniques have undergone considerable refinement, and today a variety of quantitative and semiquantitative techniques exist for the evaluation of patients with neuromuscular disorders.

Electrodiagnostic studies can provide important diagnostic information, depending on the clinical situation (Table 1). First, electrophysiologic studies can differentiate true from psychogenic weakness or simply provide objective evidence of neuromuscular disease in the patient whose clinical examination is difficult to interpret because of poor effort secondary to pain, malingering, or cognitive difficulties. Second, in peripheral nervous system disorders, electrodiagnostic studies can identify where along the peripheral motor unit (Fig. 1)

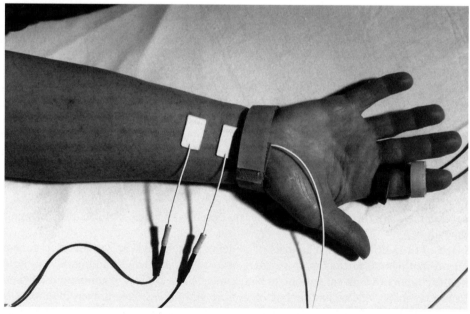

**FIG. 1.** Median sensory nerve conduction study. Stimulation by distal ring electrodes (anode and cathode) on the second digit. Proximal recording electrodes (active and reference) over the median nerve. A ground electrode is between the two sets of electrodes.

**TABLE 2.** *Components of the electrodiagnostic study*

1. Sensory nerve studies
   a. Amplitude of sensory nerve action potential
   b. Distal sensory latency
   c. Sensory nerve conduction velocity
2. Motor nerve studies
   a. Amplitude of compound muscle action potential
   b. Distal motor latency
   c. Conduction velocity
3. Repetitive stimulation responses (neuromuscular junction)
4. Needle electrode examination of the muscle
   a. Insertional activity
   b. Spontaneous activity
   c. Motor unit action potential morphology
   d. Recruitment pattern

the primary pathologic process resides, be it in the muscle, nerve, neuromuscular junction, or anterior horn cell. Such localizing information can then lead to a meaningful differential diagnosis, which may be further delimited by certain patterns of electrical abnormalities within a specific category of disease. Third, electrodiagnostic studies can assist in selecting which nerve or muscle to biopsy, thereby improving diagnostic yield. Finally, in certain situations, electrophysiologic findings can provide a measure of disease activity, elucidate the underlying pathophysiology, provide information on severity and prognosis, and identify unsuspected underlying systemic disease.

Standard electrodiagnostic studies consist of two parts, the nerve conduction studies and the needle electrode examination of muscle. Both parts together are commonly referred to as the "EMG," although technically, EMG is the acronym for electromyography, which is synonymous with the needle electrode examination (Table 2). The nerve conduction studies, in turn, consist of two main parts, the sensory nerve conduction studies and the motor nerve conduction studies. Typically, the nerve conduction studies are performed first.

## Nerve Conduction Studies

### *Sensory Nerve Conduction Studies*

The sensory portion of the peripheral nervous system consists of peripheral sensory receptors, sensory nerve axons, and the dorsal root ganglion cells that give rise to the sensory axons. The dorsal root ganglia, which are located adjacent to the spinal canal, contain the cell bodies of the sensory nerves. The dorsal root ganglion cells are "bipolar" and send a central process into the spinal cord via the dorsal horn and a peripheral process into the limb to supply a specific sensory receptor. Major nerves that convey sensory information from the periphery may contain hundreds or thousands of individual sensory axons. Although some nerves in the arm or leg are predominantly sensory, in most nerves the sensory axons run alongside motor axons in what are termed "mixed" nerves.

The sensory portions of many nerves in the arm (e.g., median, ulnar, radial, medial, lateral and posterior antebrachial cutaneous, dorsal ulnar cutaneous, etc.) and leg (e.g., sural, superficial peroneal, medial and lateral plantar, saphenous, lateral femoral cutaneous, etc.) can be studied electrophysiologically. The selection of which nerves to study depends on the clinical history, signs, and symptoms that suggest the relevant differential diagnosis. Although the specific techniques used for studying these different nerves vary, the basic principles are the same. (For a detailed description of how to perform conduction studies on specific nerves, the reader is referred to several textbooks [5–7].)

Basically, to evaluate sensory nerve function, a mixed or predominantly sensory nerve is electrically stimulated in one location while the nerve response is recorded in a distant location (Fig. 1). Nerves may be stimulated with needle electrodes implanted subcutaneously or adjacent to a nerve but more typically are stimulated percutaneously with surface electrodes on the skin. Similarly, sensory nerve responses can be recorded from needle electrodes positioned adjacent to a nerve or from surface electrodes placed on the skin overlying a nerve, although the latter are far more common for reasons of comfort.

Figure 1 shows a typical setup for a median nerve sensory conduction study. Electrical stimuli are delivered through ring electrodes wrapped around the finger, where only sensory fibers are found. A pair of electrodes (a cathode and an anode) are required to deliver the electrical stimuli. The nerve response is recorded from surface recording electrodes positioned over the median mixed nerve in the wrist. Two electrodes, an active and a reference electrode, are required for recording. A ground electrode is positioned between the two sets of electrodes.

A typical median sensory response is shown in Fig. 2. This sensory nerve action potential (SNAP) produced by a supramaximal stimulus reflects the relatively synchronous summated discharge of all individual sensory nerve axons present in that nerve. Because "supramaximal" stimuli are delivered to achieve the largest response, it is assumed that all sensory axons present have been stimulated. In different laboratories, different parameters of the sensory nerve response to stimulation are measured. The time interval in milliseconds required for the impulse to travel from the stimulus site to the recording site (response onset or peak) is measured as the "latency to onset" or "latency to peak." The sensory nerve conduction velocity is calculated by dividing the distance between the stimulating (cathode) and recording (active) electrodes by the onset latency (Table 3).

Different laboratories may use different techniques, record all or only a few of the above parameters, and may have different sets of normative data based on the technique used in that laboratory. An important indicator of laboratory quality is whether normal values for that laboratory have been established. In general, amplitudes of the sensory action potentials reflect the number of functioning sensory axons in the nerve studied, whereas measures of speed, such as the distal latencies and conduction velocity, reflect the integrity of the myelin sheath around the sensory axons. For example, neuropathies characterized by axonal loss will reveal reduced amplitudes with preserved velocities, whereas demyelinating neuropathies will display prolonged latencies and slowed velocities. Sensory conduction studies are always normal in myopathic disorders.

## Motor Nerve Conduction Studies

A "motor unit" consists of a single anterior horn cell with an axon that extends and divides into multiple terminal nerve branches to innervate numerous muscle fibers in a 1:1 fashion (i.e., one terminal branch to one muscle fiber). The neuromuscular junctions define the interface between each terminal nerve branch and the muscle fiber it supplies. An anterior horn cell may innervate from five to hundreds of muscle fibers. Macroscop-

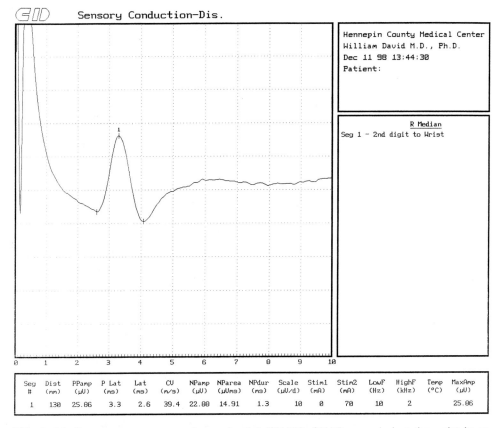

Sensory Conduction—Dis.

Hennepin County Medical Center
William David M.D., Ph.D.
Dec 11 98 13:44:30
Patient:

R Median
Seg 1 – 2nd digit to Wrist

| Seg # | Dist (mm) | PPamp (µV) | P Lat (ms) | Lat (ms) | CV (m/s) | NPamp (µV) | NParea (µVms) | NPdur (ms) | Scale (µV/d) | Stim1 (mA) | Stim2 (mA) | LowF (Hz) | HighF (kHz) | Temp (°C) | MaxAmp (µV) |
|---|---|---|---|---|---|---|---|---|---|---|---|---|---|---|---|
| 1 | 130 | 25.86 | 3.3 | 2.6 | 39.4 | 22.80 | 14.91 | 1.3 | 10 | 0 | | 70 | 10 | 2 | 25.86 |

**FIG. 2.** Median sensory nerve action potential (SNAP). SNAP recorded at the wrist in response to a supramaximal stimulation at the second digit.

ically, each muscle consists of thousands of muscle fibers and is innervated by numerous motor axons. When a given motor axon discharges, whether by voluntary activation or from electrical stimulation, all muscle fibers supplied by that motor axon discharge relatively synchronously. If multiple motor axons are stimulated simultaneously, all of their constituent muscle fibers will discharge in relative synchrony, allowing a "summated" response, the compound muscle action potential (CMAP) (Fig. 3).

**TABLE 3.** *Sensory nerve conduction studies*

| Parameter | Measure | Comment |
|---|---|---|
| Amplitude of sensory nerve action potential | "Baseline to peak" or "peak to peak" size of action potential | Amplitude reflects the number of functioning sensory axons in the nerve. |
| Distal/latency | Time interval from stimulation to onset or peak of action potential | Speed of conduction dependent on integrity myelin sheath. |
| Sensory nerve conduction velocity | Distance between stimulating and recording electrodes divided by onset latency | Speed of conduction dependent on integrity myelin sheath. |

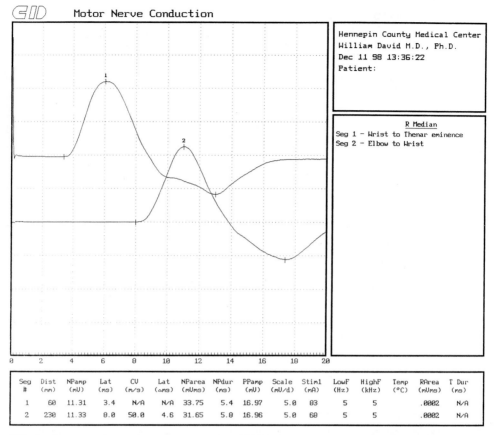

**FIG. 3.** Compound muscle action potential. CMAP response to supramaximal stimulation of the median nerve. Segment 1, wrist to thenar eminence; segment 2, elbow to wrist used to calculate the conduction velocity.

As previously described, the motor axons in a mixed nerve run adjacent to the sensory fibers. Motor axon function can be evaluated indirectly by recording the electrical response in the innervated muscle. When a mixed nerve is stimulated electrically and the nerve reaction is measured indirectly by recording the response from a muscle, only motor axons are assayed. The motor portions of many individual nerves in the arm (e.g., median, ulnar, radial, musculocutaneous, axillary, dorsal scapular, suprascapular etc.) and the leg (e.g., peroneal, posterior tibial, femoral, sciatic, etc.) can be studied in this way. As with sensory nerve testing, the sites selected for stimulation and recording have been standardized for each individual nerve to provide reproducible optimal responses to stimulation. Specific techniques for individual nerves are described in detail in several textbooks and monographs of electrodiagnostic medicine (5–8). Planning the electrodiagnostic study involves selection of which nerves to study and is directed by the specific clinical questions being addressed and the proposed differential diagnosis.

Motor nerves can be stimulated by needle or surface electrodes (Fig. 4), although the latter is almost always used for reasons of comfort. In certain situations, however, needle

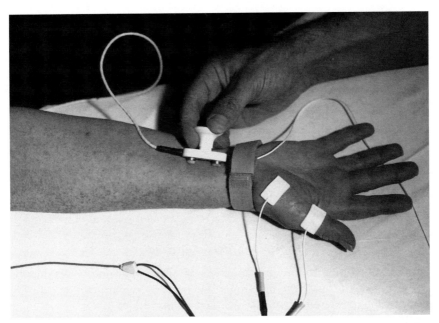

**FIG. 4.** Median motor nerve conduction study. Stimulating electrodes proximal to the wrist. Muscle response recorded with active electrode over the innervation zone of the muscle and the reference electrode over the tendon. The ground electrode is between the two sets of electrodes.

stimulation may actually be more comfortable (i.e., sciatic nerves). As discussed above, stimulating electrodes consist of a cathode and an anode. Muscle responses are measured by surface recording electrodes placed over a relevant muscle, with the active electrode positioned over the innervation zone of the muscle and the reference electrode positioned over the corresponding tendon.

The mixed nerve is stimulated several times with increasing intensity until the largest possible response is recorded. A "supramaximal stimulus" to a mixed nerve causes all the existing individual motor axons to discharge. Because each motor axon supplies numerous muscle fibers, these muscle fibers will discharge relatively at the same time. The summated discharges of all individual muscle fiber action potentials produces a large "CMAP amplitude" that is recorded by the surface recording electrodes over the muscle. Parameters of motor nerve function measured in most laboratories include the distal motor latency and the baseline to peak amplitude. Typically, motor nerves are stimulated in two or more locations, with CMAPs being recorded after stimulation at each site. By dividing the distance between stimulation sites by the difference in distal latencies, a conduction velocity of the motor fibers can be calculated (Table 4).

Different laboratories may use slightly different techniques and normative data, but in general amplitudes reflect the number of healthy motor axons and muscle fibers, whereas latencies and velocities measure the integrity of the myelin. In myopathies, distal motor latencies and conduction velocities are normal, whereas CMAP amplitudes may be normal or slightly reduced, depending on the severity of the condition. In

**TABLE 4.** *Motor nerve stimulation studies*

| Parameter | Measure | Example |
|---|---|---|
| Compound muscle action potential (CMAP) amplitude | Baseline to peak amplitude | Reflect number of healthy motor axons and muscle fibers |
| Distal motor latency | Time from stimulation to response | Measure integrity of the myelin |
| Motor nerve conduction velocity | Two sites of nerve are stimulated, conduction velocity is calculated by dividing the distance between two stimulation sites by the difference in distal latencies | Measure integrity of the myelin |

myopathic disorders, a reduced amplitude would result from loss of muscle fibers contributing to the CMAP.

### Repetitive Stimulation Studies

Repetitive stimulation studies are an extension of the motor nerve conduction techniques and are used to study the function of the neuromuscular junction. The stimulating and recording electrode setup is identical to that for a motor nerve conduction study, with the exception that the limb is immobilized by restraints with straps or arm boards to prevent shifting of the electrodes. Repetitive supramaximal stimuli (typically a volley of five to six pulses at 2 to 3 Hz) are delivered to a mixed nerve at various frequencies, and the amplitude of the CMAPs is recorded. Often, repetitive stimuli are delivered after a period of rest and again after the muscle has been maximally exercised for 10 and 45 seconds. On occasion, faster rates of repetitive stimulation may be delivered, up to 10 to 50 Hz, to identify a presynaptic disorder of neuromuscular junction transmission.

A series of CMAPs responding to 2 to 3 Hz stimulation will normally be identical in amplitude. In disorders of neuromuscular transmission, such as myasthenia gravis and Lambert-Eaton myasthenic syndrome, the amplitude of CMAPs will progressively decrease in size during with slow rates of repetitive stimulation. In myasthenia gravis, the progressive decrease in amplitude with repetitive stimulation will be most evident at 2 to 4 minutes after 45 seconds of maximal exercise. In certain presynaptic disorders of neuromuscular transmission, such as Lambert-Eaton and botulism, the amplitude of the CMAPs may increase in size after rapid rates of repetitive stimulation at 10 to 50 Hz, or with 2 to 5 Hz trains delivered immediately after 10 seconds of maximal exercise (9,10). The decreasing amplitude of CMAPs slow rates of repetitive stimulation in neuromuscular transmission disorders reflects the progressive "functional loss" of muscle fiber action potentials, contributing to the summated CMAP as a progressively larger number of dysfunctional neuromuscular junctions fail to chemically activate the underlying muscle fibers.

In muscle disease, repetitive stimulation studies are usually normal. Exceptions include the myotonic disorders wherein decreasing CMAP amplitudes may be seen with repetitive stimulation at rates above 5 Hz and periodic paralysis where abnormal increases in CMAP amplitudes may be observed with stimulation rates above 10 Hz. The repetitive stimulation study is very useful in the evaluation of patients with suspected myopathy because it can differentiate myopathy from neuromuscular transmission disorders that may otherwise appear similar both clinically and electrophysiologically.

### Long Latency Responses

Electrodiagnostic studies may include measurement of responses that have a long latency such as F and H waves. An F wave is recorded with an identical setup to a motor nerve conduction study with the exception that the position of the stimulating cathode and anode are reversed. An F wave is a late action potential (latency approximately 30 ms in the upper extremity and approximately 50 to 55 ms in the lower extremity) from a single motor unit that results from backfiring of an antidromically stimulated peripheral motor neuron. The F-wave response latency is a highly variable measure of the function of the proximal portions of a peripheral motor neurons. The H reflex, on the other hand, is analogous to a stretch reflex. A submaximal stimulation of a mixed nerve generates action potentials that are propagated centrally over the afferent sensory fibers to the α motor neuron in the spinal cord and causes a monosynaptic reflex muscle response. Although F and H waves can be useful in the evaluation of neuropathies, plexopathies, and radiculopathies, these responses are not relevant to a discussion of myopathic disorders and thus are not considered further. Interested readers are referred to the previously mentioned textbooks on electrodiagnostic medicine.

### Needle Electrode Examination of Muscle

The needle electrode examination of muscle involves recording the electrical activity of a muscle directly via a specially designed needle electrode inserted into the muscle. There are more than 400 skeletal muscles in the human body, and it is impossible to study them all. Additionally, in many disorders, particularly the myopathies, the distribution of abnormalities may be quite patchy. The needle electrode examination therefore cannot be standardized. Rather, the choice of which muscles to study is determined by the clinical signs and symptoms and the putative differential diagnoses.

In each individual case the possible diagnoses are based on the history and a careful neurologic examination, which should be performed by the electrodiagnostic medical consultant before each study. Which additional muscles to study and how many to examine will also be influenced by the findings observed in the muscles initially sampled. The needle electrode examination in suspected myopathies must be very thorough, involving sampling of multiple proximal, distal, and axial muscles in one arm and one leg. Electrical activity must be analyzed at multiple sites in each muscle. Studies are confined to one side of the body so that contralateral homologous muscles may be saved for biopsy. The needle examination requires considerable skill and experience. Normative values for the various types of data recorded will differ for each muscle and by age. A thorough knowledge of surface anatomy and of the pattern of root, nerve, and plexus innervation is essential for accurate localization and delineation of the underlying pathologic process.

The motor unit is the smallest functional unit of the motor system and consists of an anterior horn cell, its axon, and all muscle fibers supplied by the terminal branches of that axon. Different motor axons will innervate different numbers of muscle fibers. The ratio of muscle fibers to axons is termed the innervation ratio and is an estimate of the size of the motor unit. Larger motor units supply a larger number of muscle fibers and thus have a larger innervation ratio. Muscles requiring fine movements (e.g., extraocular muscles) have small innervation ratios, whereas those governing gross movements (e.g., quadriceps) will have large innervation ratios. The muscle fibers of a given motor unit are not geographically clustered but are scattered over an area of several millimeters interspersed with muscle fibers innervated by several other motor units. With voluntary effort to contract a specific muscle, smaller motor units are recruited or activated before the larger units in a stereotypic orderly fashion. Muscle fibers are of two main types, type I (rich in oxidative enzymes and fatigue resistant) and type II. All muscle fibers supplied by a given motor neuron are of the same type. Each motor unit has fiber type restriction (i.e., a given anterior horn cell will innervate only type I or type II fibers). In general, the smaller initially recruited units consist of type I fibers.

There are typically two main types of activity analyzed in a standard needle electrode examination: resting or spontaneous activity and voluntarily recruited activity initiated by effort.

### Resting or Spontaneous Activity

When a needle electrode is inserted into muscle, the muscle fibers are mechanically irritated or injured. This precipitates a burst of electrical activity that is normally less than 500 ms in duration. Prolonged insertional activity may reflect early denervation, although it can also be seen in selected myopathies (Table 5). Decreased insertional activity may be seen in chronic disorders with fibrous or fatty replacement of muscle or during attacks of periodic paralysis. Though not typically recorded in the electrodiagnostic report, some electrophysiologists will note the mechanical resistance offered by the skin and underlying subcutaneous tissues. Increased resistance may be seen in scleroderma and myxedema. Decreased resistance may be noted in Cushing's disease or steroid myopathies. Increased resistance to electrode passage can also be detected within muscle in those chronic disorders characterized by fibrous or fatty replacement of muscle (e.g., chronic myositis, dystrophy).

Normally, after the brief burst of insertional activity, a stationary electrode should detect no further electrical activity from a resting muscle. Resting muscle is typically elec-

**TABLE 5.** *Types of abnormal spontaneous activity on needle examination*

| Activity | Associated disorders |
| --- | --- |
| Fibrillation potentials (short, regular firing frequency, low amplitude triphasic action potentials) | Denervating disorders, selected myopathies |
| Positive sharp waves (biphasic shape, regular firing frequency, low amplitude) | Selected myopathies, denervating disorders |
| Fasciculations: single MUAP discharges, irregular firing rate | Amyotrophic lateral sclerosis, root compression, peripheral neuropathies, metabolic abnormalities |
| Complex repetitive discharges (complex polyphasic morphology, regular firing with "machine-like" sound, abrupt onset and termination) | Chronic neurogenic and myopathic disorders |
| Myotonic discharges (trains of fibrillation potentials and positive sharp waves with waxing and waning of amplitude and frequency producing a "dive-bomber" sound | Myotonic disorders, hyperkalemic periodic paralysis, chronic denervation, polymyositis, acid maltase deficiency |
| Myokymia (worm-like quivering of muscle associated with bursts of normal MUAPs in a fixed pattern, a "marching soldiers" sound) | Multiple sclerosis, brainstem neoplasm, polyradiculopathy, facial palsy, radiation plexopathy, chronic neuropathies |
| Cramp discharges (rapid irregular firing of MUAPs often with painful contraction) | Salt depletion, chronic neurogenic atrophy, nocturnal cramps, myxedema, pregnancy and dialysis |

MUAP, motor unit action potential.

trically silent, unless the electrode resides at the endplate region (innervation zone of the muscle) where a few specific types of normal spontaneous activity may be found. Care must be taken to avoid these regions, because such activity can confuse analysis of true abnormal spontaneous activity. Normal endplate activity can be recognized by its characteristic sound, discharge morphology, and firing characteristics. Abnormal spontaneous activity can appear in many forms (Table 5).

*Fibrillation Potentials.* Fibrillation potentials and positive sharp waves are the most common forms of abnormal spontaneous activity observed in some muscle diseases. They represent the action potentials of spontaneously discharging single muscle fibers. They have either a biphasic positive morphology or a triphasic shape with initial positivity, depending on the location of the discharging fiber with respect to the electrode. The discharges have a characteristic sound and are very regular in firing pattern. They are most often seen in neurogenic disorders (injury to a nerve, root, plexus, or generalized neuropathy or anterior horn cell disorder) but can also be seen in some selected myopathic disorders (Table 6). As such, the presence of fibrillation potentials and positive sharp waves within the context of an otherwise "myopathic" electrodiagnostic pattern will limit the differential diagnosis. Necrosis of muscle with "intramuscular denervation" has been offered as an explanation for the presence of these discharges in certain muscle diseases such as polymyositis, inclusion body myositis, toxic myopathies, the muscular dystrophies, sarcoidosis, and metabolic myopathies.

The presence of such discharges may also reflect the activity of a disease process. In polymyositis, the absence of spontaneous activity would suggest inactive disease (or advanced fibrosis), whereas the presence of many fibrillations and positive sharp waves would suggest active disease. If a patient with polymyositis develops increased weakness while on steroid therapy, the presence of abnormal spontaneous activity on electrodiagnostic testing would suggest active disease requiring more aggressive immunosuppression, whereas the absence of such spontaneous activity would be more suggestive of a steroid-induced myopathy, reflecting the need to reduce the steroid dose (11).

*Myotonic Discharges.* Myotonic discharges represent the second most common type of abnormal spontaneous activity observed in muscle disease. They may occur spontaneously or occur in response to electrical or mechanical stimulation or voluntary movement. They are composed of repetitive single-muscle fiber discharges with a waveform shape similar to that of a fibrillation potential or positive sharp wave. They fire in rapid bursts in which the amplitude of the individual discharges and the firing frequency wax and wane, producing a "dive-bomber" sound. Myotonic discharges may be seen in chronic denervating disorders but most typically are seen in certain myopathic conditions such as myotonic dystrophy, myotonia congenita, paramyotonia congenita and myositis, metabolic myopathies, and occasionally periodic paralysis (Table 6).

*Complex Repetitive Discharges.* Complex repetitive discharges, the least common form of spontaneous activity seen in muscle disorders, are irregular polyphasic discharges generated by multiple muscle fibers that ephaptically stimulate each other in a circuit. They begin and terminate abruptly and have a "machine gun-like" sound. They do not wax and wane. Complex repetitive charges are nonspecific and may be seen in a range of chronic nerve and muscle disorders such as polymyositis, inclusion body myositis, muscular dystrophies, myxedema, and acid maltase deficiency.

*Fasciculation Potentials.* Fasciculation potentials represent spontaneous single motor unit discharges and may be accompanied by a small visible twitch in the skin or muscle. Their shape is that of a single motor unit discharge. Fasciculation potentials may be benign, but when pathologic they can result from a disturbance of the motor nerve anywhere along its course. They are especially prominent in motor neuron disorders but can be seen in neuropathies, root injuries, and thyrotoxicosis. They are not common in muscle disease.

*Cramp Discharges.* Cramp discharges represent high-frequency trains of motor unit action potentials (MUAPs), often accompanied by a painful shortening of muscle. They are more common in neurogenic disorders but can also be seen in salt depletion, myxedema, pregnancy, and in healthy normal individuals. The painful muscle shortening, observed in certain metabolic myopathies (e.g., myophosphorylase deficiency), are actually electrically silent contractures, not true cramps.

Myokymia, neuromyotonic discharges, and other unusual forms of spontaneous activity have little relevance to a basic discussion of muscle disease (8,12,13).

### *Voluntary Activity*

An analysis of the electrical activity in a muscle during voluntary muscle contraction activity consists of two parts: an evaluation of MUAP morphology and an assessment of the recruitment patterns of motor unit potentials with increasing amounts of muscle contraction effort.

A MUAP is activated by voluntary effort and represents the relatively synchronous discharge of all muscle fibers supplied by a single motor unit. The MUAP results from the summated electrical activity of all individual muscle fiber action potentials that belong to a given motor unit. A typical motor unit (Fig. 5) is triphasic and is characterized by its amplitude, duration, and number of phases. The amplitude reflects the number of discharging muscle fibers located in close proximity to the recording electrode and is the

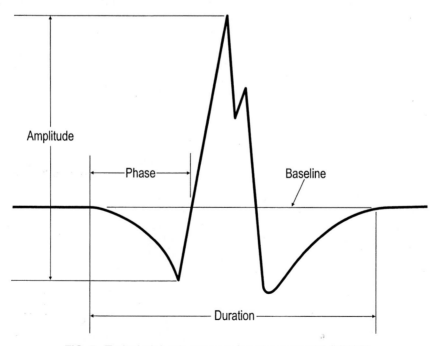

**FIG. 5.** Typical triphasic motor unit action potential (MUAP).

most variable parameter measured. The MUAP duration is measured from the initial deflection from baseline to the final return to baseline and is a reliable indicator of MUAP size. The term "phase" is used to represent the portion of the MUAP between baseline crossings. The number of phases is equal to the number of baseline crossings plus 1 and is abnormal when a certain percentage of the MUAPs is 4 or greater (the normal percentage is different for different muscles).

The amplitudes, durations, and phases of MUAPs will vary by age, muscle, and temperature. Myopathic and neurogenic disorders will impart characteristic alterations in MUAP morphology. In myopathies, there is a random loss of functioning muscle fibers. When a motor unit discharges, a smaller than usual number of muscle fiber action potentials will result, and as such, the amplitude and duration of the MUAPs will be small. Loss of distant muscle fibers principally affects the onset and termination of the MUAP, reducing the duration. Loss of fibers in close proximity to the recording electrode will result in a reduced amplitude. The remaining fibers, being spatially separated, will discharge in a less synchronized fashion, resulting in increased polyphasia. A similar set of abnormalities can be observed in disorders of neuromuscular transmission, where there is functional loss of muscle fiber activity due to failure of synaptic transmission at individual neuromuscular junctions rather than structural loss of muscle fibers.

In neurogenic processes over time, denervated muscle fibers will be reinnervated by collateral sprouts originating from adjacent healthy motor axons. This results in an increase in the number of muscle fibers supplied by these axons. When such a motor unit discharges, a high-amplitude long-duration MUAP will be recorded. The greater temporal and spatial separation of these muscle fibers will also result in increased polyphasia as a result of desynchronization.

Normally, at a small level of voluntary effort, only a few MUAPs will discharge. If increased effort is required, the body can accomplish this by either firing those active units more rapidly or recruiting additional motor units into action. Recruitment is defined as the sequential activation of additional motor units with increasing levels of effort. Typically, a single MUAP will fire no more frequently than 10 to 15 Hz before a second unit is recruited. Faster rates would be considered "rapid firing."

In neurogenic disorders (anterior horn cell, root, plexus, peripheral nerve disease), the muscle may be unable to recruit additional motor units because of a loss of motor axons. In this situation, existing units tend to fire more rapidly to achieve greater amounts of force. Thus, in neurogenic conditions, there is a reduced number of MUAPs firing rapidly. In myopathic conditions the situation is reversed. A normal complement of motor units is available, but each motor unit generates less force due to the random loss of muscle fibers. This produces smaller MUAPs. As such, even to achieve minimal levels of force, multiple MUAPs are activated to accomplish a task that only a few MUAPs could handle under normal conditions. The result is "early recruitment" at low levels of effort. This same pattern may also be seen in disorders of neuromuscular transmission. A decreased number of units firing slowly is suggestive of an upper motor neuron disorder (central nervous system processes such as stroke or spinal cord disease) or decreased effort due to pain, malingering, or other factors.

### *Quantitative Techniques*

A variety of quantitative techniques exist to supplement the needle electrode examination. These techniques have traditionally been quite laborious and time consuming, though the evolution of computer-based electrodiagnostic equipment has greatly improved this. These techniques are not widely used and are predominantly available in more sophisticated electrodiagnostic laboratories. These techniques have the advantage of increasing the sensitivity of the electrodiagnostic examination and are particularly helpful in subtle myopathies. They also provide an objective measure of dysfunction so that comparisons can be made over time and to follow treatment effects (14,15). Single-fiber electromyography is particularly useful in the diagnosis of neuromuscular transmission disorders. Quantitative MUAP analysis involves calculation of the mean duration of 20 different MUAPs. Decomposition programs or interference pattern analysis involve simplification of complex firing patterns of numerous MUAPs by a computer algorithm that extracts usable information on MUAP duration and firing frequency (16–19).

## ELECTRODIAGNOSTIC TECHNIQUES AND THE DIFFERENTIAL DIAGNOSIS OF MYOPATHY

As previously stated, patients presenting with weakness may be suffering from a disease affecting the motor neuron anywhere along its course (anterior horn cell, nerve, neuromuscular junction, or muscle). Weakness may also be central in origin (brain, spinal cord) or fictitious. By localizing the disorder in the neuraxis, a meaningful differential diagnosis can be generated.

Electrodiagnostic studies can assist greatly in this regard. Occasionally, in certain clinical situations, electrodiagnostic examinations can identify a specific disorder, such as Guillain-Barré syndrome, myasthenia gravis, amyotrophic lateral sclerosis, or diabetic neuropathy. More typically, however, electrodiagnostic examinations will suggest a category of disease, such as myopathy or neuropathy. Usually, additional electrical findings will allow one to limit the differential further within these broader categories. Although no specific individual electrical abnormality is diagnostic of any particular disease, patterns of abnormalities can be defined that are strongly suggestive of a more specific disease type.

Electrodiagnostic studies can distinguish between motor neuron disorders (e.g., amyotrophic lateral sclerosis), neuropathies, neuromuscular transmission disorders (e.g., myasthenia gravis, Lambert-Eaton myasthenic syndrome), and myopathies (Table 7). Within the category of neuropathy, any of six different electrophysiologic patterns can be defined (20), each with its own differential diagnosis. The total number of neuropathies is over 100. Each neuropathic pattern should then lead to a limited rational list of ancillary blood and urine tests that can be ordered to identify a specific diagnosis. Presynaptic and postsynaptic disorders of neuromuscular transmission can be differentiated. Within the category of myopathy, the presence or absence of specific types of abnormal spontaneous activity can help limit the differential diagnosis (Table 6).

Myopathies can vary greatly in their clinical presentation. Accordingly, the electrodiagnostic findings can vary and need to be interpreted within the context of other clinical findings. Some myopathies may demonstrate only minimal electrodiagnostic abnormalities, particularly in those where the pathologic process predominantly involves the contractile, as opposed to the electrical, elements of the muscle fiber (e.g., certain congenital and endocrine myopathies). Other myopathies reveal widespread and florid findings (e.g., polymyositis, Duchenne muscular dystrophy). Others produce episodic abnormalities (e.g., periodic paralysis). Even for a given disease, the pattern of findings may

**TABLE 6.** *Spontaneous activity in myopathies*[1]

| Fibrillation potentials | Myotonic discharges | Complex repetitive discharges |
|---|---|---|
| Myositis | Myotonia congenita | Myositis |
| Inclusion body myositis | Myotonia dystrophica | Muscular dystrophies |
| Muscular dystrophy | Paramyotonia congenita | Inclusion body myositis |
| Trichinosis | Hyperkalemic periodic paralysis | Acid maltase deficiency |
| Toxic myopathies (alcoholic, | Myositis | Debrancher myopathy |
| HMG-CoA reductase inhibitors) | Acid maltase deficiency | Schwartz-Jampel |
| Muscle trauma | Debrancher myopathy | syndrome |
| Rhabdomyolysis | Hypothyroid myopathy | |
| Acid maltase deficiency | Myotubular myopathy | |
| Debrancher myopathy | Chloroquine myopathy | |
| Hyperkalemic periodic paralysis | Diazocholesterol poisoning | |
| Nemaline myopathy | | |
| Sarcoid myopathy | | |
| Muscle carnitine deficiency | | |

[1]Modified from Ref. 22. HMF-CoA, 3-hydroxy-3-methylglutaral-coenzyme A.

vary depending on the activity of the disease. Thus, the electrodiagnostic consultant needs to interpret their findings within the overall clinical picture of each individual.

As a rule, both sensory and motor conduction studies will reveal normal latencies and conduction velocities. Motor CMAP amplitudes may be normal or slightly reduced, depending on the situation. Because most CMAPs are conventionally recorded from distal muscles, these amplitudes might be expected to be normal in proximal-predominant myopathies unless the disorder is severe or advanced. In diffuse or distal-predominant myopathies or when CMAPs are recorded from proximal muscles, amplitudes may be reduced. Repetitive stimulation studies are usually normal, although decrementing responses may be observed in myotonic disorders. The needle electrode examination classically shows an abundance of low-amplitude short-duration polyphasic units that recruit early. However, such findings may vary from muscle to muscle and from location to location within a given muscle, necessitating a meticulous search for abnormalities. Of these needle electrode examination findings, duration is the most reliable and amplitude the least reliable. Polyphasia is perhaps the earliest to appear and recruitment abnormalities are the latest. When such findings are found, the presence of specific types of abnormal spontaneous activity will further help define the differential diagnosis (Tables 5 and 7).

Often, biopsy confirmation is sought. Although biopsies are necessarily confined to one small section of one muscle, electrodiagnostic studies have the advantage of being able to assess multiple muscles and multiple sites within a given muscle. This is particularly useful in myopathies that produce a patchy distribution of abnormalities. In these situations, the electrodiagnostic examination can assist in the selection of a biopsy site. When performing a biopsy, it is advised to choose a muscle that is moderately involved. Electrodiagnostic studies can detect subclinical abnormalities and can also identify muscles that will likely be of high yield for biopsy. Because the needle electrode examination can induce histologic changes in the muscle, it is advisable to restrict the examination to one side of the body. When a promising site is then identified, the homologous muscle on the contralateral side can be biopsied. This strategy is generally effective because most myopathies are symmetric in distribution.

**TABLE 7.** *Electrophysiologic findings in disorders causing weakness*

| | Nerve conduction studies | | | | | | Needle electrode examination | | |
| | Sensory nerve studies | | Motor | | | | | | |
| Disorder | Distal latencies | Amplitude | Distal latencies | Conduction velocities | Amplitude | Repetitive nerve stimulation | Spontaneous electrical activity | MUAP | Recruitment |
|---|---|---|---|---|---|---|---|---|---|
| Myopathy | Normal | Normal | Normal | Normal | Normal | Usually normal | +/− fibs, positive sharp waves | LA, SD, Poly | Early |
| Neuromuscular transmission disorders | Normal | Normal | Normal | Normal | Normal or decreased | Decremental | Usually none | LA, SD, Poly | May be early |
| Neuropathy | Normal or prolonged | Decreased | Normal or prolonged | Normal or slow | Normal or decreased | Normal | +/−fibs, positive sharp waves | LA, LD Poly | Reduced, rapid firing |
| Motor neuron disease | Normal | Normal | Normal | Normal | Decreased | Normal | fibs, positive sharp waves | HA, LD, P | Reduced, rapid firing |

MUAP, motor unit action potential; LA, low amplitude; HA, high amplitude; SD, short duration; LD, long duration; fibs, fibrillation potentials.

## PITFALLS OF ELECTRODIAGNOSTIC STUDIES

Entire monographs have been written on the pitfalls of electrodiagnostic studies. A thorough discussion of this topic is beyond the scope of this chapter, but the reader is referred to an excellent review on this subject (21). A high-quality electrodiagnostic laboratory should be well versed on this subject and aware of how to avoid the numerous potential errors. All normative data can be affected by age and by body habitus. One needs to meticulously control temperature with external heating devices, because cool temperature will alter latencies, conduction velocities, CMAP and SNAP amplitudes, and MUAP parameters. Latencies and velocities are dependent on distances, so care must be given to these measurements. In addition, both under- and overstimulation can induce error. Inadvertent costimulation of adjacent nerves must also be avoided. Improper setting of the high- and low-frequency filters can also result in lost or altered data. The distance between the active and reference recording electrodes must be kept at the recommended value, because variations in the interelectrode distance can introduce error. Insufficient preparation or cleaning of the skin or the use of too much electrode gel can lead to shunting of current, altering both stimulation and recording. Different sets of normative data depend on specific limb positions. Results will differ depending on whether the extremity is flexed or extended. The electrodiagnostic consultant must know how to recognize anomalous innervation patterns. Normal variants can confuse results or mask abnormalities (e.g., the Martin-Gruber anomaly). An accurate needle electrode examination depends on a thorough knowledge of anatomy. Placement of the needle electrode too deep or superficial, too medial or lateral, or too rostral or caudal can result in recording from the wrong muscle.

The electrodiagnostic examination is not a standardized procedure. There are a large number of potential sensory and motor conduction studies, ancillary techniques, and muscles from which to choose. The examiner must select those tests that are appropriate to the clinical situation and that will most likely answer the questions posed. Thus, the electrodiagnostic consultant must review the medical records and perform a history and physical examination before beginning the electrophysiologic studies. Only in this way can an appropriate initial strategy be formed. The examiner must also be prepared to shift strategy in the middle of the test based on the early findings. To be most helpful, the electrodiagnostic consultant should be well versed in the differential diagnosis of neuromuscular disease and capable of analyzing the data and understanding their significance as they are obtained.

## INDICATIONS FOR OBTAINING AN ELECTRODIAGNOSTIC STUDY

Patients are referred to electrophysiology laboratories for a variety of reasons. Some are sent for evaluation of suspected focal neuropathies such as carpal tunnel syndrome, ulnar neuropathies, radial neuropathies, peroneal neuropathies, traumatic or idiopathic plexopathies, and radiculopathies. In some instances the goal is confirmation of a clinical suspicion, whereas in others it is to rule in or rule out a specific diagnosis. In other cases it is used to provide localization information (ulnar neuropathy at the wrist versus retroepicondylar groove versus humeroulnar arcade) before surgery or to judge the severity or prognosis of a focal injury. With traumatic plexopathies, serial studies may help monitor the course of regeneration, which can prove helpful in planning potential surgical intervention.

In patients presenting with suspected myopathies, neurophysiologic studies can contribute in several ways (22). As previously described, myopathies may have protean features and can present with weakness that is symmetric or asymmetric, proximal or distal, constant or episodic, or with normal strength and myalgias, exercise-induced cramping, or recurrent myoglobinuria. As such, the clinical picture may not provide a clear diagnosis. Additionally, other disorders of the peripheral nervous system can eventuate in weakness, including neuropathies, neuromuscular transmission disorders, and motor neuron disorders. Electrodiagnostic studies can differentiate among these possibilities and thereby assist in establishing a diagnosis. Electrophysiologic studies can help provide objective evidence of dysfunction in patients with suspected fictitious symptoms. When nerve or muscle biopsy is being considered, electrodiagnostic studies can provide evidence to justify (or refrain from) such procedures and, if indicated, can identify the most appropriate nerves or muscles to target. In certain situations, electrodiagnostic studies can provide information on disease activity, which may alter therapy. For example, in patients with polymyositis who experience advancing weakness despite steroid therapy, the presence of marked abnormal spontaneous activity (indicating active disease) would suggest the need for more aggressive immunosuppression. In contrast, its absence would indicate the likelihood of a steroid myopathy and the need for a corticosteroid taper. However, no individual specific electrical abnormality is diagnostic of myopathy. As such, the diagnosis depends on the presence of a pattern of electrodiagnostic findings. At times, studies may show only nonspecific changes, particularly in mild disorders or in certain myopathic processes that predominantly affect the contractile or metabolic portions of the muscle fiber.

When in doubt, a brief conversation with an electrophysiologist should provide information as to whether or not electrodiagnostic testing would likely provide answers to the specific questions being posed. The more information provided by the referring physician, the better the electrodiagnostic medical consultant can effectively plan the study. Elaboration of specific questions rather than "rule out diagnosis X" will ensure that all desired inquiries will be addressed. A direct discussion between the referring and consulting physicians is optimal.

## REFERENCES

1. Kimura J. *Electrodiagnosis in diseases of nerve and muscle: principles and practice*, 2nd ed. Philadelphia: FA Davis, 1989.
2. Brown WF, Bolton CF. *Clinical electromyography*, 2nd ed. Boston: Butterworth-Heinemann, 1993.
3. Buchthal F, Clemmenson S. On the differentiation of muscle atrophy by electromyography. *Acta Psychiatr Neurol* 1941;16:143–181.
4. Kugelberg E. Electromyogram in muscular disorders. *J Neurol Neurosurg Psychiatry* 1947;10:122–133.
5. Sethi RK, Thompson LL. *The electromyographer's handbook*, 2nd ed. Boston: Little, Brown and Co., 1989.
6. National Institute for Occupational Safety and Health, Division of Safety Research. Performing motor and sensory neuronal conduction studies in adult humans. Washington, DC: U.S. Department of Health and Human Services, Public Health Service Centers for Disease Control, 1990.
7. Oh SJ. *Clinical electromyography: nerve conduction studies*, 2nd ed. Baltimore: Williams & Wilkins, 1993.
8. Albers JW, Allen AA, Bastrom JA, Daube JR. Limb myokymia. *Muscle Nerve* 1981;4:494–504.
9. Keesey JC. AAEM Minimonograph 33: Electrodiagnostic approach to defects of neuromuscular transmission. *Muscle Nerve* 1989;12:613–626.
10. Lange DJ. Electrophysiologic testing of neuromuscular transmission. *Neurology* 1997;48[Suppl 5]:518–522.
11. Daube JR. Electrodiagnosis of muscle disorders. In: Engel AG, Banker BQ, eds. *Myology*. Vol. 1. New York: McGraw-Hill, 1986:1081–1121.
12. Auger RG, Daube JR, Gomez MR, Lambert EH. Hereditary form of sustained muscle activity of peripheral nerve origin causing myokymia and muscle stiffness. *Ann Neurol* 1984;15:13–21.
13. Stalberg E, Trontelj JV. *Single fiber electromyography*. Surrey, UK: Mirvalle, 1979.
14. Daube JR. Quantitative EMG in nerve-muscle disorders. In: Stalberg E, Young RR, eds. *Clinical neurophysiology*. Boston: Butterworth-Heinemann, 1981:33–65.
15. Sanders DB. Electromyographic evaluation of myopathies. AAEM Course C: *Update on myopathies*. Rochester, MN: American Association of Electrodiagnostic Medicine, 1992:43–53.
16. Buchthal F. *An introduction to electromyography*. Oslo, Norway: JW Capelon, 1957.
17. Daube JR. Application of quantitative methods in neuromuscular disorders. In: Halliday AM, Butler SR, Paul R, eds. *A textbook of clinical neurophysiology*. New York: John Wiley & Sons, 1987:439–458.
18. Nandeckar SD, Barkhaus PE. Multi-MUAP analysis. *Muscle Nerve* 1995;18:1155–1166.

19. Stewart CR, Nandeckar SD, Massay JM, Bilchrist JM, Barkhaus PE, Sanders DB. Evaluation of an automatic method of measuring features of motor unit action potentials. *Muscle Nerve* 1989;12:141–148.
20. Donofrio PD, Albars JW. AAEM Minimonograph 34: Polyneuropathy: classification by nerve conduction studies and electromyography. *Muscle Nerve* 1990;13:889–903.
21. Dumitru D, King JC. Nerve conduction study pitfalls, an AAEM workshop monograph, Rochester MN. 1993; 10:132–148.
22. Wilbourn AJ. The electrodiagnostic examination with myopathies. *J Clin Neurophys* 1993;10:132–148.

*Diseases of Skeletal Muscle,*
edited by Robert L. Wortmann.
Lippincott Williams & Wilkins, Philadelphia © 2000

# 18

# Muscle Biopsy

Edward H. Bossen

*Department of Pathology, Duke University School of Medicine and*
*Duke University Medical Center, Durham, North Carolina 27710*

## COLLECTION AND PROCESSING OF THE MUSCLE BIOPSY

Evaluation of muscle tissue obtained by biopsy often provides important information and is useful in making a diagnosis in patients with myopathic conditions. However, because findings are often nonspecific, once one decides to obtain a muscle biopsy, it is important to provide the pathologist with a complete history. Selecting the proper muscle to biopsy is also important. A muscle that is moderately involved by the disease process and has not been subjected recently to trauma, such as from electromyography, should be selected. Muscle groups affected by a prior condition, such as a stroke, or areas most intensely involved with disease process should not be biopsied. The damage may be too severe to distinguish more salient features.

There are two general approaches to obtaining a muscle biopsy. The first is needle biopsy, which may be used for diagnostic and physiologic studies (1–3). This technique causes the patient less discomfort than an open biopsy and permits sampling from multiple sites. Its disadvantages include the inability to identify abnormal portions of a muscle to biopsy, small individual sample size, and more difficulty in fixing the specimens properly for electron microscopy. Most pathologists prefer an open biopsy method for diagnostic purposes. This procedure allows the surgeon to see areas of the muscle that look abnormal. In addition, more tissue can be obtained than through a needle biopsy. Having a large specimen allows proper preparation for electron microscopy to be done more easily and provides sufficient tissue for other studies. Deciding which method is best depends on communication among the patient's physician, the physician performing the biopsy, and the pathologist. Regardless of the technique and unless one is concerned with only one specific analysis, sufficient muscle should be obtained to allow histologic, histochemical studies, electron microscopy, and biochemical assays. Although all these analyses may not be necessary, obtaining appropriate samples will allow them to be performed without having the patient endure another procedure.

The specimen intended for histochemistry should measure approximately 5 mm in diameter and length. This specimen should remain moist but must not be overly wet. There is a tendency to place the specimen on a very wet saline-soaked pad. This will damage the tissue if the muscle is not frozen within an hour. A tightly sealed container will be sufficient to maintain moisture if the muscle must be kept overnight in a refrigerator. A portion of this specimen or an additional specimen of similar size may be obtained and quick frozen for biochemical analyses if desired.

Ideally, the specimen for electron microscopy is clamped before it is excised. A portion of muscle no thicker than 2 mm is sharply dissected because the fixative glutaraldehyde only penetrates 1 mm. The clamp is inserted, tightened, and the muscle excised around the clamp. The clamp is then immediately placed in glutaraldehyde and allowed to fix for at least 1 hour before it is removed. Longitudinal sections approximately 1 mm in length and no more than 1 mm in width are then cut from this sample and submitted for analysis. Further details can be found in a review by Bossen (4).

## ANALYSIS OF MUSCLE TISSUE

### Light Microscopy and Uses of Stains

The fresh tissue is flash frozen at approximately −120 to −140°C, 5-μm sections cut, and a variety of stains used (5). Standard initial stains usually include a hematoxylin and eosin, a modified Gomori trichrome, adenosine triphosphatase (ATPase) at pH 9.4 and pH 4.35, nicotinamide adenine dinucleotide (reduced)-tetrazolium reductase (NADH-TR), phosphorylase, and alkaline phosphatase. A Congo red stain for amyloid may be added for patients over age 50 years. Additional stains may be performed depending on the clinical picture. For example, if there is a history of cramping, stain for phospho-fructokinase is added.

The hematoxylin and eosin stain is the standard stain for identifying general morphologic abnormalities. Normal skeletal muscle fibers are polygonal and have peripheral nuclei (Fig. 1). Fiber size and shape, necrosis, regeneration, interstitial inflammation, fibrosis, and, less commonly, vasculitis and parasites are identified with this stain. The trichrome stain identifies aggregates of mitochondria (Fig. 2) and abnormal Z-band material, including nemaline rods (Fig. 3). The NADH-TR stain is useful for fiber typing but also identifies abnormal oxidative enzyme staining within muscle fibers. This stain is

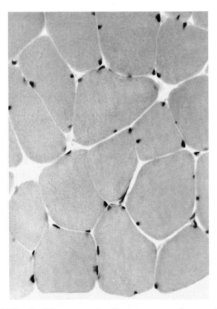

**FIG. 1.** The muscle fibers are polygonal and have peripheral nuclei. There is mild variation in fiber size. Hemotoxylin and eosin, magnification ×400.

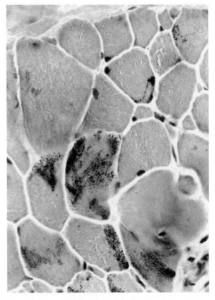

**FIG. 2.** Predominantly peripheral masses of red (dark) material produces the ragged red fiber. Trichrome, magnification ×680.

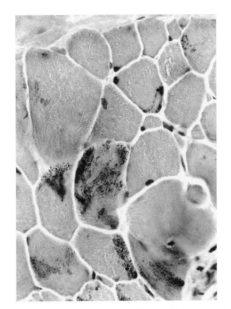

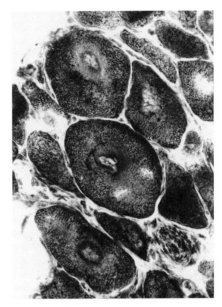

**FIG. 3**. Aggregates of dotlike and short rods of red-staining (dark) material represents nemaline rods. Trichrome, magnification ×680.

**FIG. 4**. Muscle fibers with dark-staining rims around pale zones in target fibers. NADH-TR, magnification ×520.

useful for the identification of mitochondrial aggregates, target fibers (Fig. 4), targetoid fibers, and the central cores of central core disease. The succinic dehydrogenase stain is specific for mitochondria and can be used instead of the NADH-TR. The ATPase series of stains is used for fiber typing. The myophosphorylase stain is used to identify McArdle's disease. McArdle's disease, or type V glycogen storage disease, results from a deficiency of that enzyme activity. Phosphofructokinase, myoadenylate deaminase, and cy-

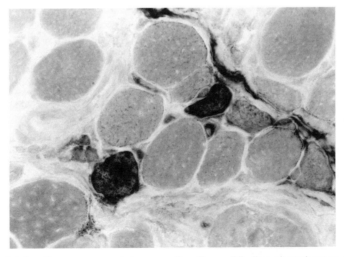

**FIG. 5**. Dark-staining fibers represent degenerating fibers. Alkaline phosphatase, magnification ×520.

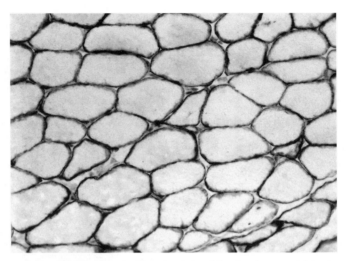

**FIG. 6.** The membrane of the muscle fiber is stained by the immunohistochemical stain for dystrophin. Magnification ×325.

tochrome $c$ oxidase stains are used to detect their respective deficiencies. The alkaline phosphatase stain can demonstrate degeneration in fibers that show little change with other stains (Fig. 5) (6). The absence of dystrophin, characteristic of Duchenne muscular dystrophy, can be detected with an immunohistochemical stain for the protein (Fig. 6) (7).

## Electron Microscopy

The specimen submitted for electron microscopy is first embedded in a plastic such as Epon, and then semithin (also called thick) sections of 0.5 to 1.0 μm in thickness are ex-

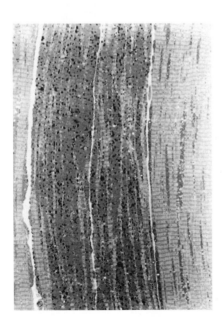

**FIG. 7.** Aggregates of pale blue (gray in this micrograph) lipid are strikingly increased in this patient with a lipid myopathy. Toluidine blue staining of Epon-embedded muscle. Magnification ×680.

**TABLE 1.** *Constituents of skeletal muscle that can be assayed through specialty reference laboratories*

Enzyme activities
  Acid maltase
  Neutral maltase
  Myophosphorylase
  Phosphorylase b kinase
  Debrancher enzyme
  Brancher enzyme
  Phosphofructokinase
  Phosphoglycerate kinase
  Phosphoglycerate mutase
  Lactate dehydrogenase
  Carnitine palmitoyltransferase
  Cytochrome *c* oxidase
  Succinate-cytochrome *c* reductase
  Rotenone-sensitive NADH cytochrome *c* reductase
  NAHD dehydrogenase
  Succinic dehydrogenase
  Citrate synthase
  Myoadenylate deaminase
Other constituents
  Glycogen
  Carnitine
    Free
      Total esterified

amined for abnormalities. Specific areas of these plastic blocks are selected for electron microscopy. Evaluation of semithin sections is useful for identifying abnormalities that cannot be seen on the thicker (5 to 6 μm) histochemical slides. Examples are the autophagic vacuoles and filaments that are characteristic of inclusion body myositis or mitochondrial abnormalities and deposits of excess glycogen or lipid (Fig. 7). These abnormalities may affect only a few fibers. Evaluation of semithin sections permits a selection of the specific fibers for electron microscopy that would most likely yield positive results.

### Assays of Tissue Contents

For certain patients, it may be necessary to have muscle assayed for levels of certain constituents or enzyme activities (Table 1). This may be indicated in the search for the cause of rhabdomyolysis, when excess lipid or glycogen is observed with special stains or by electromicroscopy or when a mitochondrial myopathy is suspected. Those analyses generally require tissue to be sent to special laboratories.

### HISTOCHEMISTRY OF NORMAL SKELETAL MUSCLE

Although normal skeletal muscle appears rather homogeneous when observed by routine histology, it is really a heterogeneous tissue composed of a variety of fiber types (Table 2) (see Chapter 2). In normal skeletal muscle there is a relatively equal distribution of type I and type II fibers. This "checkerboard" pattern is established by 28 weeks of gestation (8). The size of the fibers varies with age and sex. In the normal adult, muscle fibers are 40 to 60 μm in diameter. Mild fiber size variation can be seen in normal muscle. Part of this is true variation in fiber size, but some is because fibers cut closer to their insertion point will have a smaller profile than fibers cut in more central portions.

**TABLE 2.** *Characteristics of fiber types using various histochemical stains*

| Fiber type | ATPase pH 9.4 | ATPase pH 4.6 | ATPase pH 4.35 | NADH |
|------------|---------------|---------------|----------------|-------|
| Type I | Light | Dark | Dark | Dark |
| Type IIA | Dark | Light | Light | Light |
| Type IIB | Dark | Dark | Light | Light |

In children, the muscle fibers are approximately the same size regardless of fiber types. In adolescents and adults, type II fibers may be slightly larger than type I fibers, particularly in males.

Fiber typing is best evaluated with the myosin ATPase stain, pH 9.4 (Fig. 8). This stain reflects the activity of the ATPase in the myosin molecule itself and is little changed by most disease processes. Type I fibers are pale, and type II fibers are dark with this stain and pH. Subtyping of muscle fibers into IIA and IIB can be obtained by including ATPase stains at pH 4.6 and 4.35. Type I fibers are light at pH 9.4 and 4.6 but dark at pH 4.35. Type IIA fibers are dark at pH 9.4 but light at pH 4.6 and 4.35. Type IIB fibers are dark at pH 9.4 and 4.6 and light at pH 4.35. This is useful for physiologic studies and sometimes for deciding if there is true type II grouping rather than a mixture of type IIA and IIB fibers. The percentage of fibers that are IIB increases with age, deconditioning, and obesity (9).

Some athletes may have a fiber type distribution that would be considered abnormal. In the average patient, marked type I predominance is considered abnormal, but some endurance athletes such as marathon runners and cross-country skiers have been shown to have marked type I fiber predominance. Presumably, the greater oxidative capacity of the type I fibers contributes to their endurance. What component of fiber type distribution is a result of training, genetic composition, or both is a subject of debate. One recent study suggests an equal contribution of genetics and environment (10). Transitions from one fiber type to another, specifically IIb to IIa, have been reported with conditioning exercise (11).

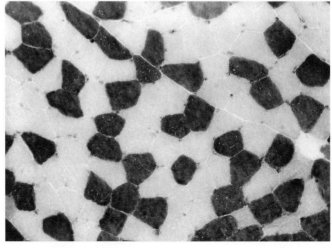

**FIG. 8.** The normal checkerboard pattern of type I (dark) and type II (light) fibers is illustrated. Reverse ATPase pH 4.35, magnification ×250.

## PATTERNS OF DISEASE

The abnormalities detected with muscle histology can be divided between two principal disease patterns, denervation and myopathy.

### Denervation

The typical findings of denervation include angulated atrophic fibers, atrophy of both type I and type II fibers, fiber-type grouping, and target fibers. The normal motor unit consists of the neuron, its axon, and the muscle that it innervates. This motor unit will be of a particular fiber type, for example, type I. Because human muscle has a mixture of type I and type II fibers, within a given muscle there will be intermixed axons that influence the development of type I and type II fibers. When a muscle fiber loses its innervation, it begins to atrophy. The previously denervated muscle fiber may be reinnervated by an axon from a motor neuron of a different type. For example, a type I fiber that has lost its innervation may be reinnervated by a type II axon. When this occurs, the muscle fiber will acquire many characteristics of the type II fiber. This process may result in "type groups," which are defined as clusters of muscle fibers of the same fiber type. For example, a type I group would consist of at least one type I fiber surrounded by other type I fibers (Fig. 9).

Denervated muscle fibers are classically angulated (Fig. 10). In contrast, atrophic fibers in myopathies are rounded. The designation of type I and type II fiber atrophy is important because pure type II fiber atrophy is more characteristic of disuse or steroid therapy but can also be seen in myopathy (Fig. 11).

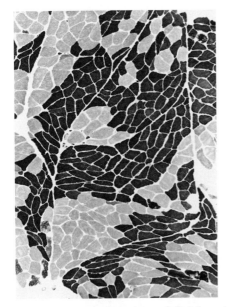

**FIG. 9**. Type grouping of type I (light) and type II (dark) fibers results from reinnervation of previously denervated fibers. AT-Pase pH 9.4, magnification ×170.

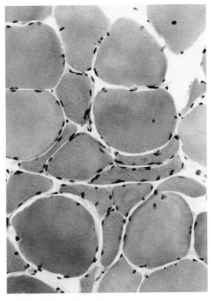

**FIG. 10**. Small groups of angulated atrophic fibers are typical of neurogenic atrophy. Hemotoxylin and eosin, magnification ×250.

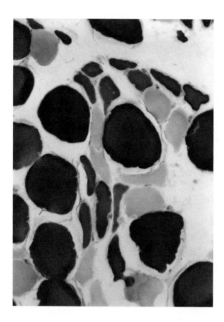

**FIG. 11.** A small cluster of angulated atrophic fibers that are both type I (light) and type II (dark). ATPase pH 9.4, magnification ×170.

Target fibers are another feature of denervation. They are best seen with an oxidative enzyme stain such as NADH-TR (Fig. 4) or succinic dehydrogenase stains. Electron microscopy of such a muscle fiber will demonstrate focal areas of disorganized myofibrils in which there is a relatively paucity of mitochondria and sarcoplasmic reticulum (Fig. 12). This produces a pale-staining central zone on cross-section of the muscle fiber stained with an oxidative stain. The mitochondria and sarcoplasmic reticulum will accumulate around this pale zone and will therefore stain more darkly. The periphery of the muscle fiber will have a normal pattern. This results in a target pattern. There is a non-

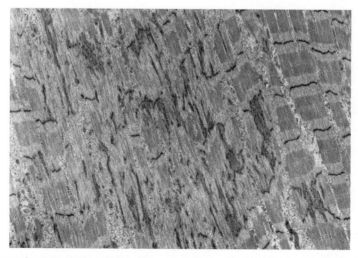

**FIG. 12.** Several sarcomeres contain disordered myofibrils with sparse mitochondria and tubules. The ultrastructural pattern is seen in the pale area of target and targetoid fibers. Magnification ×8,750.

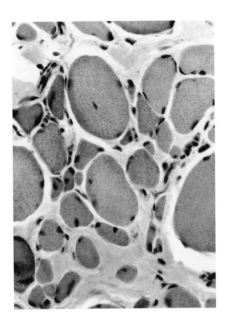

**FIG. 13**. Rounding of fibers, particularly atrophic fibers, is characteristic of myopathies. Note also the fibrosis between the fibers (endomysial fibrosis). Hemotoxylin and eosin, magnification ×400.

specific change referred to as targetoid fibers in which the dark-staining zone around the central portion of the fiber is absent. Target and targetoid fibers are almost always type 1 fibers.

## Myopathies

The general features of myopathy include rounded atrophic fibers (Fig. 13), hypertrophic fibers that may be rounded, increased internal nuclei, degeneration of muscle fibers (Fig. 14), regeneration of muscle fibers, endomysial fibrosis (Fig. 13), and fiber

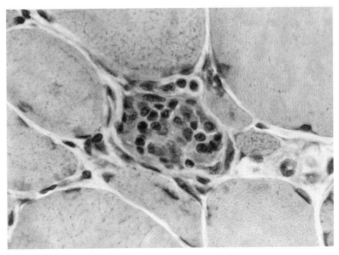

**FIG. 14**. Degenerating muscle fibers may contain macrophages, a process referred to as myophagocytosis. Hemotoxylin and eosin, magnification ×680.

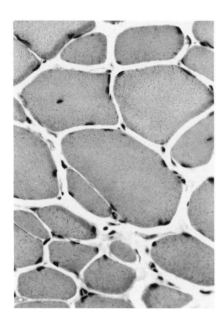

**FIG. 15.** Fiber splitting is an indication of hypertrophy and chronicity. It is a myopathic feature but can be seen in chronic denervation. Hemotoxylin and eosin, magnification ×400.

splitting (Fig. 15). The above characteristics are self-explanatory, perhaps with the exception of fiber splitting. When muscle fibers hypertrophy, at a certain point they will branch like a tree. This is called fiber splitting (Fig. 15). Many myopathic processes will present with the above characteristics and will lack more specific morphologic findings. Other biopsies will show more distinguished features that indicate a more specific disorder.

### Congenital Myopathies

Each distinctive congenital myopathy is recognized by distinguishing morphologic features. Central core disease is characterized by all or most fibers with a central pale, but not empty, zone (see Chapter 10). The muscle fibers will be predominantly type I, a common feature of congenital myopathies.

Nemaline myopathy is named for the threadlike appearance of a proliferation of a component of the Z band. These structures are red when frozen sections are stained with the modified trichrome stain. They are readily identified by electron microscopy (Fig. 3). Centronuclear myopathy is so named because most fibers have central nuclei (Fig. 6 in Chapter 10). Central nuclei are characteristic of developing muscle less than 16 weeks of gestational age. In centronuclear myopathy, 70% to 100% of the fibers will have central nuclei. Infantile myotonic dystrophy also has increased internal nuclei, but usually less than 15% of the fibers are affected. In normal muscle, up to 3% of fibers may have internal nuclei.

### Inflammatory Myopathies

Used as a general term, the designation inflammatory myopathy includes a wide range of disorders, including infectious and autoimmune disorders that are characterized by infiltration of inflammatory cells. In the case of idiopathic polymyositis, the in-

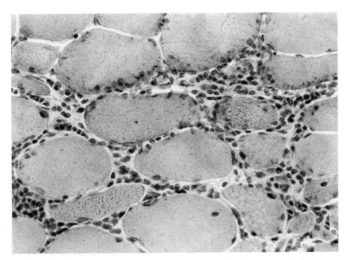

**FIG. 16.** An infiltrate of lymphocytes is seen in this case of polymyositis. Hemotoxylin and eosin, magnification ×325.

filtrates of lymphocytes and plasma cells are the characteristic feature (Fig. 16). However, the size and location of the infiltrates vary greatly, and inflammatory cells may not even be present in a particular biopsy. Inclusion body myositis is an inflammatory myopathy that has filamentous inclusions in addition to an inflammatory infiltrate. Inclusions may be seen within cytoplasmic autophagic vacuoles referred to as rimmed vacuoles because of dark-staining material at the edges of the vacuole (Fig. 17). Intranuclear filamentous inclusions are sometimes seen with electron microscopy. There are two types of filaments. One type is a little thicker than myosin and tends to be or-

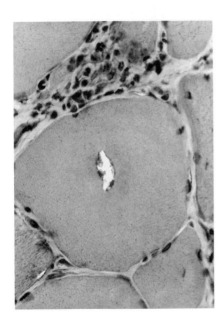

**FIG. 17.** The fiber in the center of the field contains a vacuole rimmed with dark material. This is a feature of inclusion body myositis. A lymphocytic infiltrate is adjacent to the fiber. Hemotoxylin and eosin, magnification ×520.

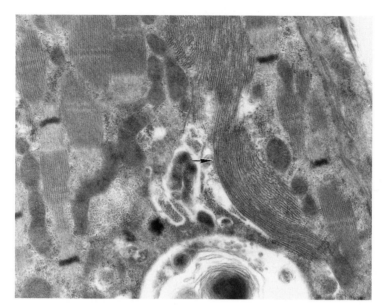

**FIG. 18**. The characteristic thick filaments of inclusion body myositis are seen. Magnification ×18,200.

ganized linearly. The second type is thinner and haphazardly arranged, similar to amyloid fibrils (Figs. 18 and 19).

Dermatomyositis may present two distinctive morphologic features. The first of these is perifascicular atrophy (Fig. 20). Fibers at the edge of the fasciculus are most susceptible to the decreased blood supply that occurs in this disease. Thus, this proba-

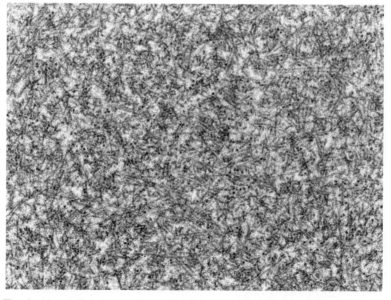

**FIG. 19**. The haphazardly arranged smaller filaments that resemble amyloid filaments are demonstrated. Magnification ×29,575.

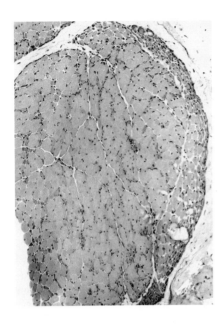

**FIG. 20**. Perifascicular atrophy is a feature of dermatomyositis. Note the smaller size of the fibers at the edge of the fasciculus. Hemotoxylin and eosin, magnification ×100.

bly represents an ischemic change. Perifascicular atrophy in the right clinical setting is diagnostic of dermatomyositis even if no inflammatory infiltrate is present in the biopsy. However, a similar change is seen in diabetes on rare occasions. The second morphologic feature characteristic of dermatomyositis is microinfarction (Fig. 21). Microinfarction also occurs in diabetes, but the clinical setting should easily distinguish between these disorders. Microinfarction can also present with a painful mass and appear clinically like a neoplasm. On longitudinal sections, the muscle may have a wavy

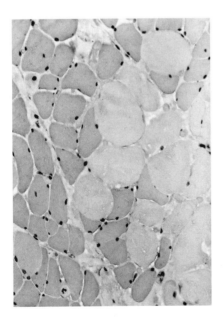

**FIG. 21**. Microinfarction is seen in dermatomyositis. The pale fibers are dead. Hemotoxylin and eosin, magnification ×325.

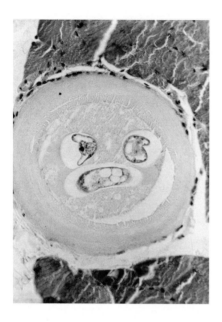

**FIG. 22**. *Trichinella spiralis* is the most common parasite seen in skeletal muscle. Hemotoxylin and eosin, magnification ×325.

look similar to that seen in recently infarcted cardiac muscle. The muscle fibers are pale and have no or indistinct nuclei. The NADH-TR of succinic dehydrogenase stains will stain the dead fibers poorly or not at all.

Granulomata may also be seen in muscle. The term granulomatous polymyositis has been applied to that observation. This almost always occurs in sarcoidosis involving muscle, although other causes of granulomata need to be excluded. These include infectious agents or a foreign body response.

Parasites in muscle can evoke an inflammatory response. The most common of these is *Trichinella spiralis* (Fig. 22). The infiltrate contains eosinophils, neutrophils, and perhaps a few lymphocytes. No infiltrate is associated with older encysted forms.

## Metabolic Myopathies

Several glycogen storage diseases may be identified morphologically. The diagnosis should be confirmed biochemically. These disorders are characterized by vacuoles in the usual preparations. The periodic acid–Schiff stain with and without diastase can be used to identify glycogen, but electron microscopy is preferable. Acid maltase deficiency, type II glycogen storage disease, presents morphologically with membrane-bound glycogen associated with lysosomal proliferation (Fig. 23). This disorder occurs in adults and children and can mimic polymyositis clinically. Adults may present with respiratory difficulty and can have the disease limited to accessory muscles of respiration. Biopsy of one of these muscles, such as the sternocleidomastoid, should be considered in adults suspected of having acid maltase deficiency. Histochemical stains are readily available for phosphorylase, phosphofructokinase, and myoadenylate deaminase deficiencies.

Lipid storage disorders are recognized by a great increase in the number of lipid droplets. Sudan black or oil-red-O stains can be used on frozen sections to demonstrate the abnormality. The droplets are also well demonstrated with plastic-embedded thick

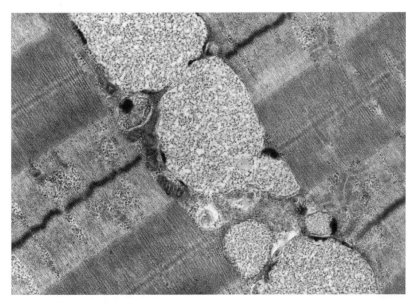

**FIG. 23**. Membrane-bound glycogen is seen in this case of type II glycogen storage disease, magnification ×24,500.

(semithin) sections (Fig. 7). Increased lipid is commonly associated with mitochondrial myopathies but may be secondary to other diseases such as renal failure and cirrhosis.

Ragged red fibers are the cardinal histochemical features of mitochondrial myopathies (Fig. 2). This change results from aggregates containing large numbers of mitochondria or abnormal mitochondria. It is important to note that not all mitochondrial myopathies have morphologic abnormalities, and in most cases only a few fibers are affected. This means that the absence of mitochondrial aggregates or abnormal mitochondria do not exclude a mitochondrial myopathy. Occasionally, abnormal mitochondria are seen in other disorders. Progressive external ophthalmoplegia, Kearn-Sayre syndrome, and inclusion body myositis are examples of diseases associated with abnormal mitochondria.

### Dystrophies

Duchenne and Becker's dystrophy are not distinctive myopathies with routine stains, but deficient dystrophin can be demonstrated with special techniques.

### Muscle Tears

Muscle tears can be mistaken for a neoplastic process. This misinterpretation can lead to great anxiety and more surgery than necessary. It is confusing because the patient, frequently a young person, will present with a mass and no memory of prior muscle pain or unusual exercise. Also, biopsies may alarm an experienced pathologist because of the multinucleation of regenerating muscle and reactive fibroblasts (Fig. 24).

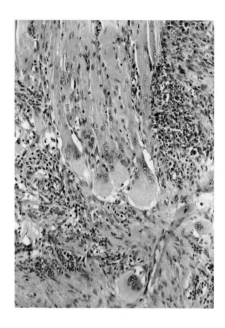

**FIG. 24**. Attempts at regeneration in a muscle tear. Hemotoxylin and eosin, magnification ×170.

## REFERENCES

1. Coggan AR. Muscle biopsy as a tool in the study of aging. *J Gerontol* 1995;50A:30–34.
2. Campellone JV, Lacomis D, Giuliani MJ, Oddis CV. Percutaneous muscle biopsy in the evaluation of patients with suspected myopathy. *Arthritis Rheum* 1997;40:1886–1891.
3. Magistris MR, Kohler A, Pizzolato G, et al. Needle muscle biopsy in the investigation of neuromuscular disease. *Muscle Nerve* 1998;21:194–200.
4. Bossen EH. Collection and preparation of the muscle biopsy. In: Heffner RR Jr, ed. *Muscle pathology*. New York: Churchill Livingstone, 1984:11–14.
5. Dubowitz V. Histology and histochemistry. In: *Muscle biopsy. A practical approach*. London: Bailliere Tindall, 1985:19–40.
6. Engel WK, Cunningham GG. Alkaline phosphatase-positive abnormal muscle fibers of humans. *J Histochem Cytochem* 1970;18:55–57.
7. Nicholson LVB, Johnson MA, Gardner-Medwin D, et al. Heterogeneity of dystrophin expression in patients with Duchenne and Becker muscular dystrophy. *Acta Neuropathol* 1990;80:239–250.
8. Martin L, Joris C. Histoenzymological and semiquantitative study of the maturation of the human muscle fibre. In: Walton N, Canal N, Scarlato G, eds. *Muscle diseases*. Amsterdam: Excerpta Medica, 1970;199:657–661.
9. Kriketos AD, Baur LA, O Connor J, et al. Muscle fibre type composition in infant and adult populations and re-lationships with obesity. *Int J Obes Relat Metab Disord* 1997;21:796–801.
10. Simoneau J-A, Bouchard C. Genetic determinism of fiber type proportion in human skeletal muscle. *FASEB J* 1995;9:1091–1095.
11. Green HJ, Klug GA, Reichmann H, et al. Exercise-induced fibre type transitions with regard to myosin, parval-bumin, and sarcoplasmic reticulum in muscles of the rat. *Pflugers Arch* 1984;400:432–438.

*Diseases of Skeletal Muscle,*
edited by Robert L. Wortmann.
Lippincott Williams & Wilkins, Philadelphia © 2000

# 19

# Rehabilitation of Patients with Muscle Weakness

Maren L. Mahowald and *Dennis D. Dykstra

*Department of Medicine, University of Minnesota Medical School and Veterans Affairs Medical Center, Minneapolis, Minnesota 55417; and *Department of Physical Medicine and Rehabilitation, Fairview—University of Minnesota Hospital and Clinics and University of Minnesota Medical School, Minneapolis, Minnesota 55455*

The rehabilitation of patients with muscle weakness is directed by the manifest functional limitations. The model of disability developed by the Institute of Medicine (Table 1) provides a good framework for understanding disability and handicap in patients with muscle disease and for developing rehabilitation strategies (Table 2) to improve or prevent the specific functional limitations related to impairments and underlying pathologies (1,2). Functional limitations are the result of impairments produced by the underlying disease pathophysiology (Table 3).

**TABLE 1.** *Institute of medicine model of disability*

| Consequences of disease | Definition | Example |
|---|---|---|
| Pathology Level of reference: cells and tissues | Measurable cellular and tissue changes caused by disease, trauma, infection, or congenital factors. Interruption or interference of normal bodily processes or structures | Inflammatory cell infiltrate in muscle; muscle necrosis, degeneration, and regeneration |
| Impairment Level of reference: organs and organ systems | Loss and or abnormality of mental, emotional, physiologic, or anatomic structure or function at the organ level; includes pain | Muscle weakness and atrophy |
| Functional limitation Level of reference: activity performance of the organism | Restriction or lack of ability to perform an action or activity within the normal range that results from an impairment: consequence at the level of the organism's activity/performance | Diminished capacity to ambulate |
| Disability Level of reference: society, task performance within a social and cultural context | Inability or limitation of ability to perform an activity within the normal range that is chronic and judged to be a cultural, social, economic and/or environmental disadvantage | Can no longer climb stairs or arise from a chair unassisted |

**TABLE 2.** *Considerations in the rehabilitation of patients with muscle diseases*

Stretching exercises to preserve range of motion and reduce contractures
Active exercise programs to improve muscle strength and endurance
Adaptive strategies and use of devices to maximize functional independence
Ventilatory support
Management of dysphagia
Nutrition

Disability is any restriction of ability to perform activities normally, whereas a handicap is any disadvantage imposed by society, the environment or one's self that prevents fulfillment of normal role functioning. Medical treatments are prescribed to affect the underlying pathology. Rehabilitation treatments are prescribed to improve function by affecting specific impairments associated with muscle diseases such as stiffness, weakness, pain, contractures, and deconditioning.

Designing a rehabilitation program for the individual patient with muscle disease requires careful analysis of the functional status. Functional limitations are analyzed in terms of specific impairments and by identifying the underlying causative pathology. The rehabilitation prescription must also be made by considering a realistic assessment of the anticipated degree of response to medical treatments, likely time course, and prognosis of the disease.

Muscle diseases may produce several different clinical scenarios that require different approaches. Patients with the relentless progression of weakness that is not responsive to medical therapy will require progressively more complex programs. Such are designed to maintain independence as long as possible and to minimize complications such as aspiration, pneumonia, contractures, and skin breakdown. Patients with the acute onset of se-

**TABLE 3.** *Impairments and functional limitations due to myositis*

| Pathology | Impairments | Functional limitations | Associated manifestations |
|---|---|---|---|
| Inflammation, muscle cell necrosis, degeneration, regeneration | Insidious onset of weakness in proximal pelvic girdle muscles | Reduced walking, arising, climbing, difficulty getting in and out of bath tub, frequent falls, and difficulty standing up waddling gait | Inflammatory arthritis Raynaud's<br><br>In dermatomyositis see heliotrope rash on eyelids, rash on dorsum of hands over mcps, pips. In some malignancy may be found in 1–4 yr |
| | Shoulder girdle muscle weakness | Reduced ADLs for dressing, grooming, eating, difficulty lifting objects overhead | |
| | Neck muscle weakness | Difficulty lifting head up from a pillow and holding head up while seated | |
| | Pharyngeal muscle weakness | Dysphagia, dysphonia, aspiration | |
| | Intercostal muscles | Shallow insufficient respirations | |
| Soft tissue and tendon contractures | Contractures | Toe walking with Achilles tendon contractures | |
| | Distal muscle weakness (in 5–10%) | Foot drop, tripping, hand dysfunction | |

ADLs, activities of daily living; mcps, metacarpal phalangeal joints; pips, proximal interphalangeal joints.

vere weakness, which may be quickly reversible or those with a more gradually reversible weakness, require early intervention designed to prevent the complications of muscle weakness followed by disease stage-appropriate restorative rehabilitation prescriptions.

## EXERCISE PHYSIOLOGY IN PATIENTS WITH MUSCLE DISEASE
### Evaluation of Muscle Function

Manual muscle strength testing is graded on the Medical Research Council 0- to 5-point scale (Table 4) (3). The utility of this scale is limited because it leads to an underappreciation of the actual motor decline (4). The change from grade 5 to grade 4 may actually reflect a 40% to 50% decline in isometric strength. More quantitative assessment of muscle strength can be measured with dynamometers or a strain gauge attached to a rigid frame to measure maximum voluntary isometric contractions. These should be used in clinical research trials because the manual muscle strength testing on the 0- to 5-point scale may be insensitive to smaller changes that are nevertheless important in functional impairments.

Serial measurements of serum markers are useful in some patients to monitor for muscle injury during an exercise program. Serum levels of enzymes derived from skeletal muscle can be assessed with creatine kinase, generally the most useful (see Chapter 14). Both MB and MM isoforms of creatine kinase are found in skeletal muscle and are elevated in serum of patients with myopathies and dystrophies (5,6). Troponin T is a regulatory protein. The troponin complex of muscle includes troponin I, C, and TnT (a small 39-kDa molecule) with cardiac and skeletal muscle isoforms. Cardiac troponin is expressed in fetal cardiac and skeletal muscle and is released into the blood during myocardial infarction, unstable angina, and other myocardial injury. It is also found in approximately one quarter of patients with polymyositis and muscular dystrophy and approximately one half of patients with renal failure. It is possible that cardiac TnT is expressed in regenerating skeletal muscle as is the MB fraction of creatine kinase (7).

Functional grades of strength for arms and legs have been used in investigations of neuromuscular disorders and are useful for following disease course (Table 5) (8). Timing activities such as how long it takes to walk 30 or 50 feet, to arise ten times from a seated position in a chair without using arm push (9), and to climb four steps are useful in monitoring treatment responses or progressive deterioration. Function level is assessed according to the patient's ability to perform activities of daily living (the self-care activities of grooming, dressing, feeding, bathing, toileting, ambulating, transfers, continence, and communication), home activities (cleaning, cooking, laundry, using the telephone, climbing stairs, managing medications), and activities outside the home (working, using public transportation, shopping, banking and money management, and social activities). The Functional Independence Measure is the standard measure used in rehabilitation units to monitor progress and determine level of services needed (10). Patient global as-

**TABLE 4.** *Medical Research Council grading system of muscle strength*

5, Normal power
4, Some weakness but the muscle is able to move against some resistance
3, Ability to move joint through normal range against gravity but not against resistance
2, Active movement only when gravity is eliminated
1, Visible or palpable muscle contraction but no joint movement
0, No evidence of muscle contraction

**TABLE 5.** *Functional grades for arms and legs*[1]

| Arms and shoulders | Hips and legs |
|---|---|
| 1. Can abduct arms from sides to touching hands above the head | 1. Is independent in walking and stair climbing |
| 2. Can raise arms to above the head only by flexing elbows or using accessory muscles (shrugging shoulders and flexing neck) | 2. Needs to use railing for stair climbing |
| 3. Can bring 8-oz glass to mouth but cannot raise hands above head | 3. Slowed walking, stair climbing using railing is slow (>12 s for 4-step climb) |
| 4. Can raise hands to mouth but cannot lift 8-oz glass to mouth | 4. Walks unassisted, can arise from a chair but cannot climb steps |
| 5. Can hold a pen and pick up coins from table but cannot raise hand to mouth | 5. Walks unassisted but cannot arise from a chair or climb stairs |
| 6. Cannot raise hands to mouth and has no useful function of the hands. | 6. Walks only with assistance |
| | 7. Nonambulatory, wheelchair bound |

[1]Adapted from Ref. 8.

sessment of health status on a 0- to 10-point scale (with 0 as poor as it could be and 10 entirely well) is perhaps the most important assessment.

### Elements of Exercise Training for Patients with Muscle Disorders

Three types of therapeutic exercise are prescribed: range of motion or stretching, strengthening, and aerobic conditioning. The exercise program is typically modified to progress from passive to active assisted range of motion when muscle strength is less than 3 of 5, to active when muscle strength is sufficient to move through the full range of motion, and to progressive resistive exercises when strength is sufficient to lift 1 to 2 pounds.

As a general rule, range of motion stretching should be carried out with each joint ten times twice a day. If strength is less than 3 of 5, positions that eliminate gravity are needed to permit movement through the full range of motion. For example, a patient unable to raise arms to 180° while standing could fully abduct the arms and clasp hands above the head when supine. With gluteal muscle weakness, the patient may be unable to lift the leg when lying on their side but can abduct the hip fully when supine. When muscle or tendon tightening limits full range stretching, an assistant can gently further the stretch to the point of mild discomfort and hold the position for 12 to 18 seconds. This is termed the static stretch. A hot shower or tub bath, local heat application, and oral analgesics before stretching may diminish discomfort. Ballistic stretching and jerking motions should be avoided. These cause soft tissue injury and increased pain. When muscle strength is 2 of 5, an assistant will have to perform all range of motion stretching, preferably once every 8 hours. When the patient has sufficient strength, an overhead pulley system will permit stretching of upper extremity joints independently.

Resistance training exercises are described in the context of the type of muscle contraction involved and the type of external resistance applied against movement. An isometric muscle contraction does not produce movement of the joint spanned by the contracting muscle and therefore does not risk muscle or tendon injury. Isotonic exercises involve muscle shortening and lengthening while overcoming an external force. A typical exercise prescription is 20 repetitions of contractions one to three times a day. Concentric muscle contraction exercises overcome external resistance while shortening the muscle. Slower concentric contractions generate more force than fast ones. Eccentric muscle contraction overcomes an external force while the muscle is lengthening. Eccen-

viation contractures. Referral to an occupational therapist is recommended for education about work simplification techniques and use of assistive devices. Finger movement is preserved throughout the course of the disease, permitting use of robotic arms, computer, and a power wheelchair.

Contractures are a severe problem because they progress more rapidly than the muscle weakness and are associated with loss of independent ambulation. Wearing ankle–foot orthoses at night and doing daily stretching routine prolongs ambulation. Consistent stretching exercises can decrease the progression of contractures and help maintain ambulation. Maximization of ambulation is attempted first with ankle–foot orthoses and progressing to a plastic knee–ankle–foot orthosis with or without a locked knee hinge. Hip-girdle muscle contracture and weakness with contracture of the Achilles tendons shifts the center of gravity. Consequently, the child walks with a wide-based gait and increased lumbar lordosis to maintain balance. Progression of lower extremity contractures and quadriceps weakness further decreases balance in standing and walking. Surgical tendon releases with intensive short-term physical therapy while the child is still ambulatory can prolong walking ability and reduce falls. If walking has already ceased, muscle strength will not be sufficient to resume walking with braces. A motorized wheelchair will be needed because upper extremity weakness will not permit independence with a manual wheelchair. Surgical tenotomy of hip flexors, tensor fascia lata, iliotibial band, hamstrings, and Achilles tendons can assist with seating problems.

Trunk muscle weakness causes scoliosis and respiratory insufficiency. Neck and pharyngeal muscle weakness leads to dysphagia and aspiration. Progressive scoliosis leads to problems with skin ulceration, back pain, sitting balance, wheelchair seating, and cardiopulmonary reserve. Bracing does not reduce the progression of scoliosis but may help with wheelchair seating. Spinal fusion can correct scoliosis and is recommended when the forced vital capacity has decreased to 45% of predicted (17). Physical therapy for mobility and strengthening is started immediately after surgery. A plastic body jacket is used while sitting for several months. Spinal fusion may prevent some of the adaptive posturing patients use to maintain balance and ambulation. When ambulation ceases, problems with obesity require careful monitoring and limitation of caloric intake.

There is an increased incidence of pneumonia when the forced vital capacity is less than 1 L. Respiratory assistance is usually needed when the vital capacity is less than 20% of predicted and hypercapnia is noted. Negative pressure ventilators such as an iron lung, a cuirass, or a rocking bed are effective initially. The cuirass permits the patient to be seated but may be ineffective in patients with significant scoliosis. As respiratory insufficiency progresses, positive pressure ventilation is used, first with oral or nasal bilevel positive airway pressure and then via tracheostomy when oropharyngeal muscle strength is inadequate to manage oral secretions or produce speech.

### Inclusion Body Myositis

Inclusion body myositis is characterized by the insidious onset of progressive symmetric weakness of proximal and distal muscles (see Chapter 4) (18). Before diagnosis, there is often a 3- to 6-year history of subtle weakness with functional limitations such as difficulty with stair climbing, reduced grip strength, and giving up leisure activities requiring leg strength. Weakness of the cricopharyngeus muscle causes dysphagia in one third of patients. Muscle atrophy may be striking in the quadriceps, iliopsoas, and long finger flexors. Treatment, if effective at all, will only stabilize the weakness or retard the deterioration (19,20). After 10 to 15 years of disease, most patients may be severely incapacitated. Rehabilitation approaches involve impairment-appropriate adaptive devices, stretching range of motion exercises, and resistive strengthening exercises. These patients will require progressive help with self-care assistive devices, home and work modifications, and education and psychological support to cope with the progressive decline in function.

Five patients with inclusion body myositis underwent a 12-week concentric heavy resistance exercise program involving both legs and one arm (21). Exercise training included three sets of 10, 15, and 20 repetitions with a 90-second rest between sets of bilateral knee extension and flexion, one elbow flexion, and wrist extension three times a week for 12 weeks. The resistance level was established as the maximum resistance the patient could overcome five times. When muscle fatigue developed, the resistance was decreased just enough to permit a few more repetitions. Each week the resistance was adjusted to accommodate strength gains. At the beginning of each exercise session there was a 3-minute warm-up on an exercycle and 10 minutes of static stretching. The strength training did not decrease generalized fatigue or improve the Barthel Index of activities of daily living. However, three of five patients noted improvement in climbing stairs, rising, and lifting objects. There were no changes in manual muscle strength testing; however, dynamic strength using a variable resistance exercise machine increased 25% to 120%. Greatest gains were seen in the muscles with the least weakness at baseline. There were no changes in muscle size, serum creatine kinase levels, or endomysial inflammation on biopsy. It is important to note that measurement of muscle strength required determination of a maximum three repetitions because manual muscle strength testing and isometric muscle strength testing were not sensitive to the changes in dynamic strength. The Barthel Index was similarly insensitive to the changes patients noted in their functional abilities.

## Other Idiopathic Inflammatory Myopathies

Polymyositis, dermatomyositis, and juvenile dermatomyositis have a course of intermittent flares with coinvolvement of other organs (heart, lung, and joints) and complications of therapy (osteonecrosis and osteoporotic compression fractures) that have an impact on disability status (see Chapter 4). Evaluation before designing the rehabilitation program involves determination of disease stage, impairments, and functional limitations. Muscle weakness usually begins proximally in the hips and then in the shoulders and anterior neck muscles. The clinical course varies. Some patients experience an acute fulminant illness lasting a few years, whereas others experience a remitting and relapsing course or a chronic stable course. Patients can recover completely or have residual mild to moderate weakness and fatigue.

Responsiveness to therapy cannot be predicted at the outset. Early-phase rehabilitation aims to preserve muscle function, prevent disuse atrophy, preserve range of motion, and prevent contractures with passive stretching exercises. Severity of the clinical problems in the acute stage is related to the severity and distribution of muscle weakness. If weakness is confined to the shoulder- and hip-girdle muscles and 50% of normal strength is preserved, patients will require minimal assistance with ambulation and daily activities. Rehabilitation therapy should focus on work simplification, pacing physical activities, gait training, and assistive devices to reduce the risk of falling and instruction for active and passive (with a helper) daily stretching exercise routine to preserve range of motion and prevent contractures. With more widespread muscle group involvement and more profound weakness, patients lose functional independence and require substantial assistance with eating, grooming, transfers, toileting, dressing, and bathing and are nonambulatory.

Neck muscle weakness limits bed mobility, transfers, and sitting endurance and is easily assisted with a soft collar. Neck muscle weakness predicts swallowing dysfunction due to weakness of the oropharyngeal muscles that may cause aspiration and pneumonia. Dysphagia occurs in 30% to 60% of patients with dermatomyositis (22). Patients with neck muscle weakness should have a swallowing evaluation. Techniques that may reduce the risk of aspiration pneumonia are described above. Respiratory muscle weakness should be monitored by measuring tidal volume with a bedside spirometer. If the diaphragm muscle becomes weak, ventilatory assistance will be necessary.

Assistive devices and adaptive strategies are recommended to compensate for muscle weakness, fall risk, and reduced endurance. Patients with hip-girdle weakness and difficulty arising from a chair are helped by an elevated seat cushion, lever-controlled booster seat, raised toilet seat, shower chairs, and handheld shower extensions. For those with arm and shoulder weakness, long-handled reachers and tooth, hair, and back brushes are useful.

With distal muscle weakness, various jar and door openers and large-handled utensils and tools are useful. Upper and lower extremity orthotics help to stabilize joints in positions for optimal function. A wrist splint with a volar shank supports the wrist and augments grip strength. With quadriceps weakness, a short leg brace with 5 degrees of plantar flexion produces an extension moment at the knee, increasing knee stabilization. However, a brace with dorsiflexion to support a weak ankle will create a flexion movement at the knee and increase fall risk if the quadriceps are weak. Canes are useful primarily for balance. Walkers may maintain ambulation if upper extremity strength is sufficient. Motorized wheelchairs or scooters are very important for maintaining community ambulation.

Patient and family education regarding the variability in clinical course, the elements of chronicity with unpredictable remissions and exacerbations, and the importance of compliance with medication and rehabilitation programs are needed for a realistic understanding of the disease process. Prognostication is very difficult because of the variability in disease severity and responsiveness to treatments. Referrals for vocational rehabilitation should be made when it becomes clear that certain functional deficits are likely permanent. Referral to rehabilitation medicine, occupational therapy, and physical therapy should be made early to design the long-term multimodal therapies that will have to be continuously revised according to the patient's condition. Psychological support is usually needed for both family and patient because of the effects on home life, work capability, sexual function, and social life.

Various additional complications of myositis have an impact on rehabilitation and recovery (23,24). Fatigue is a very distressing component that requires thorough patient education regarding strategies for energy conservation and work simplification techniques to maximize functional level. Muscle pain may limit both the stretching and strengthening exercise programs. Pain can be reduced by administering oral analgesics one half hour before exercise or prescribing a 20-minute session in a therapeutic pool at 32°C to 38°C before exercising will decrease discomfort. Gentle muscle massage and microwave therapy, which heats superficial and deep muscle, have been described as useful but have never been studied.

Osteoporotic compression fractures and avascular necrosis of the femoral head, complicating corticosteroid therapy of myositis, increase pain, cause muscle spasms, and further limit ambulation and progress in a rehabilitation program. Steroid myopathy may complicate the treatment of inflammatory muscle disease and is characterized by atrophy and an increase in muscle weakness. Pulmonary interstitial fibrosis and cardiovascular complications of cor pulmonale, cardiomyopathy, and congestive heart failure may limit the rehabilitation program.

Until recently, the typical rehabilitation approach for patients with an inflammatory myopathy included rest, thermal modalities, and passive range of motion stretching in the acute phases followed by isometric strengthening during the recovery period. Resistive strength training exercises were excluded because of the unsubstantiated belief that they would increase inflammation and muscle damage in already inflamed muscle. Data from high-intensity exercise physiology studies in normal subjects were, perhaps inappropriately, used to justify exclusion of strength training exercises. The immune response to high-intensity acute exercise in normal subjects is characterized by a transient leukocytosis and increases in natural killer cells and cytotoxic T lymphocytes (25–27). Thus, exercise could theoretically increase endomysial inflammation. Eccentric (lengthening) exercise is known to cause focal endomysial inflammation, myalgias, and increases in serum creatine kinase levels (28–30). In addition, levels of cytokines, including interleukin-1β, are elevated up to 5 days after exercise (31,32). Theoretically then, these factors could enhance muscle fiber destruction (33,34).

Interestingly, studies have shown that therapeutic resistive exercises are beneficial in the elderly with sarcopenia (33,34), in patients with neuromuscular disorders (35,36), and in patients with post-polio muscular atrophy (37). Hicks (22) demonstrated that patients with stable myositis and persistently elevated serum creatine kinase levels increased strength with isometric exercises. This occurred with no further elevation of creatine kinase levels. In another study, five patients with active myositis were treated with an alternating 2-week program of resistive and nonresistive exercises. Three of four patients had increased strength with no increase in creatine kinase levels (38).

Wiesinger et al. (39) conducted a prospective, randomized, controlled trial of a fitness and strengthening training program in 14 patients with stable active polymyositis and dermatomyositis. Outcome measures included disease activity, sense of well-being, muscle strength, and cardiorespiratory fitness. The training program consisted of a 3- to 5-minute warm-up on an exercycle with resistance increased so that heart rate was 60% of maximum, a 30-minute step aerobic exercise, and a 5-minute cool down and stretching period. Exercises were performed twice weekly for the first 2 weeks and then three times a week for the next 4 weeks. Patients were also permitted to use an exercycle at home as

**TABLE 8.** *Exercise recommendations for patients with myopathies*

| Disease stage | Exercise prescription |
|---|---|
| 1. Initial acute severe PM/DM during institution of medical treatment, G-B, critical illness weakness, late-stage dystrophy or IBM: weakness 2/5 | 1–3 times daily passive ROM stretching exercises |
| 2. Early recovery stage (beginning disease activity regression) weakness 3/5 | Daily active assisted ROM stretching exercises in positions with gravity reduced, isometric exercise of key muscle groups |
| 3. Later recovery stage (stable active disease) with weakness 4/5 | Warm up with ROM stretching exercise followed by Theraban or 1–2 lb free weights for isotonic strengthening exercises, cool down with ROM stretching routine. |
| 4. Chronic active stage | 10-min warm up and 5-min cool down with ROM stretching routine, progressive resistive strengthening exercise (Theraban, free weights or exercise machine) 3 times a week plus aerobic conditioning exercises 3 times a week. |

PM, polymyositis; DM, dermatomyositis; G-B, Guillain-Barré syndrome; IBM, inclusion body myositis; ROM, range of motion.

they wished. The control group did not undergo any exercise instruction. At the end of 6 weeks there were no increases in serum enzyme levels or disease activity. There was a 20% improvement in ability to perform activities of daily living, a 30% improvement in muscle strength, and a 12% increase in $Vo_2$max.

Thus, it appears that despite evidence that suggests exercise would have a deleterious effect in patients with active myositis, many patients may benefit from a structured exercise program. Based on these observations, aerobic conditioning exercises can be recommended for those with stable or improving muscle strength and near-normal serum enzyme levels (Table 8) (22,40).

## DISORDERS WITH ACUTE WEAKNESS

### Guillain-Barré Syndrome

Guillain-Barré syndrome is reversible in 70% of patients. Ten percent die, and the remainder have residual deficits (41). Weakness typically develops rapidly over days to a few weeks, beginning in the lower extremities with an ascending pattern. The weakness plateaus for a few weeks to months and then gradually resolves over 1 to 2 years. In the first 12 weeks of disease, up to one third of patients require ventilatory support and may develop pneumonia or deep venous thrombosis with pulmonary emboli. During this hypotonic or flaccid phase, daily passive range of motion stretching exercises are needed to prevent tendon and joint contractures, and frequent changes in positioning are needed to prevent decubitus ulcers. Approximately 40% of patients will require inpatient rehabilitation. Depending on the degree of weakness, strengthening exercises should be started early and progress from isometrics to isotonic, isokinetic, manual resistive, and progressive resistive exercises. Pain control is important to permit exercise therapy. Tricyclic antidepressants, carbamazepine, gabapentin, and narcotics may be used.

Dysautonomia with cardiac arrhythmias and orthostatic hypotension may be problematic. Bowel and bladder dysfunction may cause bladder overdistention and may be complicated by urinary tract infection. Substantial loss of muscle mass and hypercalcemia may occur during the period of immobilization. Cranial nerve involvement is associated with the need for ventilatory assistance and aspiration prevention. Patients may develop hypoxia and hypercapnia during rapid-eye-movement sleep. Therefore, they should be monitored with pulse oximetry during sleep, and bilevel positive airway pressure should be added if hypoxia is observed.

### Acute Weakness in the Intensive Care Unit

Acute weakness in the critically ill patient in an intensive care unit (42) can be due to peripheral axonal neuropathy, myopathy, neuromuscular junction dysfunction, or a combination of these. Critical-illness polyneuropathy, a sensorimotor axonopathy, is thought to be caused by inadequate perfusion of peripheral nerves during the systemic inflammatory response that develops with sepsis, surgery, trauma, or burns. Prolonged neuromuscular junction blockade can cause acute quadriplegic weakness after mechanical ventilation and the use of vecuronium for neuromuscular blockade in patients with hepatic or renal dysfunction. This is associated with a decremental response of the compound muscle action potential during repetitive nerve stimulation. Critical-illness myopathy is associated with selective degeneration of myosin filaments after several days of muscle relaxants. In some patients, a necrotizing myopathy develops when prolonged neuromuscular blockade or inactivity has been combined with high-dose corticosteroids. A polyneuropathy may be superimposed in some patients with sepsis or multiorgan failure features of critical illness.

In general, the prognosis is good if the underlying critical illness can be treated successfully. In the acute stages, rehabilitation efforts are directed at prevention of peripheral nerve compression at pressure points, daily stretching to prevent contractures, aspiration precautions, and nutritional support. As strength returns, a program of progressive strengthening and reconditioning exercise should begin.

## REFERENCES

1. Pope A and Tarlov M, eds. *Disability in America: a national agenda for prevention.* Washington, DC: National Academy of Sciences, 1991.
2. Rheumatology Rehabilitation Curriculum Committee. *ACR rheumatology rehabilitation case studies.* Atlanta, GA: American College of Rheumatology, 1999.
3. Medical Research Council of the United Kingdom. *Aids to the examination of the peripheral nervous system.* United Kingdom: Pendragon House, 1978.
4. Hays RM, Kowalske KJ. Neuromuscular disease. Rehabilitation and electrodiagnosis. 3. Muscle disease. *Arch Rhys Med Rehabil* 1995;76:S21–S25.
5. Engel AG, Yamamoto M, Fischbeck KH. Dystrophinopathy. In: Engel AAG, Franzini-Armstrong C, eds. *Myology*, 2nd ed. New York: McGraw-Hill, 1994:1130–1187.
6. Engel AG, Hohlfeld R, Banker BQ. The polymyositis and dermatomyositis syndromes. In: Engel AG, Franzini-Armstrong C, eds. *Myology*, 2nd ed. New York: McGraw-Hill, 1994:1335–1383.
7. Bodor GS, Survant L, Voss EM, et al. Cardiac troponin T composition of normal and regenerating human skeletal muscle. *Clin Chem* 1997;43:476–484.
8. Moxley RT III. Evaluation of neuromuscular function in inflammatory myopathy. *Rheum Dis Clin North Am* 1994;20:827–843.
9. Newcomer KL, Krug HE, Mahowald ML. Validity and reliability of the timed stands test for patients with rheumatoid arthritis and other chronic diseases. *J Rheumatol* 1993;20:21–27.
10. Linacre JM, Heinemann AW, Wright BD, et al. The structure and stability of the Functional Independence Measure. *Rehabilitation* 1994;75:127–132.
11. Mahowald ML, Krug H, Stevenken ME, Ytterberg SR. Exercise and other physical therapies for rheumatoid arthritis. *J Musculoskel Med* 1990;7:52–68.
12. Hagberg JM. Exercise assessment of arthritic and elderly individuals. *Balliere's Clin Rheumatol* 1994;8:29–52.
13. Ytterberg SR, Mahowald ML, Krug HE. Exercise for arthritis. *Balliere's Clin Rheumatol* 1994;8:161–189.
14. Sonies BC. Evaluation and treatment of speech and swallowing disorders. *Curr Opin Rheumatol* 1997;9: 486–495.
15. Guily J, Perie S, Willig T et al. Swallowing disorders in muscular diseases: functional assessment and indications of cricopharyngeal myotomy. *Ear Nose Throat J* 1994;73:34–40.
16. Vignos PJ. Physical models of rehabilitation in neuromuscular disease. *Muscle Nerve* 1983;6:323–338.
17. Miller FW, Moseley CF, Koreska J. Spinal fusion in Duchenne muscular dystrophy. *Dev Med Child Neurol* 1992; 34:775–786.
18. Calabrese LH, Chou SM. Inclusion body myositis. *Rheum Dis Clin North Am* 1994;20:955–972.
19. Leff R, Miller RW, Hicks J, et al. The treatment of inclusion body myositis: a retrospective review and a randomized prospective trial of immunosuppressive therapy. *Medicine (Baltimore)* 1993;72:225–235.
20. Sayers ME, Chou SM, Calabrese LH. Inclusion body myositis: analysis of 32 cases. *J Rheumatol* 1992;19: 1385–1389.
21. Spector SA, Lemmer JT, Koffman BM, et al. Safety and efficacy of strength training in patients with sporadic inclusion body myositis. *Muscle Nerve* 1997;20:1242–1248.
22. Hicks JE. Role of rehabilitation in the management of myopathies. *Curr Opin Rheumatol* 1998;10:548–555.
23. Hicks JE. Comprehensive rehabilitative management of patients with polymyositis and dermatomyositis. In: Dalakas MC, ed. *Polymyositis and dermatomyositis.* Boston: Butterworth-Heinemann, 1988:293–317.
24. Clark AE, Bloch DA, Medsger TA Jr, Oddis CV. A longitudinal study of functional disability in a national cohort of polymyositis-dermatomyositis patients. *Arthritis Rheum* 1995;38:1218–1224.
25. Field CJ, Geougeon R, Marliss EB. Circulating mononuclear cell numbers and function during intense exercise and recovery. *J Appl Physiol* 1991;71:1089–1097.
26. Gabriel J, Urhausen A, Kindermann W. Circulating leukocyte and lymphocyte subpopulations before and after intensive endurance exercise to exhaustion. *Eur J Appl Physiol* 1991;63:449–457.
27. Nieman DC, Nehlsen-Cannarella SL. The immune response to exercise. *Semin Hematol* 1994;31:166–179.
28. Clarkson PM, Byrnes WC, McCormick KM, et al. Muscle soreness and serum creatine kinase activity following isometric, eccentric and concentric exercise. *Int J Sports Med* 1986;7:152–155.

29. Jones DA, Newham DJ, Round JM, Tolfree SEJ. Experimental human muscle damage: morphological changes in relation to other indices of damage. *J Physiol* 1986;375:435–448.

30. Newham DJ, Jones DA, Edwards RHT. Large delayed plasma creatine kinase changes after stepping exercise. *Muscle Nerve* 1983;6:380–385.

31. Cannon JG, Meydani SN, Fielding RA, et al. Acute phase pre-response in exercise. II. Association between vitamin E, cytokines and muscle proteolysis. *Am J Physiol* 1991;260:R1233–R1240.

32. Fielding RA, Manfredi TJ, Ding W, et al. Acute phase response to exercise III. Neutrophil and IL-1B accumulation in skeletal muscle. *Am J Physiol* 1993;265:R166–R172.

33. Evans WJ, Campbell WW. Sarcopenia and age related changed in body composition and functional capacity. *J Nutr* 1993;123:465–468.

34. Fiatarone MA, O'Neill EF, Ryan NO, et al. Exercise training and nutritional supplementation for physical frailty in very elderly people. *N Engl J Med* 1994;330:1769–1773.

35. McCartney N, Moroz D, Ganer SH, et al. The effects of strength training in patients with neuromuscular disorders. *Arch Phys Med Rehabil* 1988;69:14–19.

36. Milner-Brown JS, Miller RG. Muscle strengthening through high-resistance weight training in patients with neuromuscular disorders. *Med Sci Sports Exerc* 1988;20:362–368.

37. Spector SA, Gordon PG, Feurestein IM, et al. Strength gains without muscle injury after strength training in patients with post polio muscular atrophy. *Muscle Nerve* 1996;19:1282–1290.

38. Escalante A, Miller L, Beardmore TD. Resistive exercise in the rehabilitation of polymyositis/dermatomyositis. *J Rheumatol* 1993;20:1340–1344.

39. Wiesinger GF, Quittan M, Aringer M, et al. Improvement in physical fitness and muscle strength in polymyositis/dermatomyositis patients by a training program. *Br J Rheumatol* 1998;37:1960–2000.

40. Villalba L, Adams EM. Update on therapy for refractory dermatomyositis and polymyositis. *Curr Opin Rheumatol* 1996;8:544–551.

41. Meythaler JM. Rehabilitation of Guillain-Barré syndrome. *Arch Phys Med Rehabil* 1997;78:872–879.

42. Members of the American College of Chest Physicians/Society of Critical Care Medicine Consensus Conference Committee. American College of Chest Physicians/Society of Critical Care Consensus Conference: definitions for sepsis and organ failure and guidelines for the use of innovative therapies in sepsis. *Crit Care Med* 1992;20: 864–874.

# Subject Index

# Subject Index

-Note: Page numbers in *italics* refer to illustrations; page numbers followed by t refer to tables-